New Menopausal Years

The Wise Woman Way

Susun S. Weed

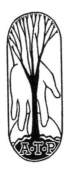

Ash Tree Publishing
Woodstock, New York

All information in this Wise Woman Ways book is based on the experiences and research of the author and other professional healers. This information is shared with the understanding that you accept responsibility for your own health and well-being. You have a unique body; the action of every remedy is unique. Health care is full of variables. The result of any treatment suggested herein cannot always be anticipated and never guaranteed. The author and publisher are not responsible for any adverse effects or consequences resulting from the use of any remedies, procedures, or preparations included in this Wise Woman Ways book. Consult your inner guidance, knowledgeable friends, and trained healers in addition to the words written here.

Copyright © 2002 by Susun S. Weed

Ash Tree Publishing, PO Box 64, Woodstock, NY 12498, USA.
Phone/Fax: 845-246-8081 www.ash-tree-publishing.com (orders)
www.ashtreepublishing.com (information)

Illustrations on pages 78, 176, 177, 244 © 2002 by Martha McGehee Teck.
Cover calligraphy and illustrations on pages xix, 20, 66, 100, 154, 158, 164, 168, 171, 194, 198, 199, 236, 253, 265 © 2002 by Alan McKnight.
All other illustrations, including borders © 2002 by Susun Weed.
Please write for permission before reproducing any graphics in this book.

Printed and bound in the United States of America; recycled, non-chlorine-bleached paper.

Publisher's Cataloging-in-Publication
(Provided by Quality Books, Inc.)

Weed, Susun S.
New menopausal years : the wise woman way / Susun S. Weed. -- 1st ed.
p. cm.
Includes bibliographical references and index.
LCCN: 2001129062
ISBN: 1888123-03-6

1. Menopause--Popular works. 2. Menopause--Alternative treatment--Popular works. I.Title.

RG186.W44 2002   618.1'75
                        QBI01-201187

May the seven directions empower this medicine work.
May it be pleasing to my grandmothers, the ancient ones.
And may it be of benefit to all beings.

So mote it be.

Acknowledgments

Many hearts and minds joined with mine to bring you this book, the original and the new. Here's where they step forward and take a bow. The trees gave themselves to make paper . . . I thank you.

Alan McKnight did the cover calligraphy, and beautiful illustrations for both editions . . . I thank you.

Peggy Goddard pasted up boards the first time around, then learned how it do it on a computer for the new edition . . . I thank you, I love you.

Betsy Sandlin edited magically in the midst of her **Change**, then edited it again ten years later, even better . . . I love you, I thank you.

Marie Summerwood kept me laughing both times, but did some serious editing of the new edition . . . I love you, I thank you.

I'd like to thank my guardian angels Keyawis Kaplan, Pierre Siead, and Gordon Cook — who offered me endless support, then, now, always . . . I love you, I thank you.

My mom, Monica Shaft, her cronies Hortense Bugbee and Kay Calvert; my aunts, Vicki Carlson and Yolanda Kozlowski; all apprentices and students and all the women who write and call and share their stories of **Change** with me . . . I thank you.

Candace Cave, Holly and David Eagle, Linda Dian Feldt, Penny King, Juliette de Baïracli Levy, Margaret Powell, Pela Sander, Ellie Sommer, Ellen Weaver, and Wonshé read the work in progress, at one time or another, and offered remedies and advice: . . . I love you, I thank you. Your wise words shifted me in subtle ways, smoothed away the rough edges, and helped reveal the beauty.

Celu Amberston, Paul Bergner, Dr. James Duke, Miriam Dyack, Lynn DeFilipo, Rosemary Gladstar, Jessica Godino, James Green, Belinda Hankins, Fern Hill, Brianna Kale, Liz Klipper, Susan Love, Gay Luce, Bruce MacFarland, Deborah Maia, Emily Millspaugh, Christiane Northrup, Melissa Oliphant, Judy Scher, Sylett Strickland, Sharol Tilgner, and Bob Walberg helped me with research, massage, and whole-hearted support . . . I thank you.

Michael Dattorre and Justine Smythe, my mate and my daughter, helped in too many ways to list. For your support of my life and my work, for your hearts, your minds, and your hands . . . I love you, I thank you.

Table of Contents

Chapter One
Is This Menopause? Preparing for the Journey   1

ॐ

Chapter Two
This is Menopause: Journey into Change   81

Chapter Three
Post-Menopause: She-Who-Holds-the-Wise-Blood-Inside 181

Introduction
Juliette de Baïracli Levy

I am very pleased to write this introduction to Susun's excellent and much-needed book for the menopausal years. I hope it will go a long way toward changing those things that threaten the health and happiness of women today. It seems to me that the beauty and power of female life is too frequently cut away with hysterectomies and mastectomies nowadays. And too many women are encouraged to become dependent on costly and harmful chemical medications derived from cruel experiments on animals.

All the herbs and remedies I would like to see for the benefit and protection of women during their menopausal years are here, all in the right place and proportions. For example, I love lavender, one of the greatest of helps to us females from childhood to old age. And there it is, on page 129, perfectly described and used. And the *Artemisias*, those lovely plants named after the goddess Artemis, protector of all women, especially those birthing, are here as well.

This book shows very well Susun's great knowledge of herbs; she is clearly an herbalist deeply informed by her quarter century of intimate dialogues with people, plants, and animals. She has been using my herbals, *Common Herbs for Natural Health* and *Herbal for Farm and Stable* for decades and helping pass on the knowledge I collected from my encounters with "man and beast." I consider her one of the mothers of herbal medicine in the United States.

It is further flattery, but true! Susun Weed is a gifted writer. Her Crone passages, in which the old woman is giving advice and encouragement, often possess poetical beauty.

Susun is very well read on matters pertaining to the life and health of women. Her references and resource lists, found throughout this book, are comprehensive and important.

This book should be in the hands of every woman, of every race, no matter what age, worldwide. I wish it the great success that it surely deserves.

What Are the Menopausal Years?

Human females are unique among all other females on two counts (at least): we menstruate (estrus bleeding in dogs is not menstruation); and we go through a second kind of puberty called menopause. We cease to be reproductively available after we've lived only half our life span. Ancient women's mystery stories, those that teach of menstruation, its beginning and end, say that our times of change are times of power: menarche, menstruation, pregnancy, childbirth, and menopause. This book focuses on the latter — the menopausal years.

Meno (*menstruation)* pause (*stops*) is, technically, the last menstrual flow of a woman's life. The years just before and just after the menopause itself are referred to as the *climacteric.* The menopausal years include two or more premenopausal years, one or more menopausal climax years, and the five years immediate post-menopause. They may begin in your late thirties or not until your early sixties. Whenever it is, remember, they call it the **Change** of Life

Menopausal **Change** is a metamorphosis (change at a cellular level). It mirrors, and may even be the matrix for, the three classic stages of initiation: isolation, death, and rebirth/reintegration. Each woman's **Change** includes these three stages, as well as three phases (before menopause, during menopause, and after menopause).

Each stage and phase of our metamorphic, menopausal **Change** is different; each has special needs and offers special challenges.

62% of the postmenopausal members of the Harvard Medical School do not use hormone replacement. 83% of American women over 50 don't either.

Wise Woman Ways
Premenopausal Years

Several years before menstruation ceases, the periods become variable (closer together, farther apart, scantier, more profuse). Spotting, flooding, cramping, and PMS-like symptoms arise or worsen, as do problems with thyroid health, fibroids, and fertility. One out of every hundred women begins her **Change** by age 35.

☞ **Nourish and tonify your entire hormonal system.** Menopausal changes occur not only in the ovaries, but also in the adrenal, thyroid, pancreas, pineal, and pituitary glands. Use mineral-rich, phytoestrogen-rich nourishing herbal infusions to keep your glands strong.

☞ **Increase the number and amount of calcium-rich foods you consume.** No single effort will repay you more richly. Calcium in the diet protects you from osteoporosis, heart disease, and emotional swings. Green leafy vegetables and yogurt are exceptionally good sources.

☞ **Experiment with phytoestrogenic herbs.** The effects of these strong plants are generally more beneficial in the early years of menopause, before hot flashes set in. They can help you maintain fertility and smooth your **Change**.

☞ **Find some regular physical activity to fall in love with.** Even gentle exercise, done regularly, helps maintain peak bone mass, strengthens the cardiovascular system, and insures deep sleep. Walking, yoga, and tai chi are practices that are easy to learn and easy to maintain well into your eighties and nineties. Start now!

☞ **Gain up to a pound a year for ten years.** Thin women have more hot flashes and an altogether more difficult menopause than heavier women. Fat cells produce estrone, a kind of estrogen. (If you won't let yourself gain ten pounds, at least stop trying to lose weight. Dieting decreases bone mass and weakens the heart.)

☞ **Plan your Crone's Time Away.** As menopausal **Change** picks up speed at the end of the premenopausal years, many women find themselves desperate to be alone, hating those around themselves and themselves. Crone's Time Away frees the menopausal woman from all social responsibility and allows her to tend to herself and her **Change**. An extended vacation, a sabbatical or a Crone's Year Away is ideal, but you can stay home and still take Crone's Time Away whenever you can create it. Plan it now. Talk about it. It will be easier to make it a reality when you need it.

Wise Woman Ways
Menopausal Climax Years

For most women, the menopausal climax (or meltdown) lasts for 2-5 years. Induced (artificial) menopause may last only 1-2 years but will be much more severe in most cases. According to Chris Northrup, MD, one out of four American women experience induced **Change**.

No matter how we achieve menopause, during the climax period, our bones may lose mass. Flashes, flushes, and night sweats become intense and frequent. Palpitations, emotional sensitivity, and sleeplessness are common. Depending on the individual woman and her response to the heightened energy that comes with the **Change**, symptoms may be multiple or next to nothing.

☞ **Take time for solitude.** If you've prepared for your Crone's Time Away, take it now. If not, figure out how to create it, or get ready to accept it when it comes (and it will) without resentment. (Children grow up, husband leaves, parents die.) Move away from care-taking others and turn your energy toward your own **Change**. Healthy women have lots of hot flashes. We all have some periods of sleeplessness and moodiness. These common complaints urge us to seek solitude, where they can become our allies of wholeness. Take one day to be totally by yourself, or a Crone's Year Away, or anything in between.

☞ **Relax and enjoy your hot flashes.** Ride them like waves, feel them in your spine, ski the edges of your flushes, honor the volcanic heat of your core. Like labor pains, hot flashes are the outward sign of metamorphosis. Like labor pains, they are worse when resisted. Herbal allies help those with unrelenting flashes relax and enjoy, too.

☞ **Spend time with a journal.** Buy a blank book and write in it, draw in it, paste articles in it. Visions and dreams are particularly vivid and intense in the menopausal climax years; keep your journal handy so you can record them. Your emotional energies are readily available during the menopausal climax years; draw them in your book. Memories abound during these years; cherish them in your journal. Write your autobiography.

☞ **Experiment with eggs, meat, and butter in your diet.** Some women find these foods, especially if from organic sources, decrease menopausal symptoms and improve overall health.

☞ **Plan your Crone's Crowning.** As months pass and the moon waxes and wanes without drawing forth your menses, you pass through the second stage of initiation, death. Your identity as Mother dies. Let yourself break all the rules. Be someone totally different than you thought you could be.

Wise Woman Ways
Postmenopausal Years

The postmenopausal years symbolically begin on the fourteenth new moon after your final menstruation. (And continue, of course, for the rest of your life.) Aching joints, heart disease, incontinence, vaginal atrophy, bladder infections, and broken bones may diminish the quality and quantity of these years. Use Wise Woman ways in the postmenopausal years to maintain healthy bones, reverse osteoporosis, keep the vagina and bladder strong and flexible, and maintain a healthy, vigorous heart and circulatory system.

☞ **Eat more vegetables, fruits, meat and grains, and lentils**. Protein is important for health and longevity, but eating it every day (especially without whole grains) may weaken your bones as well as your heart.

☞ **Move, dance, walk, stretch, go, inquire, keep active.** The essence of vitality is change. Now that you've been through the **Change**, don't stop, keep changing. Break the rules and the taboos. Become an expert on pelvic floor exercises. Take up belly dancing. Pump iron. Wear purple.

☞ **Write a legal will.** And revise it every ten years. Face your own death. Plan for your own death. This completes the second stage of your initiation.

☞ **Nourish yourself with every bite.** Aging increases our need for many nutrients while reducing our digestive ability. Make every bite count toward optimum vitality and step up digestive efficiency by using dandelion root tincture before meals. Discover new ways to serve yourself calcium-rich foods at every meal. Use herbal vinegars regularly. Gradually replace bone-depleting white flour products (bread, pasta, pretzels) with fiber-rich whole grains and whole grain products. Drink vitamin- and mineral-rich herbal infusions instead of mineral-depleting coffee, tea, and soft drinks. Try yogurt and fresh fruit instead of ice cream for stronger bones and fewer vaginal infections.

☞ **Plan your Crone's Ceremony of Commitment to Her Community.**
Any time after your second Saturn return (age 57-61), you are ready for
the third stage of your menopausal initiation: rebirth. You are She-Who-
Holds-the-Wise-Blood-Inside. You are the newborn baby Crone. After
isolation, after death, you are reborn, you rejoin the community. In isolation, you gave death to yourself as Mother, claimed all of yourself, and
revisioned yourself. It is time to share that vision, to proclaim yourself
publicly, to claim yourself as Crone, woman of wholeness.

*"I am the Crone. I feel my way along paths following the energy and warmth
that others have placed here. Trusting the dark, I am guided not by light, but
by the flowing movements I sense. I am like the water that follows, without
sight or foreknowledge, the ancient river's channel."*

My Native American teachers tell me that we are in the midst of
earth changes that will culminate around the year 2013. They say the
earth changes will bring heat, and floods, and upheaval on an enormous scale. I am struck by the fact that 50 million women will have
achieved menopause by 2013. Since we, as women, are one with the
earth, is our massive, collective **Change** Her **Change** as well? Can we
moderate Her hot flashes? Give Her ease from flooding? Soothe Her
emotional uproar? Emerge transformed together after our changes?
How will we do it? With drugs, fighting against the problems? With
nature, blessed by all we are given? Will it matter to the Earth, Gaia,
what choices I make in my menopause? What stories I tell myself?
What I tell other women?

Hormonal Changes Before, During, & After Menopause

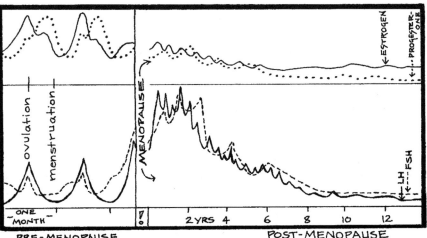

The Six Steps of Healing

(Parentheses suggest a few of the modalities of each Step.)

Step 0: Do nothing (sleep, meditate, unplug the clock or the telephone). A vital, invisible step.

Step 1: Collect information (low-tech diagnosis, reference books, support groups, divination).

Step 2: Engage the energy (prayer, homeopathic remedies, crying, visualizations, ritual, aromatherapy, color, laughter).

Step 3: Nourish and tonify (herbal infusions/vinegars, love, some herbal tinctures, life-style changes, physical activities, moxibustion).

Step 4: Stimulate/Sedate (hot/cold water, many herbal tinctures, acupuncture, most massage, alcohol). Risk of developing dependence on Step 4 remedies is influenced by frequency (how often), dosage (how much), and duration (how long).

Step 5a: Use supplements (synthesized/concentrated vitamins or minerals, special foods like royal jelly or spirulina). Supplements are *not* Step 3. There's always the risk with synthesized/concentrated substances that they'll do more harm than good: men who took fish liver oil in capsules had a greater mortality from heart disease (the oil was rancid).

Step 5b: Use drugs (synthesized alkaloids, oral and injectable hormones, high dilution homeopathics). Overdose may cause grave injury or death.

Step 6: Break and enter (fear-inspiring language, surgery, colonics, Rolfing, psychoactive drugs, invasive "diagnostic" tests such as mammograms and biopsies). Side effects are inevitable and may include permanent injury or death.

Using This Book

• Start by looking through the whole book quickly. Life is not neatly divided into chapters. Each woman will achieve her menopause in her own unique and individual way. My broad divisions of premenopausal, menopausal, and postmenopausal may not fit your experiences. *Any of the remedies may be used at any time in one's life.*

★ If you want something that works exceptionally well, or quickly, look for the stars. They mark favorite remedies, ones that I and many women have used with superior results.

• Pay particular attention to Appendix 2. The results and safety of any remedy are dependent on your ability to prepare it appropriately and use it appropriately. Note that I use **herbal vinegars** and **herbal infusions**, which are quite different from culinary vinegars and herbal teas.

• Use the remedies for your problem in order. I've arranged them from safest to most dangerous, using the pattern of the Six Steps of Healing: Step 0 is the safest; Step 6, the most dangerous.

• Use Steps 0, 1, 2, and 3 as preventive medicine. Prevention is an important, though often invisible, way of healing/wholing in the Wise Woman tradition. Deep relaxation, information exchange, energetic engagement, optimum nourishment (including touch), and exercise promote health with little or no side effects.

• If you want to remedy your problem with the least possible side effects and danger, start at Step 1. (Whether or not I mention it as a specific remedy, Step 0 is always appropriate.) After reading Step 1, pick one remedy from Step 2 and set a time limit for working with it. If your problem is unresolved within that time, decide if the time limit needs expanding or if you are ready to go to Step 3. Continue in this manner, moving to Steps 4, 5, or 6 as needed, until your problem is solved. Each step up increases the possibility of side effects and their severity, so I strongly urge you to try at least one of the Step 2 techniques, even if they seem strange to you, before going on to the remedies of Steps 3 and beyond. (Note also that time spent at Step 2 will help you choose appropriate remedies at Step 3, and so on.) When your problem is resolved, don't stop. Go back through the Steps, in reverse, before resting at Step 0.

• You can continue to take remedies from a previous Step after moving on, but be cautious about the use of Step 4 remedies in combination with Step 5 remedies. Motherwort tincture and vitamin E (5a) may be fine together, while valerian and an antidepressant (5b) may not. (See next section: "Using Herbs Safely.")

• If you deem it necessary to heal through Step 5 and/or 6 (and real healing can and does take place with the aid of drugs and surgery) and have not yet tried any techniques from Steps 2 and 3, do so immediately. Engaging the energy, nourishing and tonifying will aid and abet the healing powers of the more dangerous healing ways and help prevent or moderate their side effects.

• Note that Appendix 2 lists food/herb sources of all vitamins and minerals needed during the menopausal years. If you are currently taking supplements, this is a good time to stop and switch to optimum sources of nourishment: seaweeds and nourishing herbal infusions.

• Use the index to help you find more information on an herb you are using. Wise Woman teaching flows in spiraling cycles, so this book is not a formal garden with a *Materia Medica*, but rather a wildflower garden with different information on one plant appearing here and there throughout the book.

• I have included German, French, and Chinese names for many herbal allies.

• Trust your own sense about what's right for *you*. Use this book in conjunction with your own inner Wise Woman. Seek second and third opinions. Respect the uniqueness of your body, your intentions, and your feelings.

May it be in beauty; may it be in a sacred way.

Using Herbs Safely

Plants feed us, clothe us, house us, heal us, and kill us. There's no way around it, when you use herbs, you need to be alert and aware. Here are some ways to be sure you're using herbs safely.

• Identify all plants you intend to use by botanical name (e.g., *Leonurus cardiaca*). Only buy herbs that are labeled with the botanical name. The botanical name is specific to only one plant, while common names overlap and vary. "Sage" refers to at least five plants in at least two different families, but *Salvia officinalis* only means garden sage.

• Use only one herb at a time. Learn all you can about that one herb. Read books; experiment on yourself, others, pets; listen to your elders' stories. If you discover that your herbal ally likes to work with partners, pair her up with other herbs one at a time.

• Seek out the worth of the weeds on your doorstep. Learn about, eat, or use as a remedy, one wild food/medicine that grows in your yard or nearby lot this year. When you make your own medicines and healing foods you eliminate one of the possible dangers of crude herb use: mistaken identity (or right label, wrong herb). Not that you can't make mistakes, but you're more likely to catch your own mistake than someone else's. When you make your own medicines and healing foods, they are fresh, full of energy, and in tune with you and your environment. You'll also feel better as you become more aware of the vitality and abundance of nature expressing herself everywhere.

• Begin with gentle nourishing and tonifying herbal infusions and vinegars. Watch carefully for side effects during the first 24 hours the first time you use any new plant. Don't worry if it takes your system a couple of tries to figure out how to digest a new food/herb; that's normal. Use herbal tinctures after you have some grounding in the use of herbs as foods and infusions. Start with the smallest recommended dose and build up slowly if needed.

• Build up a foundation of trust in the healing effectiveness of plants by using remedies for minor problems before tackling serious concerns.

• Gather or join a support group of people interested in self-care and home remedies and consult them when you feel uncertain.

• Respect the power of plants; those strong enough to act as stimulants, sedatives, and near-drugs (such as opium) affect the body and spirit in powerful ways and may be useful only in minute doses.

• Respect the individuality of every plant, every person, and every situation. Everything changes.

• Remember that you become whole and healed in your own unique way, as you will. Plants can help in this process. People can help in this process. (Animals, too.) But each individual body/spirit does the healing/wholing itself. Don't expect plants to be cure-alls.

• Respect the difference between herbs used in Step 3 — nourishing and tonifying herbs — and those used in Steps 4 and 5 — stimulating, sedating, and toxic herbs.

Nourishing herbs are the safest of all herbs; side effects are quite rare. Nourishing herbs may generally be taken in any quantity for any period of time. They are foods, just as leafy greens, garlic, and carrots are. They provide high-level nutrients, including vitamins, minerals, trace minerals, starches, simple and complex sugars, bioflavonoids, carotenes, and essential fatty acids (EFAs). The nourishing herbs in the *New Menopausal Years the Wise Woman Way* are: alfalfa, borage, calendula, chamomile, chickweed, cornsilk, comfrey, elder blossoms or berries, fennel, fenugreek, lemon balm, mallows, nettles, oatstraw, plantain, raspberry, red clover, seaweeds, sweet briar (rose hips), St. Joan's wort (*Hypericum*), slippery elm, and violet.

Tonifying herbs act slowly in the body and have a cumulative, rather than immediate, effect. They are most beneficial when they are used in small quantities for extended periods of time. Side effects are slightly more common with tonics. (Note that many herbalists equate stimulating herbs with the tonics, leading to misuse and unwanted side effects.) The more bitter the tonic tastes, the less you need to take of it. Bland tonics may be used like nourishing herbs, in quantity. Nearly half of the herbs in the *New Menopausal Years the Wise Woman Way* are tonics, including: birch, black cohosh, blackstrap molasses, chasteberry, dandelion, dong quai, echinacea, false unicorn, ginseng, hawthorn, horsetail, lady's mantle, motherwort, peony, sarsaparilla, spikenard, wild yam, and yellow dock.

Sedating/Stimulating herbs cause a wide variety of usually rapid reactions, some of which may be unwanted. Long-term use can lead to dependency, so sedating/stimulating herbs are best used in moderate doses for fairly short periods of time. Side effects are frequent; there may be loss of tone or a rebound/manic effect when the herb is no longer taken. Some parts of the person may be stressed in order to help other parts. The sedating/stimulating herbs in the *New Menopausal Years the Wise Woman Way* are: catnip, cinnamon, ginger, hops, kava kava, licorice, liferoot, myrrh, passion flower, poplar, primrose, sage, skullcap, uva ursi, valerian, vervain, willow, and wintergreen.

Potentially poisonous herbs are potent medicines; they activate intense effort on the part of the body and spirit. Potentially poisonous herbs are best taken in tiny amounts for very short periods of time. Unexpected side effects are common when these herbs are used without regard for their power. Increase your herbal knowledge and sense of security when contemplating use of a potentially poisonous herb: consult other herbals and experienced herbalists. It is especially important to check on the possible side effects of these herbs if you are allergic to any foods or medicines. The potentially poisonous herbs in the *New Menopausal Years the Wise Woman Way* are: cayenne, cotton root, goldenseal, poke root, rue, sweet clover (*Melilot*), and wormseed.

Green blessings.

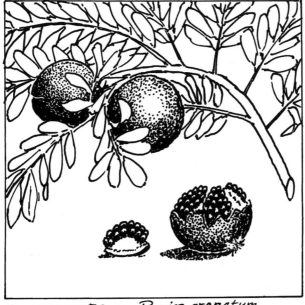

Pomegranate — *Punica granatum*

Foreword
Wonshé (Sher Willis)

I first read this book at the time of my own quickening as Crone. I was experiencing biological changes, shifts in my rhythm that I had never known, yet somehow remembered. These changes were deep, primal; they called me to respond to everything from a visceral place. I was a volcano ready to erupt, a bird destroying her own nest, an island about to form. Friends and practitioners insisted I was too young (not yet 40) to be menopausal. I felt like a woman, pregnant for the first time, who has never seen another pregnant woman.

Then *Menopausal Years the Wise Woman Way* came to my hands. Susun's words affirmed my **Change**, brought my opposites together, showed me how to use all my healing options wisely, and offered me an unsurpassed opportunity to recreate my wholeness.

As a midwife, and keeper of the blood mysteries, I see a profound parallel between the experiences of menopause and those of childbearing. As Crone, or as Mother, we generate power from the archetypal and elemental source of all life: female sexual energy.

With the help of this *New Wise Woman Ways for the Menopausal Years*, we can use this energy to resanctify ourselves, to re-wild ourselves, and to break free from the unnatural definitions of menopause that would domesticate and disempower us.

As an herbal resource alone, it is of extensive value to every reader. And it is more than just a book about menopause. It speaks to our entire planet — literally, symbolically, scientifically, poetically, authentically — from the heart of a wise woman. It is perhaps the single most important book for women — and men — to read as we shift into the twenty-first century and the time of the "earth changes." Woven throughout the text is the ancient truth of the new millennium of our planet: potent image of woman reflecting the spirit and the truth of Earth as Earth reflects the truth and spirit of woman.

Thank you sister. Thank you Susun. Now I understand what menopause is: a time to generate female sexual energy beyond fertility, a season to **Change** with Earth, and an initiation.

Preface

February cold rainbows glint in mooncaught snow. My birthday. This is the face of an aging woman who looks at me, clear-eyed, from my mirror. This is a face which has known some weathers: smiles line the mouth and eyes, worries are gathered between the brows, and forty-six winters glitter silver lights (like the rainbows in the snow under the full moon) from my crown. Forty-six is surely not old yet. But just as surely getting old. Old woman. Getting to be an old woman.

Now my monthly bleeding is precious. Dear. Soon I will go without it. The anxious wait for blood to signal that I am *not* pregnant turns on its head and becomes an anxious wait for blood to show that I *am* still fertile. This companion of more than thirty years is preparing to leave; I feel her restless stirrings, the way her attention wanders, how irregular she's become. I know my life will be different when she's gone.

Different? How? Without my monthly bloody show will I be a woman? Is this not what made me a woman when I thought I was but a girl? All I know of myself as woman is the ripening of the egg, the building of the nest, the giving unto/into life.

"Great granddaughter, it is time to prepare for your journey. I am Grandmother Growth. I, my plant friends, and my stories have come to guide you on your menopausal journey, your metamorphosis to Crone, woman of wholeness."

Crone? Old woman! **Change?** The **Change!** Menopause! When my ovaries abandon me to the ravages of old age: brittle bones! uncertain heart! withered sexuality! wrinkles! grey hair! No!

Why do I wake at night sweating? Bad dreams? Too many covers? Hot flash? Hot flash! But I'm too young. I'm bleeding. It can't be. I'm not ready. Hot flash? How can I keep up my work? Maintain my responsibilities? Hot flash! Oh no.

"I bring you the ancient women's mystery stories. Take the time to listen to me. Slow down. Take time off so you can hear the old, old memories beginning to chant in your bones, drum in your heart, pulse in your veins, transform your energy."

The Crone reaches out her hand. The air crackles with heat and power, a sudden sweat starts up along your sides, between your thighs, around your neck, along your spine. The sensation is intense.

"Open your hands; release your expectations. Take my hand. Let me awaken memories of wise old women, crazy old women, peaceful, joyous, strong, invisible old women, whose trail you can find and walk, whose songs you can hear and sing. Journey with me into Change, sing with me the forgotten melodies, come with me along this old, old trail. Come. baby Crone, come."

Modern Western doctors and the media tell me I'm on my way over the hill; that I should prepare for the inevitable downhill slide. "Your ovaries are calling it quits," they tell me. "Soon you'll be a useless old woman. Your bones will break, your heart will fail, and all because you're lacking estrogen. Of course, we can supply you with it . . . for a price. And any price is worth paying for your share of estrogen. It may cost you your breasts and your uterus, but at least you'll still be a woman."

Grandmother, what is happening? Everything seems so strange. I thought I was comfortable with myself in many forms, but I don't know who I am anymore. What is overcoming me? What am I becoming?

"Sweet child, the wise woman achieves menopause, it does not overcome her. Through the gate of menopause the wise woman steps into her final glory, her crowning as Crone. Daughter, sister, listen well: the time and place in which you live seeks to deny you your last crown. Few leaders and healers of your day honor the Crone. Instead, they try to beguile you with the flowery wreath of the Maiden or the Mother's lush harvest headdress, telling you that growth into your deep maturity, into your Cronehood, is not worthwhile, not desirable; you must stay young. They hope to scare you away from this powerful Change, to convince you it's a deficiency state, of all things. Come with me and learn the true nature of your metamorphosis to Crone, woman of wholeness."

Grandmother Growth, if I go with you, if I sing with you, if I ally with your plant friends, will it be an easy journey?

"Not even I can promise you that, granddaughter. The journey of each woman into and through menopause is unique. If you encounter harsh weather or unexpected setbacks . . . well, that is the truth of the journey."

Ovary, ovary, talk to me. What are you doing? Are you tired? Out of juice? energy? eggs? Ovary, ovary, both of you, say something for yourselves. Are we still in this together?

"Woman, it is well that you sit in silence and harken to our words. Here in your ovaries there are memories. In the womb of your mother we gathered these memories, memories passed down from mother egg to daughter egg for hundreds of thousands of years. It is true that our stock of eggs grows low. This is as it should be, for our store of memories is full.

"Just as we have released ripened eggs each month, flooding your system with hormones so you could conceive and gestate, now we begin to release memories and the hormones needed to gestate memories. Take the time to ripen and swell these memories and you can give birth to the past (which, incidentally, changes the future).

"With our help, you have held out the hand of **giving life** for many years. Let it rest now. Come to know the hand of **giving death**. Grasp the hand of Grandmother Growth, grasp the fact of your own death. And, thus anchored in reality, give death to yourself as Maiden, give death to yourself as Mother, and birth yourself as Crone, woman of wholeness, who enfolds and holds within herself Maiden, Mother, and Crone, life and death."

Grandmother Growth suddenly appears, and drops a quartz crystal into my upturned palm.

"Now, great granddaughter. Take my hand. Yes, release the crystal, let it roll into the stream. Let go of yourself as Maiden. Take my hand."

Her gaze holds my eyes, which are suddenly wet with tears. Something small and cool slides into my palm. *"Take my hand."* I glance down quickly to see light shimmering in my hand.

"Let go of the moonstone, too. Nest it into the earth at the base of this tree. Let go of yourself as Mother. Take the hand of Grandmother Growth and open your eyes, wide. Look here. What do you see?"

Yes, this is the face of an aging woman who looks at me, clear-eyed from my mirror. Now I am 55. A woman walking toward herself as Crone. A woman humming the long-forgotten songs of menopause. An aging woman with many questions, and a few more answers.

February cold rainbows glint in mooncaught snow. My birthday. For years I have talked about and researched menopause. I have experienced it myself: descended to the underworld, and returned.

"It is time to share."

It is time to share what I have uncovered, discovered, recovered, learned, lived, understood. I offer, through these words, the guidance of my own heart and inner wisdom as well as the results of my studies.

"Take my hand."

Yes, take my hand, and walk a ways with me, deeper into the mystery as we share the *New Menopausal Years the Wise Woman Way.*

SSW
Laughing Rock Farm
8 February 1992/2001

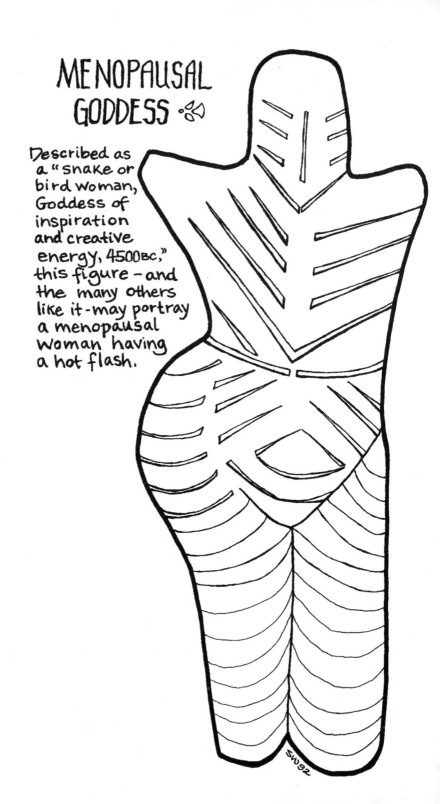

MENOPAUSAL GODDESS

Described as a "snake or bird woman, Goddess of inspiration and creative energy, 4500BC," this figure – and the many others like it – may portray a menopausal woman having a hot flash.

SW92

Is This Menopause?
Preparing for the Journey

"Is today not the best day to begin?" asks Grandmother Growth. "If you are old enough to ask 'Is this menopause?,' you are old enough to plan your journey to the old woman you are growing into. Let us gather what we need. It is time to begin your journey into Change."

"Is this menopause?" is a self-answering question. As soon as you ask, consider the process begun. Something is changing or you wouldn't be asking. Irregular periods? An occasional hot flash? If you are over forty, you are definitely beginning your menopausal years. (Menopausal changes begin for some women even earlier.)

"Is this menopause?" It is the rare woman who menstruates every 28 days until one month she simply doesn't any more. For most of us, menopause is a process that takes many years, not a specific, knowable end-point.

"Is this menopause?" In linear time, in the minds of many MDs and gynecologists, menopause is a single event, a definite end: the last menses. Everything before that last drop of blood is called "peri-meno-pause," and everything after that last drop of blood is "postmenopausal." To this way of thinking, there are no menopausal women. Only peri- or postmenopausal women. This is like defining puberty as the first drop of blood and nothing more.

To the wise woman, to the woman experiencing menopause, menopause is a spiraling process over time. One that changes and shifts even as it courses through us, so we never know what to expect from day to day during the **Change**.

"Is this menopause?" you surmise as you skip a cycle, then bleed normally for a year.

"Is this menopause?" you ponder, struggling to understand your new sexual preferences and appetites.

1

"Is this menopause?" you desperately hope as the blood pulses out of you in torrents.

"Is this menopause?" Since you asked: Yes, it is. And there are preparations you can make *now* that will help ease your journey of **Change**, of metamorphosis, of initiation as a fully mature woman.

"Is this menopause?" you wonder, taking off your sweater when everyone else seems chilled.

"Is this menopause?" you guess as you start to bleed 13 days after your last menses.

Yes, this is menopause. Your menopausal years have begun. Ally with hormone-helpful herbs, now. They'll moderate menopausal flooding and stabilize the ending of your menstrual cycles. They'll nourish and tonify the glands in transition at menopause, so you can encounter your flashes (of heat! of insight!) with more serenity.

"Is this menopause?" you think as you awaken, in a panic, sweating, and toss off the covers.

"Is this menopause?" you wonder as you contemplate your first grey hairs . . . your first serious wrinkles . . . the softening texture of your skin . . . the way your breasts and belly are growing larger and giving in more and more to the downward tug of gravity.

"Is this menopause?" you suspect as you find yourself sleeping less yet flowing with creative juices.

"Is this menopause?" you ask, noticing that you're digesting everything (food, people, events) differently.

"Is this menopause?" you whisper, feeling bone-tired, deathly tired, deeply exhausted.

This is menopause and you are not alone. This is menopause no matter what your doctor says. You are beginning your **Change** and you can change with grace and humor. Let herbs and other foods rich in essential fatty acids help you **Change**. They'll moderate cardiovascular disturbances (flashes, flushes, sweats), strengthen your liver, and help keep your energy levels high and your heart healthy.

Let calcium- and mineral-rich herbs and foods give you deeper sleep, more even emotions, and strong old bones. (The more bone you build before your menses stop, the more you'll have as a crone.)

The physical/menstrual/emotional/sexual changes that accompany menopause may be frightening. Let Grandmother Growth help. She knows the ways of women's mysteries. She lives the ways of the Wise Woman, healing and wholing person and planet. She offers stories about **Change**. New ways to understand the menopausal years, and new visions of Old Woman, She-Who-Holds-the-Wise-Blood-Inside.

"Shall we begin?"

Menstrual Irregularities

"Take heed granddaughter," murmurs *Grandmother Growth. "You are growing and changing. Sometime soon you will achieve your menopause. Take time now to listen to your inner wise woman. Lend your inner ear to the voice of your uterus, your ovaries (if they have been removed, listen to their energies, for they still remain). Lend your heart to their urgent messages.*

"Your blood is moving in new ways, dear woman," sings *Grandmother Growth. "Resistance will only make you tired. Allow the movements and changes inside you to spill out. There is no separation between your life and your Change. Let go now of your routines, your habits, your need for control. Give yourself up to this Change, this metamorphosis, the seeming chaos. I promise you, it will only be for a short while."*

You may very well feel the first tremors of your **Change** in increasing menstrual changes. Your menstrual cycles may become erratic. You may find yourself passing large clots when you bleed. You may spot. It is the rare woman who simply stops having her regular periods, never to bleed again (though it does happen).

Irregular intervals between menses is the norm as you enter the menopausal years. The remedies offered here don't imply that we ought to have regular menses during the menopausal years. The erratic movements of our cycles help us transform our self-image from fertile woman/Mother to wise grandmother/Crone.

Large blood loss at menstruation, an extended, dribbling menstruation, spotting at mid-cycle or other times — all are normal during the menopausal years, when non-ovulatory cycles allow the blood-rich lining of the uterus to grow until its weight induces a flow/flood.

Hysterectomy is the orthodox solution to heavy bleeding and can be a "life-saving" measure. But most menopausal women have only one or two episodes of heavy (or extended) bleeding during their **Change**, so removal of the uterus is usually overkill. The remedies offered here for women who are flooding (and for those with fibroids) are given in the hope of saving not only your life, but your uterus as well, that you may ever be a womb-one.

The quotes are from real women; may they help us remember that each woman's experience of menopause is uniquely her own.

Erratic Intervals Between Flows

"I never know when to expect my flow now. Sometimes it comes in two weeks, sometimes in six."

Step 1. Collect information . . .

Don't be surprised if your menstrual pattern changes noticeably sometime in your forties or late thirties.

The onset of menstruation at puberty is triggered by the production of estradiol, the most powerful of the estrogens. Estradiol production increases (sometimes smoothly, sometimes erratically) throughout the years of puberty, growing stronger through the late teens and peaking during the mid-twenties. The onset of menopause is triggered by the cessation of estradiol production. This may happen abruptly, but for most women, it occurs erratically — with lots of **Change**. One could truthfully say that *all* women are menopausal, that is, on the downhill side of estradiol production, after the age of thirty.

As estradiol production declines you may skip a cycle or two, find your menstrual bleeding scanty, or have heavier periods than you've ever had, sometimes two weeks apart. How can you tell what's normal and what's not?

Missing periods is fine. Missing periods for months (even for a year) and then getting them again is also fine. Very little blood and very much blood, even with big clots, is fine if it seems and feels like menstruation to you. (As in saying, when the blood shows: "Oh, that's why I was so irritable . . . constipated . . . weepy . . . you name it. . . .")

If the amount of blood is usual for you but the pattern is weird, that's menopause. If the cycle is usual for you but the amount of blood isn't, that's menopause. If you seemingly skip a period and then have a real drencher several weeks later, that's menopause. If you bleed for a month or spot at ovulation, that's menopause.

So, how can you distinguish the normal "abnormalities" of menopause from real abnormal bleeding needing attention and treatment?

Listen to your body. Pay attention to your dreams. Trust your own wisdom. Talk to other women. Keep records. I charted my menstrual cycles and my hot flashes on a Lunar Phases card (from Susan Baylies, 511 Scott King Rd., Durham, NC 27713. www.snakeandsnake.com) and recommend it highly. The thirteen months of moons on each card (one year) allow you to see your patterns, even during the chaos of menopause. You may find a certain regularity to your irregularity. Note: For help with birth control while having erratic menses, see page 61.

• **It is always wise to seek the opinion of someone experienced in women's health care if you are bothered by erratic or profuse menses.**

Step 2. Engage the energy . . .

• Try **lunaception** if your menses are highly erratic. Sleep where the **full moon** can shine on your face. If that isn't possible, sleep in a totally dark room except for the three nights when the moon is full. On those nights, turn on a small light and sleep with it on all night. Then resume sleeping in the dark until the next full moon. Repeat for as many cycles as it takes to regulate your menses (generally 3-6 moon-ths).

Sleeping in the dark increases melatonin production, reducing breast cancer risk. Low melatonin levels are strongly linked to cancer. Any light shining while we sleep — streetlights or nightlights, even the light from a digital clock — disrupts melatonin production. For health's sake, sleep in the dark; except when the moon is full!

• **Breathe deeply.** Do a full body relaxation before going to sleep.

• It takes a lot of energy to journey through menopause and you may feel "unreasonably" tired. **Take time for yourself when you bleed, even if you never have before; plan your Crone's Time Away.**

Step 3. Nourish and tonify . . .

• Get in the habit of drinking **nourishing herbal infusions every day**. They tonify and nourish your ovaries, uterus, adrenals, nerves, and liver, helping you move more easily with your **Change**. I have 2-4 cups of **red clover** blossom (page 161), **oatstraw** (page 239), **nettle** (page 241), or **comfrey leaf** (page 60) infusion daily. (Learn how to make infusion on page 254.) Comfrey leaf, unlike the root, is safe for regular internal use.

★ Slow-acting **chasteberry** is highly recommended for women bothered by menopausal irregularities. A dropperful of tincture, in a small glass of water 3-4 times a day usually brings results in 2-3 months. Long-term use, even for years, is considered quite safe. Many women, especially those dealing with fibroids, endometriosis, and after-forty fertility, call it a miracle. Chasteberry seemed helpful at first to me, but increased the severity of my "meltdown" phase menopausal symptoms.

• Nothing tones the pelvic area and helps maintain regular menstruation — up to the very last period — like regular sexual stimulation and release (**orgasm**), alone or with a partner. **Pelvic-floor exercises** (page 188), are a close second, though.

★ Essential fatty acids (EFAs) are critically important in regulating menses, protecting the heart, and keeping the vagina lubricated. A daily tablespoon or two/15-30 ml of **fresh wheat germ oil** or **cod liver oil** was used by savvy grandmothers fifty years ago. Modern grandmoms are more likely to use **flax seed oil, evening primrose oil, hemp oil**, or **borage oil**. Unfortunately, all these oils go rancid very quickly. Instead of buying the oil, I buy **flax seeds** and grind them (or **plantain seeds**) in an electric coffee mill immediately before use. About 1-2 tablespoons/15-30 mg per day is a "dose." Large amounts will be laxative.

• Tincture of **liferoot blossoms**, 5 drops taken daily, helps tonify the sites where reproductive hormones are produced: ovaries, uterus, adrenals, liver, and pituitary.

• **Four Roots Tonic** (page 259) warms, regulates, and gently heals the uterus and ovaries. It is especially useful when premenstrual distress accompanies irregular cycles. CAUTION: Dong quai can increase the menstrual flow and is best avoided by women who bleed heavily, especially those with fibroids or endometriosis. If you are one of those women, make it *Three* Roots Tonic; it will be just as helpful.

Step 4. Stimulate/Sedate . . .

★ Too much animal fat (and the estrogen-like pollutants concentrated in it) in our diets can contribute to menopausal symptoms. If you eat **meat**, cut back on the amount, and choose wild, free-range, or organic as much as possible. If you're vegetarian, you may be surprised to find yourself *wanting* meat as menopause progresses. All animal fats, including our own fat, can be converted into estrogens by our bodies. Too much animal fat taxes the liver and adrenals, increasing menopausal distress. But too little starves the tissues, leading to chronic problems. For optimum health, I eat butter in moderation, eggs as desired, and meat two or three times a month.

• **Cinnamon** (*Cinnamomum zeylanicum*) bark invigorates the blood, helps regulate the menstrual cycle, and checks flooding. The usual dose is a cup/250 ml of infusion sipped, 5-10 drops of tincture once or twice a day, a gnaw on a cinnamon stick, or cinnamon powder sprinkled on everything you eat. (*Everything?!*)

• **Acupuncture** is very effective in regulating erratic menses.

Step 5b. Use drugs . . .

• Birth control pills are used to regulate the intervals between "menses." But women taking the pill don't actually menstruate (they have "breakthrough bleeding") so it is difficult to determine when the last (forever) menses, that is, menopause, occurs. In addition, the risk of detrimental side effects from hormones increases with age.

Step 6. Break and enter . . .

"After the last planned pregnancy, the uterus becomes a useless, bleeding, symptom-producing, potentially cancer-bearing organ and therefore should be removed."   — RC Wright, MD, gynecologist, 1988

• The modern scientific remedy for women with premenopausal problems such as erratic periods is dramatic and invasive: remove the uterus (hysterectomy)! Then, they say, there is no need for about birth control and it makes it much safer for you to take estrogen therapy. However, a hysterectomy is major surgery, and while loss of your uterus will not necessarily make you ill, retaining it will contribute significantly to your sexual, emotional, and physical health.

Flooding

"I would contrive to get two super tampons inside and I'd use two thick pads as well, but I couldn't make it through the night, and when I went to the bathroom, I'd leave a trail of blood behind."

Step 1. Collect information . . .

Heavy bleeding (flooding) during the menopausal years — or prior to them — has a variety of causes: fibroids, endometriosis, and high levels of hormones, most notably high progesterone. Since it is a drop in the progesterone level that signals the uterus to contract and expel the menses, when progesterone levels stay high during the cycle, the endometrium continues to grow and reaches an unprecedented density and richness. It actually grows so dense that it crowds itself out of the uterus. When that finally happens, you have a "late" period that comes in floods, gushes, clots, and the occasional long slow bleed (not profuse, but it may go on for a month or more). **If you are bleeding profusely, go immediately to Step 4.**

Some healthy menopausal women report bleeding for as long as 40 days. Midwives note that it isn't so much the amount of blood a woman loses as her individual physiological response to the blood loss. Weakness, dizziness, paleness, and mental confusion signal danger.

Except in an emergency, hysterectomy is rarely the best answer for women who flood during menopause. Most women I spoke to reported only one episode of heavy or extended bleeding during their menopausal years. Only a few had two or more such incidents.

Loss of blood always means loss of iron. That usually leads to iron deficiency. And iron deficiency increases blood loss. To protect against flooding, **keep iron levels high**. (See pages 9 and 251.)

Flooding sometimes signals uterine and ovarian distresses such as an irritation or infection from an IUD, cysts, adenomatous hyperplasia, cervical/uterine/endometrial polyps, or, rarely, cancer. Of these, only cancer is directly life-threatening. (Remedies for women with cysts, polyps, hyperplasia, and reproductive cancers will be in *Down There, The Wise Woman Way*, to be published in 2005.)

Seek knowledgeable advice and health care from an experienced person if your period lasts more than a month, if you have pain or bleeding with intercourse, or if your flooding is accompanied by persistent low back/pelvic pain.

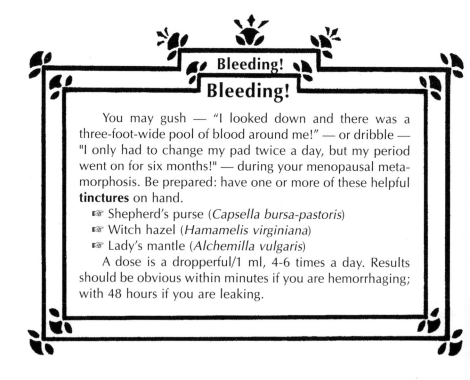

Bleeding! Bleeding!

You may gush — "I looked down and there was a three-foot-wide pool of blood around me!" — or dribble — "I only had to change my pad twice a day, but my period went on for six months!" — during your menopausal metamorphosis. Be prepared: have one or more of these helpful **tinctures** on hand.

☞ Shepherd's purse (*Capsella bursa-pastoris*)
☞ Witch hazel (*Hamamelis virginiana*)
☞ Lady's mantle (*Alchemilla vulgaris*)

A dose is a dropperful/1 ml, 4-6 times a day. Results should be obvious within minutes if you are hemorrhaging; with 48 hours if you are leaking.

Step 2. Engage the energy . . .

★ Emotional stress, says Christiane Northrup, MD, makes heavy irregular bleeding worse. Try Susun's Favorite Relaxation (page 130). Breathe.

★ There are many homeopathic remedies against menopausal flooding.

☞ *Lachesis*: flooding blood is very dark, thick, and strong-smelling; pain is more intense at the beginning of the flow; feelings of rage.

☞ *Sepia*: periods come frequently; bleeding is heavy or painful; menses are accompanied by backache, constipation, or depression.

☞ *Belladonna:* flooding with bright red blood and clots; you're swollen, ultra-sensitive, and/or headachy before and during bleeding.

☞ *China:* flooding with dark clots; exhaustion.

☞ *Crocus sativa:* flooding with clots but without pain.

☞ *Ipecacuanha:* flooding is bright red and continuous; you may have cramps, feel weak, and/or vomit.

☞ *Natrum mur.:* flooding brings tears, exhaustion, depression; periods irregular and prolonged; cramps, headache, constipation.

☞ *Sabina:* severe cramping, weakness, clots accompany flooding.

☞ *Secale:* flooding without clots, but with severe cramps.

☞ *Sulfur:* for the woman who floods and has drenching sweats with her hot flashes.

Step 3. Nourish and tonify . . .

★ **Lady's mantle** (*Alchemilla vulgaris*), the alchemical weed, controlled menstrual hemorrhage in virtually all of more than 300 women in a European study. When taken after flooding began, lady's mantle took 3-5 days to be effective. And when 10-30 drops of the fresh plant tincture were taken 3 times a day for 1-2 weeks before menstruation, lady's mantle tincture prevented flooding altogether.

★ The single most important element for the woman who bleeds heavily is **iron**. Try to consume 2 mg or more of iron from foods and herbs each day that you flood; 1-1.5 mg daily on days you aren't bleeding. Expect to feel more energetic and alive within two weeks. Flooding is usually noticeably diminished at the next menses.

My three favorite sources of usable iron are **cooked dandelion leaves** (which contain more than 5 mg in 1 ounce/30 grams), **molasses**, and **yellow dock root** (which promotes iron uptake). I prepare dandelion or yellow dock roots as a vinegar (2 tablespoons/30 ml a day) or tincture (20-40 drops twice a day). Other iron sources: page 251.

It is best to take iron throughout the day, not all in one big dose, as most bodies can absorb only a little at a time. To further enhance absorption, take your dandelion or yellow dock with something acidic like orange juice or milk. Both acid and protein increase iron uptake. **Avoid** tofu, soy drinks, soy protein powders, bran, calcium supplements (over 250 mg), coffee, black tea, and large amounts of egg yolks. They impair or prevent iron absorption.

★ **Bioflavonoids** strengthen the capillaries and provide estrogenic factors; together these effects help decrease flooding. (See page 248.)

★ A lack of prostaglandins can contribute to menopausal flooding. (And a surplus contributes to menopausal flashing!) Seeds rich in gammalinoleic acid (GLA) — such as **flax** (*Linum usitatissimum*), **borage** (*Borago officinalis*), **black currant** (*Ribes nigrum*), and **evening primrose** (*Oenothera biennis*) — are precursors to and helpers of prostaglandin production. Results from use are generally noticeable within two months; if not, discontinue use.

• **Flax**, also known as linseed, contains an oil unsurpassed in health benefits, but only if it is absolutely fresh and taken uncooked. Those wise in the ways of oils believe commercially pressed flax oil is rarely fresh enough. Instead they grind a tablespoon of organic flax seeds (which are inexpensive, usually about $2 a pound) in a little electric mill and cook them in muffins or pancakes or sprinkle them on breakfast cereal or lunch salads or anywhere else, so long as you consume the seeds promptly after grinding them. (Drink a glass of water or a mug of nourishing herbal infusion at the same time, please.)

If you don't have a grinder (or electricity), soak a tablespoon of flax seeds overnight in water and drink the whole thing, chewing the seeds very well, the next morning. Hemp, plantain, borage, black currant, and evening primrose seeds may be ground or soaked also.

If you don't want to bother and think you'll just take the already expressed (and usually encapsulated oil), stop! That's Step 5a, and you aren't there yet! Try some other remedies first.

★ **Chasteberries**, ground and added to food, or taken as a tincture (25-30 drops 3-4 times a day) promote progesterone production and decrease flooding. Women whose menstrual flow is normally heavy, and women with fibroids may wish to begin using chasteberry (*Vitex*) before problems occur, as its effects may take months to manifest.

★ **Wild yam** root tincture, 20-30 drops daily for the two weeks preceding the expected onset of menses, can supply enough progesterone precursors to decrease or eliminate flooding.

• **Astringent uterine tonics** offer help for women who bleed profusely. Herbs such as raspberry leaves, garden sage, and black haw bark are astringent and provide weak estrogens. If your period is generally heavy or if you have fibroids, start using infusions of these herbs (singly or in combination) as soon as possible, as they work slowly. Consume a cup or more a day, at room temperature or cooler, for best effect.

• **Carotenes** are a large class of compounds with many health benefits, including the building of healthy new blood cells. Brightly colored foods, especially those that are red, orange, yellow, and dark green are sources of carotenes (more on page 248), but only if they are *cooked*. (And best if they are cooked with oil or fat.) If flooding is part of your journey through menopause, make it a goal to eat carotene-rich foods at every meal. Or drink a cup of **nettle** infusion 3-4 times a day, which helps keep your energy level up too. (I do both.)

Step 4. Sedate/Stimulate . . .

• **Acupressure points** are used to sedate flooding in an emergency. One is located above the center of the upper lip (right under the nose); the other is right at the top of the head. Press very firmly on either point for one minute out of every fifteen until the bleeding stops.

★ **Shepherd's purse** (*Capsella bursa-pastoris*), tincture made from the fresh seed pods, leaves and stalks, is a cherished ally for women with uterine hemorrhage. It is especially recommended for women who bleed for many days, as well as for those who are flooding. A dropperful under the tongue, repeated every 10-15 minutes, can slow or stop flooding within hours, sometimes in minutes. If results are not noticeable within 24 hours, use another remedy.

   Women with fibroids say daily use of shepherd's purse tea or infusion reduces flooding. This may be continued safely for months.

★ **Witch hazel** (*Hamamelis virginiana*) bark/leaf tincture is another favorite with women who deal with flooding. Unlike shepherd's purse, which contracts and closes down the uterus (an effect which can increase flooding with the first dose), witch hazel contracts the blood vessels. A dropperful of tincture usually diminishes flooding within a few hours and brings it to normal within two days. Women with heavy periods may wish to use witch hazel infusion (1-3 cups a day) instead, for its tonic effect on the uterus.

• **Blue cohosh** (*Caulophyllum thalictroides*) or **trillium** (*Trillium* species) root tinctures are also used to stop hemorrhage. One, not both, may be used up to four times a day (20-30 drops) for several days.

• CAUTION: Avoid tinctures and capsules of **blood-thinning herbs** such as red clover (*Trifolium pratense*), alfalfa (*Medicago sativa*), cleavers (*Galium aparine*), pennyroyal (*Hedeoma pulegioides*), willow bark (*Salix*), wintergreen (*Gaultheria procumbens*), and ginkgo (*Ginkgo biloba*).

• CAUTION: **Dong quai** and **motherwort**, two herbs widely used by menopausal women, **may increase flooding**.

★ **Acupuncture** treatments are extremely helpful for women with severe menopausal flooding. Daily treatments during the flooding commonly stop acute blood loss. Frequent treatments during the luteal phase help prevent further flooding.

• Sipping strong **cinnamon** tea (a teaspoonful of the powder in a cup of boiling water) or using 5-10 drops of tincture every fifteen minutes can slow flooding and relieve uterine cramping. CAUTION: Do not use cinnamon oil internally.

Step 5a. Use supplements . . .

★ Capsules of certain seed oils are taken to increase prostaglandin production. This can reduce flooding, but increase joint inflammation. If the oil is rancid, it could increase the risk of cancer and heart disease. A dose of borage, black currant, evening primrose, flax, or hemp seed oil is 4-8 capsules daily. It may take six or more weeks before results are evident. CAUTION: Restrict use to three months or less.

• **Vitamin B$_6$**, by helping us assimilate iron, minimizes anemia from flooding, and thereby reduces flooding. A dose is 25-50 mg per day. CAUTION: Poisoning can result from taking 100 mg B$_6$ daily for more than 6 months. (See Appendix 1 for herbal sources of this nutrient.)

★ Avoid aspirin, Midol, large doses of ascorbic acid (vitamin C supplements), and other blood-thinning agents (see Step 4); they increase flooding.

Step 5b. Use drugs . . .

• **Progesterone** is an alternative to surgery for women with uncontrollable, life-threatening flooding. Synthetic progesterone (progestin) is highly effective if taken orally during the luteal phase (last two weeks of the menstrual cycle). Alternately, an injection of Depo-Provera may be used. So-called "natural progesterone" is useless in this regard, as are creams containing wild yam. Avoid them.

Step 6. Break and enter . . .

★ An IUD (intra-uterine device) can cause or increase flooding. If you have one, now's the time to have it removed. (See Menopause and Birth Control, page 61.)

• Surgical remedies for flooding involve dilating the cervix and inserting an instrument to remove the blood-rich lining from the womb. In many instances, flooding ceases and menopause continues uneventfully.

☞ **Aspiration curettage**, like a clinical abortion, removes a thin layer of the endometrium. It can be done under local anesthetic and without a hospital stay. This procedure is far less risky to you and your uterus than the more common D&C. Tests for cancer can easily be done on the aspirated material if need be. The endometrium regrows naturally.

☞ **D&C** (dilation and curettage) is the standard modern medical treatment for women with menstrual hemorrhage. After dilation, a serrated spoon-like instrument is inserted into the uterus and used to scrape away a layer of the endometrium. This is done under general anesthesia and requires a hospital stay. The endometrium regrows.

☞ **TCRE** (trans-cervical resection of the endometrium) completely removes the endometrium. It rarely regrows. This may be done under local anesthesia. Over 90 percent of the women who chose this treatment over a hysterectomy report relief from heavy bleeding. Long-term results are unknown.

• CAUTION! Hysterectomy is the preferred orthodox treatment for menopausal women with severe flooding. More than 25 percent of all hysterectomies done in the USA are done to control flooding. Menopausal flooding doesn't last forever; hysterectomy does.

★ Note: **If you elect to have a hysterectomy**, 30-60 drops of **echinacea** tincture several times a day for the week preceding and the several weeks following surgery will strengthen the immune system and help prevent infection.

Uterine Fibroids

"Finally, when my fibroid grew to the size of a twelve-week pregnancy, I asked my uterus to tell me what was happening. I heard these words: 'I want to be pregnant, I want to carry a child.' I've never had a child, nor really wanted one, but I could recognize that my womb did want it. The more I welcomed my 'child,' the more my fibroid shrank. It's still there, and still noticeable, but it feels less threatening, definitely easier to live with."

Step 1. Collect information . . .

Uterine fibroids, also called fibroid tumors, myomas, or leiomyomas, are solid muscle tissue growths in the uterus. They occur so frequently (in up to half of all women over forty) that they could be considered a normal irregularity. The causes of uterine fibroids are unknown, but it seems likely that estradiol (the strong estrogen made during the fertile years) promotes their growth.

Uterine fibroids which have been asymptomatic may respond to high estrogen levels during the menopausal years and cause aggravating symptoms including pelvic heaviness, low back pain, pain with vaginal penetration, incontinence, bowel difficulties, and hemorrhage. Women of color are three to nine times more likely to have fibroids than white women, and theirs will grow more quickly.

Occasionally a fibroid will become as large as a grapefruit, or even a cantaloupe (medical literature reports a 100 pound/45.5 kilo fibroid!), but the majority (80 percent) remain as small as a walnut. If you have no symptoms, but are told during a routine pelvic exam that you have fibroids, don't worry. You don't have cancer. (Tumor means a swelling or a growth, not cancer. Fewer than one-tenth of one percent of all fibroids are malignant.)

Small fibroids rarely cause symptoms and often disappear spontaneously, so they need cause you no concern. Large fibroids can exert pressure on the bladder, bowels, and sensitive pelvic nerves, causing a variety of symptoms including dull pelvic pain, bloating, frequent urination, constipation, infertility, and severe menstrual pain and flooding. While large fibroids are more difficult to resolve than small ones, many women have shrunk theirs without resorting to hysterectomy, the standard treatment for most menopausal women in the USA. (More hysterectomies are done because of fibroids than for any other reason.)

Here's the good news. Uterine fibroids usually disappear after menopause! (Unless you take hormones.)

"Over the more than 14 years I have been in clinical practice, not many health problems have eluded successful treatment as consistently as uterine fibroids. Women seeking an alternative to drug or surgical treatment . . . will not find an easy, reliable alternative. . . ."   — Tori Hudson, ND, 1999

Step 2. Engage the energy . . .

• **Reiki** treatments have been helpful to some women with large fibroids.

• Fibroids may be thought of as **too much energy** staying in the uterus. Here's one way to move it: Sit or recline comfortably and pay attention to your breath. Imagine that you are breathing out of your womb and out of your vagina. Breathe into your vagina and into your womb. Pause a moment and feel the breath spiral inside the uterus. Breathe out. Pause a moment. Breathe in. Continue for at least ten breaths.

• The "root chakra" (lowermost energy center in the body, which includes the uterus, cervix, perineum, prostate gland, and bladder) is strongly connected with **anger**. Unwanted growths in these organs may be seen as unexpressed, or stored, anger and countered by allowing the anger to discharge safely. Supportive therapies such as Pathwork or Bioenergetics can help you touch these feelings and move them.

Step 3. Nourish and tonify . . .

• One woman's fibroids (and menstrual cramps) disappeared within three months of beginning a vigorous **exercise** program. Another found it increased her bleeding a lot. Exercise does help insure regular ovulation, and regular ovulation seems to discourage fibroids.

★ **Lignans**, found in all whole grains, are anti-estrogenic phytoestrogens. Consuming three or more servings of whole grains daily not only reduces the size of fibroids but offers protection from several cancers as well (breast, endometrial). (Women with fibroids seem to have an increased risk of these cancers.)

Lignans are present in decreasing order in: flax seed, rye, buckwheat, millet, oats, barley, corn, rice, and wheat.

★ Beans have lots of anti-estrogenic phytoestrogens. Not just soy beans, but pinto beans, navy beans, pea beans, aduki beans, Anasazi beans, Appaloosa beans, baked beans, black beans, and any other bean you can think of. Lentils, all sizes and colors, work the best of all the beans. Like whole grains, used daily, beans can reduce the size of fibroids and reduce cancer risk.

• **Red clover** is a member of the bean family. A quart of red clover blossom infusion once a week is an excellent source of anti-estrogenic phytoestrogens. CAUTION: More than that, or red clover in capsules, or as a tincture may increase the size and bleeding tendencies of fibroids.

★ Strengthening the liver with herbs such as **dandelion, milk thistle** seed, or **yellow dock** root helps it metabolize strong estrogens into weak ones, thus reducing fibroids.

• The glycerine macerate of *Sequoia gigantica* buds is recommended by Swiss herbalist Rina Nissim for women dealing with uterine fibroids. She uses 50 drops, 1-3 times daily, in a small glass of water.

★ Rina Nissim also suggests an **anti-estrogenic brew** for women with fibroids. It contains equal parts tinctures of: black currant buds or leaves (*Ribes nigrum*), gromwell herb or seeds (*Lithospermum offici-nalis*), lady's mantle herb (*Alchemilla vulgaris*), chaste tree berries (*Vitex agnus-castus*), yarrow flowers (*Achillea millefolium*), and wild pansy flowers (*Viola tricolor*). Dosage: a teaspoonful/5 ml upon arising. Expect noticeable results within 2-4 months. This is such a beautifully conceived formula, that, like a superb soup recipe, any ingredients may be omitted without destroying the integrity of the whole. In fact, any one of these herbs — used as a simple — would be extremely beneficial to premenopausal women dealing with fibroids.

★ **Vitex** (chasteberry) tincture, 25-30 drops twice daily, often shrinks small fibroids within two months. But long-term results come from long-term use — up to two years.

• Ask someone to burn moxa over the area of the fibroid while you envision the heat releasing the treasures in your uterus. What is locked up in this fibroid? What can you give birth to? (It's OK to birth anything, even a monster.) Do this 4-6 times a week for at least six weeks.

Step 4. Sedate/Stimulate . . .

★ **Acupuncture** treatments can shrink fibroids.

★ **Poke root**, used internally as a tincture (1-10 drops per day; start small) and externally as a belly rub oil, has gained an increasing reputation as a profound helper of women with fibroids and endometriosis. Considered poisonous, poke root preparations may be hard to find (one source is Red Moon Herbs, see page 246). But they're easy to make! (How to: page 255).

★ **Cotton root bark** (*Gossypium*), primarily known as an extremely effective abortifacient, is a specific for stopping flooding due to fibroids. Use 1/2 cup/125 ml of infusion every half hour as needed, or a dropperful of the tincture every 5-10 minutes until hemorrhage stops. (See also previous section on stopping flooding, especially information on shepherd's purse and witch hazel.)

• Warm **castor oil** packs on the belly, or **ginger compresses** (soak a towel in hot ginger water) relieve pain and help shrink the fibroids.

★ CAUTION: **Avoid** dong quai, especially in capsules, or limit use to tincture, no more than 10 drops a day.

Step 5b. Use drugs . . .

• The role of **progesterone** apropos uterine fibroids is hotly debated. One side holds that fibroids result from estrogen dominance, or lack of progesterone. They advocate the use of progesterone creams.

The other side makes, to my mind, the better case: that progesterone is the culprit, not the cure. During pregnancy, when progesterone production is greatest, fibroids grow; after menopause, when progesterone levels decrease, they atrophy. To reduce fibroids, avoid progesterone, especially in supplemental forms, and actively reduce your estrogen load by eating whole grains, beans, and lentils on a daily basis.

• An injection of Depo-Provera, a synthetic progesterone, is used to stop excessive, life-threatening bleeding from fibroids.

• Large fibroids may be reduced by reducing the amount of estradiol and other strong estrogens in the blood, that is by avoiding birth control pills, estrogen replacement, and hormone replacement. Because some agricultural chemicals mimic the effects of estrogen in the body, use of organic foodstuffs may also reduce fibroids.

• Lupron (leuprolide acetate), a drug which induces "artificial menopause," may be used during the menopausal years by women with problematic fibroids to quickly lower their estradiol levels. More than half of the women who take it experience significant decrease in the size of their fibroids within 8 to12 weeks. The high cost of this treatment is a prohibitive factor for many women. And continued use is not possible. Fibroids return (to about 90 percent of their original size) when the drug is withdrawn (if natural hormone levels remain high). Lupron is frequently used to shrink fibroids before surgery.

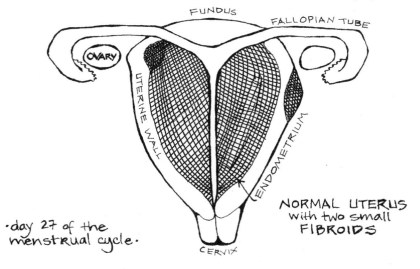

FUNDUS

FALLOPIAN TUBE

OVARY

UTERINE WALL

ENDOMETRIUM

·day 27 of the menstrual cycle·

NORMAL UTERUS
with two small
FIBROIDS

CERVIX

Step 6. Break and enter . . .

• Major advances in surgical treatments for women with fibroids were brought into use in the beginning of the new millennium. Educate yourself. Read about these new surgical procedures, talk with women who have tried them. If you decide one could work for you, take the time to find a surgeon who is skilled in the specific treatment you want.

☞ **Hysteroscopic resection**: Removes fibroids from within the uterus with the aid of a scope and a laser or electrical knife. Especially effective when the fibroids are pedunculated.

☞ **Uterine embolization**: The blood vessels serving the fibroid are closed off by the injection of various substances. Especially useful for women in their menopausal years.

☞ **Supracervical hysterectomy**: The uterine body is cut away, leaving only the cervix.

• When surgery removes only the fibroids, leaving the uterus, it is called **myomectomy**. Myomectomy requires a talented and sensitive surgeon. It is considered dangerous because it often causes significant blood loss. *Laser myomectomy* and *laparoscopic myomectomy* procedures reduce this risk. Fibroids regrow 15-30 percent of the time after a myomectomy.

• **Hysterectomy** is recommended by many Western physicians as the best treatment for menopausal women with fibroids. The image of the uterus as worthless to a woman past the age of childbearing is a strong one in their minds. Certainly there are times when hysterectomy is called for, but when we consider that, by the age of sixty, more than one-third of American women will have given up their wombs to the surgeons, we must ask if there are not better options. *The presence of non-symptomatic fibroids is never sufficient reason, to my mind, for a hysterectomy.*

When there are symptoms, it is worthwhile to work carefully through all the Steps of Healing before deciding on surgery. Of my students and apprentices who have had hysterectomies because of fibroids, and there have been many, those who "did their homework" — that is, helped themselves before and after their surgery with all the tools at their disposal — seemed to fare much better than those who did not.

• Hysterectomy carries grave side effects: half the women who have one experience loss of sexual desire, urinary problems, or a precipitous menopause (even when the ovaries are retained). Adhesions can form on the intestines after a hysterectomy, eventually constricting them and sometimes necessitating emergency surgery or causing death.

• Many surgeons insist that removal of the ovaries is a wise thing to do as part of the hysterectomy. Nothing could be further from the truth. The lifetime risk of ovarian cancer is 1 in 70, and there are important functions that the ovaries perform even after menopause. With very few exceptions, no woman is healthier without her ovaries. So, even if you elect a hysterectomy, **keep your ovaries**.

• If you choose **surgery** to remedy your fibroids, use these remedies as well to protect your health and improve healing time from the operation:
  ☞ Use 25 drops of echinacea root tincture 1-3 times a day, for three days before the operation and seven to ten days after.
  ☞ Try acupuncture treatments, before and after surgery.
  ☞ Avoid blood-borne diseases by donating some of your own blood to be used during the surgery.
  ☞ One woman created a ritual for "giving my uterus away rather than giving up on my uterus."
  ☞ Rub calendula oil on your belly to help prevent adhesions.

Spotting

"I used to feel a little twinge of pain when I would ovulate. Then one month there was a spot of fresh blood. This has gradually increased, and now I spot for several days around ovulation."

Step 1. Collect information . . .

Vaginal bleeding other than a menstrual flow is called spotting. The amount of blood may be barely enough to stain the underwear or it may be enough to require a minipad.

Like flooding, spotting and staining are normal manifestations of menopause, as well as indicators of possible reproductive distress.

Causes of spotting include menopause, ovulation, unsuspected miscarriage or spontaneous abortion, cervical infections, polyps, cervical dysplasia, irritation or infection from an IUD, cancer, and hyperplasia.

Seek help if more than two years have passed since your last period and you begin to spot or stain. Also seek help if your staining continues for more than ten days.

Step 2. Engage the energy . . .

• There are two primary homeopathic remedies for women with menopausal spotting: *China* is for the woman who also floods, feels weak, and is often depressed. *Pulsatilla* is for the woman who is highly emotional.

Step 3. Nourish and tonify . . .

★ **Red raspberry leaf** is the ally of choice for the menopausal woman who is spotting for no known reason. Try at least two cups/500 ml of the infusion daily. Add some mint to lighten the taste, if you wish.

• **Ginger root** tea warms and nourishes the entire pelvis. Try a cup/250 ml a day, sweetened with honey, for several weeks. Regular menses may be re-established, or the spotting may temporarily increase, then stop.

Step 4. Sedate/Stimulate . . .

• Cinnamon is a specific remedy for spotting. (See page 6.)

★ **Wild yam** root tincture (10-15 drops) or a full cup of tea can prevent and halt mid-cycle spotting by contributing to progesterone production. So can **chasteberry**.

Step 5b. Use drugs . . .

• Birth control pills may be prescribed to control spotting. This is not advised for women older than forty.

• Women who are bothered by erratic spotting during menopause may elect to take synthetic progesterone for ten days. Progesterone creams are not advised, but taking herbs with progesterone precursors may help; they are listed on page 74.

Step 6. Break and enter . . .

• Because spotting can indicate serious problems, many MDs prefer to do a D&C or an endometrial biopsy (to rule out cancer). The remedies suggested for use before a hysterectomy (page 19) are helpful here, too.

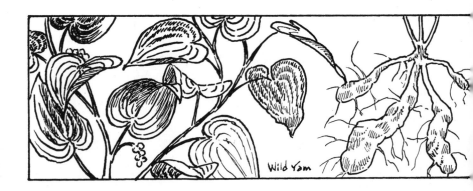
Wild Yam

Menstrual Cramps

"The hot flashes didn't slow me down, but the menstrual cramps did. I remember cramps like this when I was a teen. I vaguely remember hot water bottles, my mother's tender touch, thick novels, time alone to dream, to envision how my life would flower."

Step 1. Collect information . . .

The amount and intensity of your menstrual cramping may very well change during your **Change**. The major problem menopausal women face in dealing with cramps is that most herbs and many drugs which relieve cramping also increase flooding. Steps 2 and 3 offer some that don't.

Step 2. Engage the energy . . .

• Menstrual cramps remind us to take time alone.
• Sit in a hot bath and flow, melt, dissolve, relax, release, let go.

Step 3. Nourish and tonify . . .

★ **Liferoot** is one of my favorite remedies for menopausal women dealing with intense cramps, especially if accompanied by severe fatigue, nausea, and faintness. A small dose (5-10 drops) of the tincture of the fresh liferoot flowers, taken daily during the luteal phase (from ovulation to menstruation) for at least 3-6 months has "worked wonders" for many women who were totally incapacitated by menstrual distress. This remedy may be difficult to purchase. Mail order sources are listed on page 246. Or make your own. (Directions on page 255.)

★ **Black haw** and **cramp bark**, both *virburnums*, are superb allies for menopausal women with cramping and flooding. The tincture of either is an astringent tonic, powerful antispasmodic, and rich source of hormonal precursors. A dose is 10-20 drops, in water, as often as needed.

• **Garden sage** tea is hormone-rich and astringent, and, like all mints, a remedy for menstrual cramps. Most mints — such as catnip and pennyroyal, common and highly effective remedies for cramps — increase flooding, and are best avoided during the menopausal years. Smoking a **catnip** cigarette is, however, a highly effective way to diminish cramps and is unlikely to promote excessive bleeding.

Step 4. Sedate/Stimulate . . .

• If you're cramping but not flooding, try **ginger tea**.

• A dose of 5-15 drops of **motherwort** tincture is a great choice for menopausal women with menstrual cramping. The dose may be repeated, but it is better not to use this remedy on a daily basis, as it may increase circulation and provoke flooding.

★ **Valerian** root tincture, 30 drops repeated as needed, eases menstrual pain dramatically. Valerian makes many women sleepy and a few hyperactive.

Step 5b. Use drugs . . .

• Aspirin eases menstrual cramps but can provoke flooding. So can Midol. **Willow** bark (*Salix*) tincture is as effective as aspirin in relieving cramps but less likely to cause flooding. Best in vinegar.

Step 6. Break and enter . . .

★ A Crone's Year Away will disrupt every part of your life, breaking down carefully established patterns. It's time for a **Change**.

Cessation of Menses

"I was bleeding when the news came that he had been killed. I stopped within the hour and I haven't had a period since. I was 38 then; I'm 62 now."

Step 1. Collect information . . .

Menopause is the cessation of menses. In some books, it is nothing more than that, and what I call the "menopausal years" gets demoted to "perimenopause" (a word I intensely dislike, having seen it arrive just as women were claiming the power of their menopausal years). The Crone does not menstruate. If your periods stop during your menopausal years, no remedy is needed. Even if they start again, and stop again. . . .

I have met quite a few women in their late forties who are eager to have a child and want to prevent the cessation of their menses until they achieve their goal. A woman at one of my workshops said she had a child at 53, three years after her last period. To our wail of outrage and surprise, she laughed and advised: "Stay away from new lovers during menopause!"

When not associated with menopause, lack of menstrual flow (indicating, usually, lack of ovulation as well) is called amenorrhea, and constitutes a severe health risk. Bone loss during one premenopausal month without menses is the equivalent of one year's bone loss postmenopausally. The most common reasons for the menses to disappear before menopause (besides pregnancy) are lack of body fat (from eating disorders or heavy athletic training) and stress. These remedies may be used by women of all ages.

Step 2. Engage the energy . . .

• If menses cease due to loss and grief, try homeopathic *Ignatia*. If after a severe emotional shock, try *Natrum mur.*

Step 3. Nourish and tonify . . .

★ **Nettle** leaf infusion has reportedly returned the monthly flow to women drinking it regularly, even in their sixties!

• If menses stop due to lack of body fat, increase the amount of olive oil and butter in the diet to at least 4 tablespoons a day. And read the section on **weight gain**, starting on page 35.

• If emotional upheaval has stopped your menstrual cycles, seek **supportive counseling** or a therapy group to help you work with your grief, anger, and repressed memories.

★ **Dong quai** (*Angelica sinensis*) root tincture, especially when combined with white peony root (*Paeonia albiflora*) and licorice (*Glycyrhiza glabra*), is a superb remedy for women whose menses cease unaccountably. Let a daily dropperful or two nourish your "palace of the child" and help you establish regular cycles. CAUTION: Avoid dong quai if you are prone to flooding, or have fibroids.

Step 4. Sedate/Stimulate . . .

• **Acupuncture** treatments can be quite useful in re-establishing normal menstrual/hormonal cycling.

• Strong **pennyroyal** (*Hedeoma pulegioides* or *Mentha pulegium*) tea, a cupful/250 ml or more a day, for the three days of the new moon, can stimulate menstrual bleeding and restore regular cycling.

Step 5a. Use supplements . . .

• Supplements of **vitamin E**, 200-600 IU daily, have helped women restore ovulation and menstruation. Consistent use brings best results.

Step 6. Break and enter . . .

• Ten or more sessions of Rolfing (body work focused on breaking patterns held in the fascia between the muscles) can restore menstrual cycles for women not yet in the menopausal years.

Building Better Bones

"It is a bone-deep Change you are going into, my beloved," counsels Grandmother Growth. "You must open to your very marrow for this transformation. No cell is to remain untouched. You are to open more than you ever dreamed you could open, more than you have opened in birth or in passion. You open now to the breath of mortality as it plays the bone flute of your being. What can you do but dance to the haunting melody, develop a passion for an elegant posture and a long stride?

"Ah, yes," Grandmother Growth smiles rather wantonly. "It would do you well to develop a taste for fermented milk, and for dark leafy greens, cooked well, tarted with vinegar and mated with garlic. These things will build strong flexible bones to support you as Crone."

Did you know that your bones are always changing? Every day of your life, some bone cells die and some new bone cells are created. From birth until your early thirties, you can easily make lots of bone cells. So long as your diet supplies the necessary nutrients, you not only replace all the bone cells that die, you have extra cells to use for lengthening and strengthening your bones.

After the age of 35, new bone cells are more difficult to make. Sometimes there is a shortfall: more bone cells die than you can replace. In the orthodox view, this is the beginning of osteoporosis, the disease of low bone mass. By the age of forty, many American women have begun to lose bone mass; by the age of fifty, most are told they must take hormones or drugs to prevent further loss and avoid osteoporosis, hip fracture, and death.

Women who exercise regularly and eat calcium-rich foods enter their menopausal years with better bone mass than women who sit a lot and consume calcium-leaching foods (including soy "milk," tofu, coffee, soda pop, alcohol, white flour products, processed meats, nutritional yeast, and bran). But no matter how good your lifestyle choices, bone mass usually decreases during the menopausal years.

For unknown reasons, menopausal bones slow down production of new cells and seem to ignore the presence of calcium. This "bone-pause" is generally short-lived, occurring off and on for five to seven years. I noticed it in scattered episodes of falling hair, breaking fingernails, and the same "growing pains" I experienced during puberty.

I didn't see it in a bone scan, because I didn't have one, and won't. Why not? Because bone scans don't find women who are at risk of broken bones, alert them to the danger, and help them engage in preventative strategies. They find women who have low bone density (osteoporosis) and scare them into taking drugs whose long-term effects are unknown. According to Dr. Arminée Kazanjian, bone scans "mislabel most women. The majority of those who will ultimately suffer fractures will not get appropriate treatment because the focus is on [those] with low bone density, most of whom will *not* suffer fractures." No correlation between bone density and bone breakage has been established, according to Susan Brown, PhD, director of the Osteoporosis Information Clearing House, and many others.

The Wise Woman Tradition focuses on healing the whole person, not fixing a problem (osteoporosis). The Wise Woman tradition does not try to cure diseases, but to create a healthy/whole/holy being. When we focus on disease, we lose sight of wholeness.

Osteoporosis is a better indicator of breast cancer risk than of fracture risk. The postmenopausal women with the highest bone mass are two-and-a-half to four times more likely to be diagnosed with breast cancer than those with the lowest bone mass.[1] Hormones which maintain bone mass adversely affect breast cancer risk. Women who take estrogen replacement (ERT) even for as little as five years, increase their risk of breast cancer by twenty percent; those who take hormone replacement (HRT) increase their risk by forty percent in five years.[2]

Women who take ERT/HRT, even those who take calcium supplements too, still experience bone changes, suffer spinal crush fractures, and are more at risk of fractures when they discontinue hormone use. The U.S. Preventative Services Task Force 1996 Report says: ". . . few studies have been able to demonstrate directly that these interventions [calcium supplements and estrogen] reduce fractures."

Wise women build strong bones with nourishing herbal infusions. These exceptional sources of bone-building minerals prevent bone breaks better than supplements.[3] The minerals in leafy green herbs seem to be ideal for keeping bones strong.[4] Dr. T. C. Campbell, professor of Nutritional Biochemistry at Cornell University, who studied the diet in rural China where the lowest known fracture rates for midlife and older women are found, says, "The closer people get to a diet based on plant foods and leafy vegetables, the lower the rates of . . . osteoporosis."[5]

Calcium-rich plants and moderate exercise build strong flexible bones. Hormones and calcium supplements build thick, rigid bones that break easily. ERT/HRT do not increase bone cell creation; they only slow (or suppress) bone cell death and removal by osteoclasts. Use of nourishing herbal infusions and vinegars, fermented milk, and exercise improves health by feeding the bone creator cells (osteoblasts). When hormones are stopped, there is a rebound effect and bone loss jumps. Women who take hormones for five years or more are as much as four times more likely to break a bone in the year after they stop than a woman of the same age who never took hormones.

If you take hormone or estrogen replacement at menopause and continue for the rest of your life, you can reduce your risk of post-menopausal fractures by 40-60 percent. If you take frequent walks, eat a quart of yogurt a week, and drink nourishing herbal infusions regularly, you can reduce your risk by 50 percent. That's about the same reduction. The first is expensive and dangerous. The second, inexpensive and health promoting. Unless taking drugs appeals to you, I suggest you "just say no" to bone scans and osteoporosis scares.

It is never too late to build better bones, and it is never too soon. Your best insurance for a fracture-free, strong-boned cronehood is to build better bones before (during and after) menopause. The more exercise and calcium-rich green allies you get now, the less you'll have to worry about as you age.

"A woman has lost half of all the spongy bone (spine, wrist) she'll ever lose by the age of 50, but very little of the dense (hip, hand, forearm) bone. Attention to bone formation at every stage of life is vital; there is no time when you are too old to create healthy new bone."

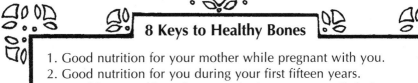

8 Keys to Healthy Bones

1. Good nutrition for your mother while pregnant with you.
2. Good nutrition for you during your first fifteen years.
3. Monthly menses throughout your fertile years, especially before 30.
4. Special attention to maintaining high levels of protein, fat, minerals, and vitamins from herbs and foods in your diet when menses cease during pregnancy, lactation, during and after menopause.
5. Regular rhythmical movement, the faster the better, daily.
6. Consistent practice of yoga, tai chi, or any strengthening, opening, flexibility-building discipline.
7. Chop wood, carry water.
8. Eat yogurt.

Calcium

"Osteoporosis is much less common in countries that consume the least calcium. That is an undisputed fact."   *—T. C. Campbell, PhD. 1993*

Step 1. Collect information . . .

Calcium is, without a doubt, the most important mineral in your body. In fact, calcium makes up more than half of the total mineral content of your body. Calcium is crucial to the regular beating of your heart, your metabolism, the functioning of your muscles, the flow of impulses along your nerves, the regulation of your cellular membranes, the strength of your bones, the health of your teeth and gums, and your vital blood-clotting mechanisms. Calcium is so critical to your life that you have a gland (the parathyroid) that does little else than monitor blood levels of calcium and secrete hormones to insure optimum levels of calcium at all times.

When you consume more calcium than you use, you are in a positive calcium balance: extra usable calcium is stored in the bones and you gain bone mass (insoluble or unusable calcium may be excreted, or stored in soft tissue, or deposited in the joints). When you consume less calcium than you use, you are in a negative calcium balance: the parathyroid produces a hormone that releases calcium stores from the bones, and you lose bone mass.

To insure a positive calcium balance and create strong, flexible bones for your menopausal journey, take care to:

☞ **Eat three or more calcium-rich foods daily.** See Appendix 3.

☞ **Avoid calcium antagonists.** See page 29.

☞ **Use synergistic foods to magnify the effectiveness of calcium.** See page 32.

☞ **Avoid calcium supplements.** See page 30.

Step 2. Engage the energy . . .

• The homeopathic tissue salt *Silica* is said to improve bone health.

• What does it mean to you to support yourself? To be supported? To stand on your own? To have a backbone in your life?

Step 3. Nourish and tonify . . .

• What do we need to make strong flexible bones? Like all tissues, bones need **protein**. They need **minerals** (not just calcium, but also potassium, manganese, magnesium, silica, iron, zinc, selenium, boron, phosphorus, sulphur, chromium, and dozens of others). And in order to use those minerals, **high-quality fats**, including oil-soluble vitamin D.

• Many menopausal women I meet believe that protein is bad for their bones. Not so. Researchers at Utah State University, looking at the diets of 32,000 postmenopausal women, found that women who ate the least protein were the most likely to fracture a hip; and that eating extra protein sped the healing of hip fractures. Acids created by protein digestion are buffered by calcium. Traditional diets **combine calcium**- and **protein**-rich foods (e.g. seaweed with tofu, tortillas made from corn ground on limestone with beans, and melted cheese on a hamburger). Herbs such as **seaweed**, stinging **nettle, oatstraw, red clover, dandelion,** and **comfrey leaf** are rich in protein and provide plenty of calcium too. Foods such as **tahini, sardines, canned salmon, yogurt, cheese, oatmeal,** and **goats' milk** offer us protein, generous amounts of calcium, and the healthy fats our bones need. If you crave more protein during menopause, follow that craving. CAUTION: Unfermented soy (e.g., tofu) is especially detrimental to bone health being protein-rich, naturally deficient in calcium, and a calcium antagonist to boot.

• Bones need lots of minerals not just calcium, which is brittle and inflexible. (Think of a chalk, calcium carbonate, and how easily it breaks.) **Avoid calcium supplements**. Focus on getting generous amounts of calcium from herbs and foods and you will automatically get the multitude of minerals you need for flexible bones.

• Because minerals are bulky, and do not compact, we must consume generous amounts to make a difference in our health. Taking mineral-rich herbs in capsule or tincture form won't do much for your bones. (One cup of nettle tincture contains the same amount of calcium — 300 mg — as one cup of nettle infusion. Many women drink two or more cups of infusion a day; no one consumes a cup of tincture a day!) Neither will eating raw foods. I frequently come across the idea that cooking robs food of nutrition. Nothing could be further from the truth. **Cooking maximizes the minerals** available to your bones. Kale cooked for an hour delivers far more calcium than lightly steamed kale. Minerals are rock-like, and to extract them, we need heat, time, and generous quantities of plant material.

★ **Green sources of calcium are the best.** Nourishing herbs and garden weeds are far richer in minerals than ordinary greens, which are already exceptional sources of nutrients. See Appendix 3, page 261.

★ But calcium from green sources alone is not enough. We need calcium from white sources as well. Add a quart of **yogurt** a week to your diet if you want really healthy bones. When milk is fermented or changed by *Lactobaccillus* organisms, the lactose is removed and the calcium, other minerals, proteins, and fats are more easily digested. This carries over, enhancing calcium and mineral absorption from other foods, too. (I have known several vegans who increased their very low bone density by as much as 6 percent in one year by eating yogurt.) Organic raw milk cheeses are another superb white source.

★ **Horsetail** herb (*Equisetum arvense*) works like a charm for those pre-menopausal women who have periodontal bone loss or difficulty with fracture healing. Taken as tea, once or twice a day, young spring-gathered horsetail dramatically strengthens bones and promotes rapid mending of breaks. CAUTION: Mature horsetail contains substances which may irritate the kidneys.

Step 4. Stimulate/Sedate . . .

★ Beware of **calcium antagonists**. Certain foods interfere with calcium utilization. For better bones avoid consistent use of:
- ☞ Greens rich in **oxalic acid**, including chard (silver beet), beet greens, spinach, rhubarb.
- ☞ **Unfermented soy** products, including tofu, soy beverages, soy burgers. (See page 163.)
- ☞ **Phosphorus-rich foods**, including carbonated drinks, white flour products, and many processed foods. (Teenagers who drink sodas instead of milk are four times more likely to break a bone.)
- ☞ Foods that produce acids requiring a calcium buffer when excreted in the urine, including coffee, white sugar, tobacco, alcohol, nutritional yeast, salt.
- ☞ **Fluoride** in water or toothpaste.
- ☞ Fiber pills, **bran** taken alone, bulk-producing laxatives.
- ☞ **Steroid** medications, including corticosteroids such as prednisone and asthma inhalers. (Daily use reduces spinal bone mass by as much as ten percent a year.)
- ☞ **Restricted calorie diets**. Women who weigh the least have the greatest loss of bone during menopause and "neither calcium supplements, vitamin D supplements, nor estrogen" slow the loss. Among 236 premenopausal women, all of whom consumed similar amounts of calcium, those who lost weight by reducing calories lost twice as much bone mass as women who maintained their weight.

• Although chocolate contains **oxalic acid**, the levels are so low as to have only a negligible effect on calcium metabolism. An ounce/3000 mg of chocolate binds 15-20 mg of calcium; an ounce of cooked spinach, 100-125 mg calcium. Bittersweet (dark) chocolate is a source of iron. Recent research has found chocolate to be heart healthy. (See page 211.) As with any stimulant, daily use is not advised. Chocolate is an important and helpful ally for women. Guilt about eating it is damaging to your health and interferes with your ability to hear and respond to your body wisdom. If you want to eat chocolate — do it; and get the best. But if you're doing it every day — eat more weeds.

• **Excess phosphorus** accelerates bone loss and demineralization. Phosphorus compounds are second only to salt as food additives. They are found in carbonated beverages, soda pop; white flour products, especially if "enriched" (bagels, cookies, cakes, donuts, pasta, bread); preserved meats (bacon, ham, sausage, lunch meat, and hot dogs); supermarket breakfast cereals; canned fruit; processed potato products such as frozen fries and instant mashed potatoes; processed cheeses; instant soups and puddings.

★ To **avoid phosphorus overload** and improve calcium absorption:
☞ Drink spring water and herbal infusions; avoid soda pop and carbonated water.
☞ Eat only whole grain breads, noodles, cookies, and crackers.
☞ Buy only unpreserved meats, cheeses, potatoes.
☞ Avoid buying foods with ingredients; they are highly processed.

• **Excess salt leaches calcium.** Women eating 3900 mg of sodium a day excrete 30 percent more calcium than those eating 1600 mg.[6] The main sources of dietary sodium are processed and canned foods. Seaweed is an excellent calcium-rich source of salt. Sea salt may be used freely as it contains trace amounts of calcium. Salt is critical for health; do not eliminate it from your diet.

• **Increase hydrochloric acid** production (in your stomach) and you'll make better use of the calcium you consume. Lower stomach acid (with antacids, for example) and you will receive little bone benefit from the calcium you ingest. Some ways to acidify:
☞ Drink **lemon juice** in water with or after your meal.
☞ Take 10-25 drops **dandelion** root tincture (or any herbal bitters) in a little water before you eat.
☞ Use calcium-rich **herbal vinegars** in your salad dressing; put some on cooked greens and beans, too.

Step 5a. Use supplements . . .

• **I really wish you wouldn't** use calcium supplements. They expose you to dangerous side effects (page 31), and increase fractures. An

Australian study that followed 10,000 white women over the age of 65 for six and a half years found "Use of calcium supplements was associated with increased risk of hip and vertebral fracture; use of Tums antacid tablets was associated with increased risk of fractures of the proximal humerus."[7]

• If you insist on supplements, go for calcium-fortified orange juice or crumbly tablets of calcium citrate. Chewable calcium gluconate, calcium lactate, and calcium carbonate are acceptable sources.

• CAUTION: Dolomite, bone meal, and oyster shell supplements usually contain lead and other undesirable minerals. Avoid.

• For better bones, take 500 mg magnesium (not citrate) with your calcium. Better yet, wash your calcium pill down with a glass of herbal infusion; that will provide not only magnesium but lots of other bone-strengthening minerals, too.

• Calcium supplements are more effective in divided doses. Two doses of 250 mg, taken morning and night, actually provide more usable calcium than a 1000 mg tablet.

Step 5b. Use drugs . . .

• Even if you take hormone therapy (ERT or HRT) you must get adequate calcium to maintain bone mass, according to researchers at Columbia University. That's 1200-1500 mg a day (a cup of plain yogurt, two cups of nettle infusion, a splash of mineral-rich vinegar, plus three figs is about that). As you increase your intake of calcium-rich foods/herbs, gradually cut back on your hormone dose if you wish.

Calcium Supplement Cautions

◊ Calcium supplements increase bacterial adherence in the bladder and urinary tract, increasing likelihood of infections and cystitis.

◊ Kidney stones have been precipitated in those who took large daily doses of calcium supplements (2500 mg or more) and drank too little water.

◊ There is much folklore, and even some slight scientific evidence, linking arthritis to use of calcium supplements.

Step 6. Break and enter . . .

• Bone density tests are frequently used to push women into taking hormones or drugs. If your bone density is low, use the remedies in this section and schedule another test (for at least six months later) before agreeing to such therapies.

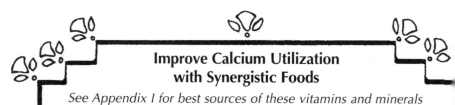

Improve Calcium Utilization with Synergistic Foods

See Appendix I for best sources of these vitamins and minerals

◊ Calcium and **vitamin D** work together. Approximately half the women who suffer hip fractures are low in vitamin D.[8] Get it from the sun, or from foods and herbs. In terms of fracture rates among 10,000 white women 65 and older: "There was no evidence of a protective effect from vitamin D supplements."[9]

◊ **Vitamin K** helps a bone protein called osteocalcin to undergo a chemical alteration that allows it to become part of the bone. Even when calcium and vitamin D levels are high, insufficient vitamin K allows "significant skeletal weakening" according to researchers at Tufts University who looked at the diets of 73,000 women.

High levels of vitamin K correlate strongly with lower risk of hip fracture.[10] The effect is strongest for women not taking hormones. For better bones, eat at least 110 mg of vitamin K a day. Best sources are (in order): nettle (760 mg), kale (620 mg), parsley (540 mg), collards (440 mg), spinach (380 mg), green cabbage (340 mg), watercress (310 mg), Brussels sprouts (235 mg), broccoli (180), comfrey leaves, and mustard greens. A 1/2 cup serving supplies at least 100 mg of vitamin K.

◊ **Magnesium** and **potassium** neutralize acids, sparing calcium from this task and protecting bones. Those whose diets are richest in these minerals are the least likely to have weak bones. Calcium-rich herbs and foods are usually magnesium- and potassium-rich as well.

◊ **Boron** increases bone mass, both as a synergist with calcium and as a nourisher to hormone production. In one study, blood levels of estrogen in postmenopausal women taking boron supplements began to rise within a week, and were equivalent within the month to those of women on ERT.

◊ **Lactose** and other natural sugars boost calcium absorption.

Dairy for Your Bones?

If I want to start an argument in a group of menopausal women, all I have to do is say "milk." Osteoporosis — does it cause it or prevent it?

Both. Neither. Real (yes, raw) milk from free-ranging animals is one of the the most healing substances I've ever used. I've seen it help women reverse severe bone loss, overcome life-threatening allergies, reduce asthma, and a put a variety of cancers into remission. New research finds dairy calcium a key player in switching the body's fat cells from storing calories to burning them.[11]

Of course, I am blessed; very few women have access to real milk. Fortunately, all of us have easy access to the next best thing: **yogurt**.

The health benefits of live-culture yogurt (when made from organic milk if possible) are amazing, especially for menopausal woman. Regular ingestion improves digestion of calcium from all sources, helps prevent cancer and strengthens immune system functioning. Women who eat a quart of yogurt a week have 75-80 percent fewer bladder and vaginal infections than those who eat none. And yogurt eases the nerves, like a cool, soothing touch on your overheated brow. Ahhh. . . .

When you buy yogurt, choose one containing only milk and culture. Avoid those with dried milk, whey, milk solids, and other processed ingredients. Better yet, make your own. See page 259. One cup/250 ml of plain yogurt supplies 400 mg of calcium, 33 percent of your daily need (1200 mg).

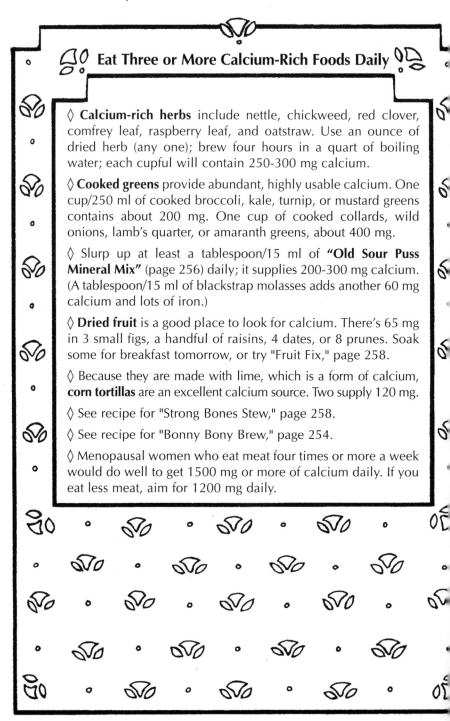

🌿 Eat Three or More Calcium-Rich Foods Daily 🌿

◊ **Calcium-rich herbs** include nettle, chickweed, red clover, comfrey leaf, raspberry leaf, and oatstraw. Use an ounce of dried herb (any one); brew four hours in a quart of boiling water; each cupful will contain 250-300 mg calcium.

◊ **Cooked greens** provide abundant, highly usable calcium. One cup/250 ml of cooked broccoli, kale, turnip, or mustard greens contains about 200 mg. One cup of cooked collards, wild onions, lamb's quarter, or amaranth greens, about 400 mg.

◊ Slurp up at least a tablespoon/15 ml of **"Old Sour Puss Mineral Mix"** (page 256) daily; it supplies 200-300 mg calcium. (A tablespoon/15 ml of blackstrap molasses adds another 60 mg calcium and lots of iron.)

◊ **Dried fruit** is a good place to look for calcium. There's 65 mg in 3 small figs, a handful of raisins, 4 dates, or 8 prunes. Soak some for breakfast tomorrow, or try "Fruit Fix," page 258.

◊ Because they are made with lime, which is a form of calcium, **corn tortillas** are an excellent calcium source. Two supply 120 mg.

◊ See recipe for "Strong Bones Stew," page 258.

◊ See recipe for "Bonny Bony Brew," page 254.

◊ Menopausal women who eat meat four times or more a week would do well to get 1500 mg or more of calcium daily. If you eat less meat, aim for 1200 mg daily.

Weight Gain

"Pack your bags for the journey," Grandmother Growth advises softly. "Your Change may be rough in places, so cushion yourself. Your Change may have some hard edges, so let your contours round. Your wise blood is stirring and you are learning to let it move without attaching fear to its meanderings. In the same way, you can gracefully allow your natural weight gain. Struggling with your weight or dieting is bad medicine for you now, resulting only in thin bones that break easily, extreme hormone shifts that will keep you from sleeping and thinking, and an inner fire reduced to ashes or burning out of control. Pack your bags, slowly, dear one. There is no rush," sighs Grandmother Growth, closing her eyes and sinking into a nap.

The best ally you can have on your menopausal journey is ten "extra" pounds. I know you don't want to hear this. I understand how difficult it is to desire ten extra pounds (or accept it happening to you, as it does to most menopausal women). You may have spent much of your life trying to get rid of ten extra pounds. The ultimate failure as a woman nowadays is not to be infertile, but to gain weight.

When thin and young is the standard of beauty, any menopausal woman might find it difficult to maintain a positive self image as she sees herself becoming a thick-waisted, silver-haired Crone.

I had some killer hot flashes, but the most difficult part of menopause for me was gaining weight. I knew it was going to happen; I knew it was supposed to happen. But I never thought it *would* happen. I read the studies; I knew that most healthy women, thin or thick or in between, gained ten to fifteen pounds during their menopausal years. But not me, I thought. I eat superbly. I exercise: an hour and a half of yoga every week, tai chi, and my ordinary farm chores (moving and splitting firewood, throwing bales of hay, hauling water, chasing goats). Not me.

Yes, me. I watched my image in the mirror take on a shape more and more closely approximating the Venus figurines of pre-history. And my modern prejudices surged to the fore: "Yuck. You look disgusting. You're overweight. It isn't healthy. Lose weight!" I knew it wasn't true. But despite years of feminism and consciousness-raising on every -ism, from ageism to weightism, there was my culture yelling at me in my own mind every time I looked in the mirror.

Now I looked like my aunts. Now I looked like a woman. It was as strange and unfamiliar as the sprouting of my breasts and pubic hair at puberty. I remember standing in my clothes closet at the age of thirteen, wistfully and resentfully removing my favorite little-girl dresses, none of which fit.

Not looking in the mirror didn't help. (I didn't have to resist looking at the scale. I don't own one.) My clothes didn't fit. First it was my blouses: my buttons gaping and my t-shirts straining. Then it was my pants: Tight waistbands became absolutely impossible. My size fluctuated wildly from morning to night, growing bigger as the day went on. For several months, I walked around the house with my pants unfastened from dinner until bedtime, a menopausal symptom my sweetheart was completely in favor of.

Fortunately, I knew that dieting would not improve my health, and could easily harm me. But without the loving acceptance I felt from my lover, I might have faltered and given in to the desire to resist this change with all my might. I might have given up on being proud to look like a postmenopausal woman: like Margaret Mead, Eleanor Roosevelt, Susan B. Anthony.

I wish every menopausal woman could have someone to tell her each evening when she disrobes, how goddess-like, how voluptuous, how attractive and desirable she is, and to say with her: "The best ally I can have on my menopausal journey is ten extra pounds."

Of course, I don't mean ten pounds of ordinary fat. You want ten pounds of healthy fat supported by healthy muscle and bone. And you want to gain that weight very, very slowly. Ideally about a pound or two a year during menopause. Remember, you are cushioning yourself for the journey. Love yourself as you get "in shape" for **Change**.

Step 1. Collect information . . .

• Fat cells convert androstenedione, a substance produced by the adrenals and the ovaries, into estrone, the primary postmenopausal estrogen. Women who gain weight during menopause have less severe hot flashes, an easier **Change**, and denser bones, according to Jeanine O'Leary Cobb, past editor of *A Friend Indeed, the Newsletter of Menopause*, and menopause investigator.

• Despite pronouncements that extra fat is a health risk, weight gained during the menopausal years is not associated with any increase in mortality risk.[12]

• And losing it will not improve your health.[13,14]

• In fact, weight loss can lead to thyroid malfunction, severe gall bladder problems, increased insulin-resistance, and weakening of the cardiovascular and immune systems.[15]

• If you don't have a sweetie to tell you your bigger body is bodacious, read:

☞ *Radiance: The Magazine for Large Women*, PO Box 30246, Oakland, CA 94604

☞ *Healthy Weight Journal*, PO Box 620, LCD1, Hamilton, ON; L8N 3K7, Canada. 800-568-7281

☞ *You Count, Calories Don't*, Linda Omichinski. Box 102A, RR#3, Portage La Prairie, MN; R1N 3A3, Canada. 800-565-4847

☞ *Loving Your Midlife Body*, Linda Moore Browning, Health Forum for Older Women, Winter 1999

Step 2. Engage the energy . . .

"The first time I saw pictures of my postmenopausal self I was frightened by my size!"

• Give yourself permission to **take up more space**. Allow your needs to be uppermost. Enlarge your view of yourself. Enlarge your world.

• If you don't already do an hour or more of yoga, tai chi, or some other **meditative physical exercise** weekly, begin . . . now.

• Go to an art gallery, or get a book from your library, and find a picture of an attractive woman with a **round proud belly**. Meditate with her. Become her for a moment. Feel the energy in your belly. Feel the wise blood stirring within your belly. Stirring and simmering and sending its heat up along the energy pathways of your body. Be proud of yourself and your belly.

• Say a short prayer of thanksgiving, or sing a song, or light a candle, or observe a moment of silence before you eat. Affirm that the food will bring you **health** and **pleasure**.

Step 3. Nourish and tonify . . .

• Give up dieting. Eat the widest variety of whole foods possible. Don't make any foods absolutely forbidden. What you eat everyday has the most effect. The best way to stop worrying about weight gain is to eat ten or more servings of fruit and vegetables, three or more servings of whole grains, and a cup of yogurt daily.

• To insure that you add hormonally-helpful, bone-strengthening, empowering fat, include one serving of a high calorie phytoestrogen-rich food and three servings of super mineral-rich foods in your daily diet.

☞ **High-calorie hormone-rich foods** include olives, olive oil, organic butter, freshly ground *flax* seeds, homemade *beer*, alcohol-free beer, nuts and fresh nut butters.

☞ **Super mineral-rich foods** include nourishing herbal *infusions* of nettle, oatstraw, red clover, or comfrey leaf; *cooked greens* such as kale, collards, lamb's quarter, amaranth, mustard; *seaweeds*; whey; whole grains including oats, millet, wheat, and brown rice; bitter-sweet *chocolate*.

• Beer is traditionally brewed from hops and sprouted whole grains. The fermentation creates easily assimilated B vitamins and liberates minerals. One beer a week will slowly increase your weight, improve your memory, soothe your nerves, and improve your immune system. A cup of hops tea with a spoonful of barley-malt sweetener is an alcohol-free alternative.

Step 4. Stimulate/Sedate . . .

• Most herbal remedies sold for weight loss include stimulants which can disturb heart function, and diuretic and laxative herbs which can cause excessive fluid loss and disrupt electrolyte balance. This may lead to life-threatening events during the menopausal years, when heart and adrenal functions are unstable. Avoid all "weight-loss" herbs.

• If you are determined to lose weight during your menopausal years, here are some safe strategies.

☞ Eat a substantial breakfast and a large lunch and **skimp on dinner**. Absolutely avoid midnight snacks.

☞ Eat a cup/250 ml of fresh **chickweed** daily or take a dropperful of the fresh plant tincture in some water during or after every meal (at least four times a day).

☞ Gently simmer a handful of dried or fresh **bladderwrack** (*Fucus*) **seaweed** for 15 minutes in enough water to cover. Strain. Drink a cup before each meal for no more than three months.

☞ Eat a bowl of hot soup at the beginning of the meal. You will feel more sated and eat less. Cold soups and drinks do not have the same effect.   .

• **Keep active.** But you don't have to buy any spandex. Five-minute periods of exercise, done several times a day, every day, are better than one long session once a week. Weight lost as a result of increased physical activity is safer than weight lost through diet manipulation. **Lift weights.**

• Depression can be associated with intense cravings for starchy foods. If we satisfy these cravings with mineral-rich foods (including chocolate), the depression will be "treated" and will dissipate. If we attempt to satisfy these cravings with mineral-deprived white flour and white sugar, the depression will deepen. (See depression, pages 111-117.)

Step 5b. Use drugs . . .

• Appetite-suppressant drugs upset your metabolic rate and make it harder and harder for you to maintain a normal weight with a normal diet. Avoid all drugs and herbs and supplements of any kind that claim to suppress your appetite.

Step 6. Break and enter . . .

• Science is ready to help you deny your increasing wisdom and power by liposuctioning fat from your derrière and adding it to your face to plump out wrinkles.

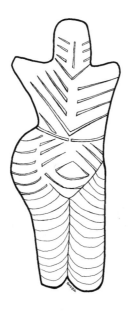

PMS Forever?

"Counting days will not get you through this Change, my love," warns Grandmother Growth. "You are on the way to transformation; do not expect predictability. Do not become alarmed when you experience yourself in totally new ways. You are changing, getting ready for a new birth, getting ready to be initiated into the third stage of your life as a woman. Your wise blood and your wise hormones are shifting in their courses. They may flood, wash away their usual routes, rearrange their known boundaries, cause you pain, entice you to solitude. Let it happen; fasten your seat belt and get ready for the ride of your life!"

Over the years you've probably gotten to know the changes you'll experience in the days just before your menstruation begins. Perhaps it's water retention, sore breasts, constipation, diarrhea, bloating, or emotional uproar — the symptoms are different for every woman. But, whatever they are, they disappear with the onset of menstruation. During your menopausal years, you may have premenstrual symptoms for weeks or months, until menstruation arrives to relieve them. One woman described menopause as "PMS that goes on for years."

My premenstrual symptoms were always minor, until I entered my menopausal journey, when those minor annoyances seemed magnified, and new ones appeared. That's normal. The thing about the **Change** is that it is a change. Menstruation doesn't just disappear, it likes to make a dramatic exit. Here are some remedies then, for premenopausal premenstrual distresses — ones you know and ones you may get to know. (Depressed premenstrually? See pages 111-117.)

Water Retention

"I tried everything to ease the swelling in my fingers and ankles. My daughter suggested nettle infusion, but I hated the taste of it. I finally froze some into ice cubes and put them in everything I drank. Within a week my ankles were trim again."

Step 1. Collect information . . .

Fluid retention is also called bloating or edema. If you have a tendency toward this, strengthen your kidneys with nettle infusion. If your legs and feet are retaining fluid, strengthen your heart with motherwort tincture. If you get bloated in the evening for no reason, that's menopause.

Step 2. Engage the energy . . .

• Listen to a recording of running water, or, better yet, sit beside a gurgling brook or a noisy river. Feel the waters inside you moving, flowing, sliding. . . .

• Sleeping with a lavender dream pillow is said to help correct a tendency toward water retention.

Step 3. Nourish and tonify . . .

★ My favorite herbal ally for women with water retention is **dandelion**. Take 10-20 drops of the tincture of the spring-dug root with meals and watch the edema recede. Continue for as long as you like. Dandelion not only helps remove excess fluid from the cells, it nourishes and tones the liver, improves digestion, and contains plant hormones that help ease your **Change**.

★ Frequent use of **nettle** infusion, a cup or more a day, rapidly relieves (and helps prevent further episodes of) water retention. Nettle is a superb nourisher of the kidneys and adrenals.

• Chinese women use **dong quai** root, cooked with other herbs, to relieve premenstrual bloat. It does this by "warming" the womb, which may increase menopausal symptoms.

Step 4. Stimulate/Sedate . . .

★ Bloating is aggravated by use of mineral-poor salt in the diet. Replace your table salt with **sea salt**.

• Limit your consumption of sweet fluids, such as sodas, fruit juices, and sweetened teas. The more sweet fluids you drink, the harder your kidneys have to work, and the more easily fluid builds up in the cells. Instead, drink nourishing herbal infusions, unsweetened herbal teas, and water. Limiting fluid intake seems like a way to forestall water retention, but may actually aggravate it.

• In order of increasing potency, these common foods will help you let go when you feel bloated: **asparagus**, **corn** (and corn silk tea), **grapes**, **cucumber**, **watermelon** (and tea from the seeds), parsley, celery, black tea, and **green tea**. Use these foods freely; or try a small amount of corn silk tincture.

★ Exercise and massage stimulate movement of all the fluids in your body.

Step 5a. Use supplements . . .

• Large doses of **ascorbic acid** (vitamin C) increase fluid output, but stress the kidneys, increasing the likelihood of future water retention.

Step 5b. Use drugs . . .

• Chemical diuretics leach potassium, contributing to osteoporosis. Counter this by eating substantial amounts of potassium-rich foods. Nettle infusion or dandelion tincture are herbal diuretics that contain large amounts of potassium. Regular use may cause lovely side effects like increased energy and improved digestion.

Step 6. Break and enter . . .

• Catheterization, short-term or in-dwelling, empties the bladder when you are unable to void on your own. Daily drinks of cranberry juice, blueberry juice, or uva ursi infusion help prevent bladder infections, a frequent side effect of this treatment.

Sore Breasts

Step 1. Collect information . . .

Breast tenderness premenstrually is normal: cells in the breasts that have been readied for pregnancy reach a peak of reproduction, stretching tender tissues, just before menstruation gets under way. Sore breasts may also be due to water retention, or benign lumps which enlarge as menstruation nears (and shrink afterward). Uncomfortable feelings in the breasts may increase in some women during their menopausal years. For others, menopause brings relief at last from chronically tender nipples and breasts.

Want to learn how to massage your breasts? Have a lump that worries you? My book *Breast Cancer? Breast Health! The Wise Woman Way* will help you take good care of your breasts.

Step 2. Engage the energy . . .

• Meditate on your breasts when they feel ultra-sensitive. Sit quietly and follow your breath. As you breathe out, imagine air, or water, or energy, or milk flowing out of your breasts. With each breath out, let this nourishing, healing, moving energy flow out of your breasts and into the world. Feel your breasts relaxing as they pour out abundance with each breath. Finish by breathing in and opening your eyes.

Step 3. Nourish and tonify . . .

★ Women whose diets are rich in calcium (1300-1500 mg a day) from dietary sources have less breast tenderness.

★ One of my favorite remedies for women with breast tenderness is the common weed **cleavers**, or goosegrass (*Galium mollugo*). A dose of the tincture of the fresh flowering and seeding plants is 30-60 drops, taken up to four times a day for several days if needed.

• Herbal allies for women whose breasts are tender and sore include 10-20 drops **black cohosh** tincture, or 20-40 drops **vitex** tincture, or 5-10 drops **liferoot** tincture twice a day for the two weeks preceding your bleeding. Or try chewing on a little piece of licorice or dong quai root or bittersweet **chocolate** daily during those two weeks.

Step 4. Stimulate/Sedate . . .

• Does consumption of caffeine-rich foods aggravate your breast tenderness? Eliminate soft drinks, coffee, and black tea for six weeks and see.

★ Use large **cabbage** leaves, steamed whole until soft, to compress swollen, sore breasts.

★ Very tiny doses of **poke** root tincture (1-4 drops, use fresh root tincture only) pack a wallop when it comes to easing breast pain. Poke (*Phytolacca americana*) is a renowned anti-cancer herb, too.

• **St. Joan's/John's wort oil**, gently stroked onto aching breasts, penetrates the nerve endings and relieves pain.

• Breasts engorged with excess fluid? Try cleavers or any of the herbal remedies for relieving water retention, starting on page 40.

Step 5a. Use supplements . . .

• To reduce breast tenderness, increase your intake of calcium, magnesium, and B vitamins. Whole grains and oatstraw infusion supply all three in abundance. Other good sources are listed in Appendix 1.

Step 5b. Use drugs . . .

• If your breasts are still painful after trying all the previous remedies, low doses of hormones (progesterone or birth control pills) may help. CAUTION: Some women say taking birth control pills made their breast tenderness worse.

Step 6. Break and enter . . .

• Cancel your appointment for a mammogram if your breasts are swollen and tender. The image won't be as clear then.

Digestive Distress

Step 1. Collect information . . .

As the mix of hormones in your blood changes during your pre-menopausal years, you may notice the effects on your gastrointestinal tract both directly — estrogen is a gastrointestinal stimulant and varying levels may swing you from loose stools to dry ones — and indirectly, as the hormonal load places ever heavier demands on the liver.

Hormones have a strong effect on the motility of the intestinal tract. When your levels of estrogen and progesterone change (as they do throughout menopause, during pregnancy, and before menstruation and birth), your bowel patterns change, too.

Your liver is, among other things, a recycling center. It breaks down hormones circulating in the blood when they are no longer needed and makes their "parts" available for the production of more hormones. During the menopausal years some hormones (such as LH and FSH) are produced in such enormous quantities that your liver may struggle to keep up with its recycling work, and have little energy left over for digestive duties. Help yourself with these Wise Woman Ways.

Step 2. Engage the energy . . .

★ Bless your food out loud before you eat; say grace; thank the plants and animals who nourish you; breathe in and feel grateful.

★ My mother's favorite way of preventing digestive distress and ensuring regularity is to eat at regular times and go to the toilet at regular times. You'd be surprised how effective this is.

• First thing in the morning, get yourself a cup of hot water (or herbal tea) and bring it back to bed. Sip it slowly, and gnaw gently on your bottom lip. Then lie on your back and bring your knees up, feet flat on the bed; place your palms on your belly and breathe deeply. Gently begin to rub your belly (in spirals): up on the right, across the middle, and down on the left. Soon you will feel the movement gathering momentum. Sit up slowly and head for the toilet.

Step 3. Nourish and tonify . . .

★ **Yellow dock root** vinegar or tincture is a wonderful ally for menopausal women with digestive distress. Daily doses of 1 teaspoon/5 ml vinegar or 5-10 drops of tincture eliminate constipation, indigestion, and gas. Yellow dock is especially recommended for the woman whose menopausal menses are getting heavier.

★ **Dandelion** is everyone's favorite ally for a happy digestive system and a strong liver. It relieves indigestion, constipation, gas, even gallstone pain. How to use it? Have a glass of dandelion blossom wine. Eat the omega-3-rich leaves in salads. Enjoy the phytoestrogenic roots as a vinegar or tincture (a dose is 1-2 teaspoons/5-10 ml vinegar or 10-20 drops tincture taken with meals) or as a coffee substitute.

★ Any **rhythmical exercise**, especially walking, relieves digestive gas and improves intestinal peristalsis (the involuntary movement of food through the intestines). Chinese wisdom says the liver loves movement.

• Motherwort, fenugreek, or chasteberry tinctures, taken daily, strengthen digestion and ease menopausal digestive woes. Or try a cup of **garden sage** tea. Or some herbal bitters before meals.

★ If constipation occurs due to a lessening of the moistening, lubricating cells in the colon, **slippery foods** such as slippery elm bark powder, oats, seaweed, flax seed, and seeds from wild *Plantago* (or cultivated psyllium) are wonderful allies. Adding a teaspoon/5 ml of any, or better yet, all of them to a cup/250 ml of rolled oats and cooking until thick in 3 cups/750 ml of water is a delicious way to prepare this remedy.

★ My favorite remedy to relieve digestive and gas pain is **plain yogurt**. Sometimes even a tiny mouthful will bring instant relief. Acidophilus capsules work, too. I use both when dealing with chronic constipation or severe diarrhea.

Step 4. Stimulate/Sedate . . .

• White flour products slow the digestive tract; so does too much grain-fed meat. Whole grain products, well-cooked beans, wild meats, and cooked greens speed it up.

• Add more **liquids** and **soft foods** to your diet — applesauce, yogurt, nourishing soups, herbal infusions — to help relieve constipation. Chew your food slowly and savor it. Drink lavishly between meals.

• Menopausal women will want to *avoid the use of bran* as a laxative, as it interferes with calcium absorption. Instead try **prunes**, prune juice, or **figs**. (See "Fruit Fix," page 258.)

★ **Ginger** tea with honey is a warming, easing drink when your tummy is upset. Ahhh. Try the fresh root grated and steeped in boiling water, or put a tablespoon of the powdered stuff from your spice cupboard in a cup of hot water and enjoy.

• Crushed **hemp seed** (*Cannabis sativa*) tea — rich in essential fatty acids — is a specific against menopausal constipation.

• CAUTION: **Herbal laxatives** such as aloes, *Cascara sagrada*, rhubarb root, and senna are addictive and destructive to normal peristalsis. Except in rare cases (such as relief of constipation for those using morphine or codeine, or confined to a bed), I do not advise their use.

Step 5a. Use supplements . . .

• Constipation and digestive distress are common side effects from taking iron supplements. A spoonful of molasses with 10-25 drops of yellow dock root tincture in a glass of warm water is a better way to increase iron and improve elimination.

Step 6. Break and enter . . .

• Enemas and colonics are last-resort techniques. They do not promote health and may strip the guts of important flora. Regular use of enemas is highly habit-forming. For the sake of your health, avoid them.

Emotional Uproar

Step 1. Collect information . . .

Premenstrual, pregnant, premenopausal, and menopausal women rage and weep. Like it or not, you'll probably find your emotions harder to control as you enter your menopausal years. Men given hormone therapy (against prostate cancer) weep and rage too!

Step 2. Engage the energy . . .

★ **Take time for yourself** when you find yourself crying, yelling, raging, depressed, out of control. Create your own sacred space, even in a closet, where you can be alone, without responsibilities, where you can be safe to have every one of your feelings.

• Begin (or deepen your commitment to working with) a **journal** as a way to care for yourself and your emotions. The **Change** is an opportunity to value your emotional self and to nourish all of your feelings, from grief to bliss, rage to outrageous.

• Universal healing energy can help when your emotions are roaring. Channel it through your hands to your heart or womb; hold yourself.

Step 3. Nourish and tonify . . .

★ My remedy of choice for women dealing with premenstrual emotional uproar is **motherwort** — the calm, fierce-hearted mother who helps you find your center in the wildest of emotional storms. A dose of 5-15 drops taken several times when you're upset will bring calmer feelings quickly. A dose of 10-30 drops taken twice a day for a month can help prevent mood swings.

★ Let a cup of **garden sage tea with honey** restore your emotional center and soothe your irritated nerves. It is even said to cure insanity and relieve hysteria. In Chinese herbal practice, honey is used (in tea, not cooked) to soften the energy of the liver when it is hardened by rage, frustration, and anger.

★ Pamper yourself. Get a **massage**. Cuddle with someone you love.

★ Moods don't swing so much in women who nourish their nerves and even out their blood sugar levels with lots of **calcium**.

• Slow-acting **liferoot** flower tincture (5 drops) or slower-acting **vitex** berry tincture (25-40 drops), taken daily for a week or two premenstrually for several months will help you unravel your emotional snarls.

• **Black cohosh** root tincture eases menopausal flashes and is said to cure hysteria, too. Try 10-20 drops once or twice a day for a month.

• Keep a piece of **licorice** or **ginseng** root handy to chew on when you feel like chewing someone's head off.

Step 4. Stimulate/Sedate . . .

• **Valerian** root, as a bath or tincture (15-20 drops as needed) is a powerful sleep-inducing sedative that also eases uterine cramps. Avoid long-term use.

Step 5b. Use drugs . . .

• Feeling moody? Mood-altering drugs, legal (tranquilizers, antidepressants, alcohol, coffee, cigarettes) or illegal (cocaine, opium), create dependence.

Step 6. Break and enter . . .

• Psychoactive plants (such as marijuana, psilocybin mushrooms, and mescaline), when taken in a safe setting, with a clear intention, offer radically different results than mood-altering drugs. Instead of dependence, they foster self-worth, helping the individual to break open new neural pathways and establish easier flows of emotions and energy through both the physical and subtle bodies.

Fibromyalgia

"Dear woman," Grandmother Growth's voice seems to float in the deepening twilight, echoing, reverberating, ringing in your ears. "Bring me your soreness. Bring me your pain. Bring your aches to me. Bring your burdens. Bring all you can no longer stand, can no longer bear, can no longer carry, can no longer shoulder, can no longer be responsible for. Give it to me. Put it down. Let us sit in council together and listen to the stories your pain tells. Menopause is a journey which requires you to pack light. Heavy things — bitterness, regret, vengeance, clinging to pain — will make your travels wearisome and bring you down. Take only the stories. Leave the rest behind. Burn the soreness in your hot flashes. Let it leave you. This is the Change. Let it change you, dear woman; let it change you."

Step 0. Do Nothing . . .
• Many women dealing with fibromyalgia have less pain if they sleep in a completely dark room or wear a sleep mask.

Step 1. Collect information . . .
The chronic pain disorder I called "sore all over" ten years ago is now called fibromyalgia. Ninety percent of the 4-6 million Americans dealing with this debilitating, frustrating condition are women, and many of them are menopausal.

Fibromyalgia is not a disease but a range of symptoms. (Soreness at eighteen specific tender points is the current diagnostic.)

In addition to widespread chronic pain on both sides of the body, above and below the waist ("But you don't hurt in all those places at once. The pain moves around."), there may be headaches, profound fatigue, severe cognitive difficulties, bowel and pelvic pain, low fever, sleep disturbances. Fibromyalgia mimics aspects of multiple sclerosis, Parkinson's disease, arthritis, hepatitis C, hypothyroidism, lupus, polymyalgia rheumatica, and early dementia.

Because the variability of symptoms makes diagnosis difficult, and there is no blood or laboratory test to verify it, many women with fibromyalgia are told their distress is "all in your mind." And it is!

Latest research indicates that those with fibromyalgia have restricted blood flow to the brain.[16] This limits the transmission of brain signals throughout the central nervous system and reduces the levels of neuro-chemicals including serotonin (modulates pain sensations) and growth hormone (in adults, used to repair muscle microtraumas).[17,18] Women with fibromyalgia have three times more pain-registering chemicals in their brains.[19]

But it isn't all in your mind (alone). Menopause can leave you feeling beaten on. Muscles respond to hormonal changes by feeling sore and cranky. Sleep loss can make you ache. (Non-restorative sleep is a hallmark of fibromyalgia. See pages 128-134 for help.) And lack of calcium, magnesium, and other minerals makes your bones ache.

Pay special attention to the Wise Woman ways of Step 2 — including Alexander and Feldenkrais techniques, hypnotherapy, archetypes, symbolic/somatic therapies, craniosacral therapy, sacred dance, visionary practices, and meditation. Techniques which engage the energy were, according to many women, the most successful in helping them mitigate fibromyalgia. "I changed anxiety to curiosity," said one.[20,21]

Step 2. Engage the energy . . .

★ Join a **support group**. This may help more than you'd think.

• Daily use of homeopathic *Rhus toxicodendron* reduced fibromyalgia pain by 25 percent. Homeopathic *Arnica* eases sore, aching muscles.

★ Women with fibromyalgia are often **survivors** of trauma. What are you sore (upset, angry) about? Where do these things live in your body? With the help of an experienced bodyworker, listen to those places.

★ Go back to your Mother. **Float** in the ocean. Lie belly down on the earth. Naked. Let her ease you. Let her heal you.

• Listen to a **relaxation** tape. Have someone show you how to do the yoga position called the "Corpse Pose." Learn how to bring yourself to a deep state of inner quiet and peaceful mind. (See page130.)

• A low-intensity EEG (electroencephalogram) biofeedback system, the Flexyx Neurotherapy System, is receiving attention as a new and promising way to help those with fibromyalgia reduce pain and decrease symptoms.

• The Jaffe-Mellor technique seeks to "neutralize the energetic signatures of any energy that takes advantage of a patient's compromised immune system." They claim to have virtually eliminated fibromyalgia in 75 percent of those treated. (Info: www.jmt-jafmeltechnique.com)

"People with fibromyalgia aren't just sensitive to pain; they also find loud noises, strong odors, and bright lights aversive." —Daniel Clauw, MD, Director: Chronic Pain and Fatigue Research Center, Georgetown University

Step 3. Nourish and tonify . . .

★ Consistent use of nourishing herbal infusions, especially **comfrey** leaf, **oatstraw**, and stinging **nettle**, in place of coffee, tea, and sodas is the single most effective remedy I know of for women with fibromyalgia. Regular consumption of **yogurt** is a close second, though.

★ Avoid vegetable oils. Their omega-6 fatty acids promote inflammation, soreness, stiffness, and pain. Use olive oil only. Increase omega-3 fatty acids by snacking on sardines and swigging cod liver oil.

• Gentle exercise — **walks**, **yoga** or **tai chi** — keeps muscles flexible and strong without trauma. Start with three minutes a day; gradually build up to four sessions of five minutes each. Persist; the reward is worth it.

• **Magnesium** is needed to moderate pain response in muscles and connective tissues. Large amounts are available from legumes, whole grains, leafy greens and nourishing infusions such as oatstraw or nettle.

★ **Moxibustion**, or needleless acupuncture, is safe, easy to do at home for yourself, and gives fast relief to sore joints and aching muscles. And its tonic action acts to lessen future pain. Buy a moxa "cigar" at a health food store or Chinese pharmacy. Bring the glowing end (after lighting it) near the painful area and move it around in small slow spirals until the heat becomes too intense. (This may take a few minutes or many.) Pain relief often lasts for twelve or more hours.

Step 4. Stimulate/Sedate . . .

★ Tinctures of **willow bark** (*Salix* species) or **Spirea** (1-2 dropperfuls/1-2 ml is a dose of either) are highly recommended by women dealing with fibromyalgia. Their active ingredients are almost identical to aspirin, and they have the same anti-spasmodic, anti-pain effect.

★ **St. Joan's wort** (*Hypericum*) tincture — not capsules, not the tea — is a superb muscle relaxer. A 25-30 drop dose not only stops, but also prevents muscle aches. I have used it as frequently as every twenty minutes (for ten doses). St. Joan's wort prevents soreness when taken after exercise; and even better if taken before. Prevents jetlag, too.

★ Regular **massage** stimulates the circulation of blood and energy, relieves pain, reduces fatigue, and eases stiffness. Avoid deep tissue massage; it increases pain. Light strokes and gentle myofascial releases are more helpful. Chiropractic manipulations are of little benefit.

• Massage with heated stones and other **heat treatments** work wonders for some women. For others, **cold** treatments work better (but not too cold, and not for too long either, please).

★ **Ginger compresses**, hot or cold, stir up circulation and mobilize the body's own healing agents to ease your pain. I grate several ounces of fresh ginger into simmering water, cook it gently for ten minutes, then soak a cloth in the liquid and apply that to the sore area. Or you may want to chill the wet cloth in the freezer for a few minutes first.

★ The National Institutes of Health lists fibromyalgia as one of the few conditions that **acupuncture** can relieve.

Step 5a. Use supplements . . .

• Some women said they knew someone who had benefited from taking **SAM-e** or **5-HTP** (5-hydroxytryptophan — a precursor to serotonin), but no study has found either helpful for those with fibromyalgia. Both are easily degraded by heat or light, and interact poorly with *Hypericum*.

• Lack of sleep can quickly aggravate symptoms of fibromyalgia. **Melatonin** at bedtime, the lowest dose you can get, may help. Or, paradoxically, it may make matters worse.

Step 5b. Use drugs . . .

★ Essential oil of **lavender** was recommended by several women who have dealt with fibromyalgia for many years. Dilute with jojoba or olive oil and use as a rub on the sore places.

• Orthodox treatment of fibromyalgia relies heavily on drugs, primarily **antispasmodics**, **antidepressants** and **muscle-relaxers**. But Celebrex, Vioxx, Valteran, amitriptyline (Elavil), fluoxetine (Prozac), vanlafaxine (Effecor), trazadone (Desyrel), alprazolam (Xanax), and cyclobenzaprine (Flexeril) can adversely affect the liver and disrupt the immune system. Instead, you could use herbal antispasmodics, page 195.

• Nonsteroidal anti-inflammatory drugs (NSAIDs) such as ibuprofen do not reduce fibromyalgia pain for most women; but they help some.

• Tramadol (Ultram) is a drug which addresses both the altered brain chemicals and the pain signals of those with fibromyalgia.

Step 6. Break and enter . . .

• Beware invasive diagnostic tests. Many women report enduring endless rounds of tests trying to put a name to their pains with no success and at the price of physical, mental, and emotional distress.

• Injections of lidocaine, a drug that temporarily numbs nerves, are effective in relieving fibromyalgia pain for some women. Injections of capsaicin (from cayenne) relieve pain by destroying nerve endings.

Thyroid

"Relax your jaw," commands Grandmother Growth as her strong fingers carefully encircle and sensitively touch your throat. "Do you know there's a butterfly in here?

"A butterfly that can literally change how you perceive the world. As you change, it changes, too. During menopause its pulsation is slower. Its ability to give voice to the truth increases, becomes insistent.

"Be still, dearest granddaughter. Turn off the radio, the TV, the stereo, the phone." Her voice is firm and strong. "Then listen carefully to the murmurs and screams of your own truth. Accept your psyche's need to turn in, to grieve, to rage. You will emerge stronger and wiser."

Step 0. Do nothing . . .

• Ryan Drum, herbalist and thyroid specialist, strongly urges all women with thyroid problems to try "indulgent bed rest." A protracted period of quiet, even complete withdrawal, is the best preliminary treatment to improve thyroid functioning, especially during menopause.

• Menopause changes the rhythms of all your endocrine glands, including the thyroid. I suspect periods of slow thyroid activity are normal during the menopausal years. If you think your thyroid is in trouble, take your time before getting tested or treated. It might get itself out of trouble on its own (or with just a little help from you). Unless your symptoms are severe, it is considered safe to wait a year before seeking diagnosis or treatment.

Step 1. Collect information . . .

The thyroid is the largest of the hormone-producing glands. It works with the pituitary, parathyroid, adrenals, and ovaries to moderate metabolism, protein synthesis, and bone density.

When the thyroid produces too little or too much of its hormones problems arise.

When too little is produced (hypothyroid), the inner fires burn more slowly. Symptoms include a persistent feeling of chill; lowered basal body temperature; lethargy, lack of energy, sleepiness; weight gain; dry, falling hair; brittle nails; leathery, puffy, thick skin that may be itchy, rashy, or scaly; poor memory; depression; constipation; unresolved joint pain; persistent dry vagina (not just too dry for intercourse). In extreme cases, the thyroid enlarges; this is called goiter.

When the level of thyroid hormones is too high (hyperthyroidism), inner fires rage: weight loss may be rapid, blood pressure rises, muscles begin to tremble, emotions range from apprehensive to overexcited, and bowel movements become loose and frequent.

If the thyroid is also attacked by the immune system, the diagnosis is Hashimoto's (hypo) or Graves' (hyper) disease. Women may have both simultaneously, or Graves' may progress to Hashimoto's. These diseases "may be a whole body attempt to enforce a slowing down of activity," says Dr. Drum. (See Step 0.)

• Does your thyroid need nourishment and attention? Absolutely! Undetected thyroid problems occur in 1 out of 70 women. One in 10 women is currently diagnosed with a thyroid disorder. And some specialists believe 1 out of 3 women have undetected hypothyroidism.

• Hypothyroidism may be a contributing factor in most non-infectious diseases, including osteoporosis, breast cancer, heart disease, arthritis, and reproductive problems. Menopausal and postmenopausal women who live long, active lives take care of their thyroids.

• How can you tell if your thyroid is okay?
   ☞ Take the **iodine challenge**. Paint tincture of iodine on a small patch of skin on your inner arm. If it disappears within an hour, you need more iodine (and your thyroid is probably unhappy).
   ☞ Test your **basal body temperature**. For four mornings in a row, first thing, as soon as you awaken, take your axillary (armpit) temperature while resting quietly. The average of the four readings should be between 97.8 and 98.2. For a more accurate test, take readings daily for two lunar cycles. (Ovulation, viral infection, and consumption of alcohol within 12 hours of taking your temperature can change basal readings regardless of thyroid function.)

• Thyroid tests that measure TSH (thyroid stimulating hormone) are more likely to reveal hypothyroidism than tests that measure T3 (triiodothryronine) and T4 (thyroxine).

• For more information contact: The **Thyroid Society**, 7515 S. Main St., Suite 545, Houston TX 77030, (713) 799-9909 or The American **Thyroid Association**, Townhouse Office Park, 55 Old Nyack Trnpk, Suite 611, Nanuet, NY 10954-2454.

Step 2. Engage the energy . . .

★ Wear a scarf with beautiful butterflies on it around your neck. Envision one of the butterflies fanning your thyroid with its wings.

★ Speak your truth, no matter how difficult.

"Situational hypothyroidism is a normal, desired, helpful, wise-body response to severe trauma, excessive unresolvable stress, and grief." — Ryan Drum

Step 3. Nourish and tonify . . .

★ **Nettle seed** (1/4 teaspoon/1 ml a day) is an excellent thyroid tonic, but you'll have to harvest it yourself (or buy from Carla Jo, p. 56). **Red clover** infusion or **ginseng** root extract are thyroid allies sold widely.

• Adrenal exhaustion disturbs the thyroid. Nourish your adrenals with **nettle leaf** infusion for 6-13 weeks and feel your thyroid smile.

★ **Lemon balm** (*Melissa officinalis*) is a possible ally for those with overactive thyroids; it reduces thyrotrophin production. Tea of the dried leaves, 1-3 cups a day, is preferred; avoid capsules or tinctures. Lemon balm loses its valuable essential oils rapidly; store it tightly sealed.

• Eat foods rich in **iodine**, **manganese**, and **tyrosine**, the major elements needed for optimum thyroid health. Seaweed supplies the first two; look for tyrosine (an amino acid) in aged cheeses and meats, alcoholic beverages, yeast-containing foods, bananas, almonds, avocados, pumpkin, and sesame seeds. (CAUTION: Avoid tyrosine-rich foods if you are taking an MAO inhibitor.)

Thyroid Helps Heart

A healthy thyroid means a healthy heart. Women with low levels of thyroid hormones are twice as likely to have a heart attack as women with normal levels.

When thyroid levels are low

☞ cholesterol goes up   ☞ plaque builds up in blood vessels
☞ LDL levels rise   ☞ homocystine becomes elevated
☞ blood-clots increase   ☞ diastolic blood pressure rises

★ **Kelp**, such as **wakame**, **kombu**, or **nereocystis**, is the herb of choice to help those with an underactive thyroid, or those with partial thyroidectomies. Forget pills or capsules; use high-quality powdered kelp or snack on dried pieces: 3-5 grams per day, or at least one ounce (dry weight) each week, added to cooked food. Results may take as long as 3-4 months to become evident. Persevere!

★ Herbalists 5000 years ago used *Fucus* seaweed to increase levels of thyroid hormone. It tastes strong, and acts strongly. If you are already taking thyroid hormone and want to stop, this is the ally for you.

An aggressive withdrawal protocol used by Ryan Drum adds 3-5 grams of *Fucus* to the daily diet and halves the amount of hormone taken each week; careful monitoring is essential. The conservative approach adds one gram of *Fucus* to the diet for a month, halving the medication. Two grams of *Fucus* are taken the second month and the medication is again halved. This is continued for five months.

If results are positive, continue taking five grams of *Fucus* a day to control symptoms. If negative, discontinue.

• **Avoid raw cabbage** family plants — including broccoli, Brussels sprouts, cauliflower, collards, kale, and mustard greens. They interfere with iodine uptake, and contribute to hypothyroidism.

Step 4. Stimulate/Sedate . . .

• **Iodine** stimulates the thyroid into action. Edgar Cayce recommended liquid Atomidine, one drop a day for five days, a rest for five days, then a drop a day for five more days. Stop for two weeks, then repeat.

★ **Bugleweeds** (*Lycopus virginicus*, *L. europaeus*) have antithyrotropic abilities, perfect for those dealing with hyperthyroid or Graves' disease. Dried leaf tea, 1-3 cups a day, is effective. Tincture, capsules, are not.

• Dr. Christopher recommends **poke root tincture** as a thyroid stimulant. Start with one drop a day; increase by one drop every 2-3 days up to 8-10 drops. Doses over 15 drops a day can damage the kidneys.

★ From my yoga teacher: The **lion pose** (tongue actively and fully extended) stimulates thyroid functioning, as do sessions of **Ujai breath**.

• Decades of exposure to **halides** — such as fluoride (in water and toothpaste), chlorine (in water), and bromine (released into the air from burning coal) — may cause thyroid problems. Ease your uptake by drinking spring water and conserving electricity (so less coal is burned).

• Decades of exposure to **radioactive iodine** also stresses the thyroid. Since the 1950s, iodine 131 has been released daily from all nuclear facilities, power plants, and weapons facilities. I can't avoid this, but I can protect myself by eating plenty of seaweed. Kelp, especially khombu, prevents absorption of radioactive iodine and removes it from tissues.

★ Cigarette and cigar smoke, whether inhaled directly or secondhand, diminishes thyroid functioning. So does the combination of alcohol use and food deprivation.

Step 5a. Use supplements . . .

• Iodine supplements (potassium iodide) are not absorbed or utilized as well as the biomolecular iodine present in seaweeds.

• Armour thyroid is natural thyroid hormone extracted from pigs. Some people strongly prefer it to the synthetic thyroxine.

• Capsules of powdered kelp have a reputation for causing thyroid problems. There appears to be little substance to this; but I avoid herbs in capsules as a general rule anyway.

Step 5b. Use drugs . . .

★ Barbiturates, sulfa drugs, antidiabetic agents, **estrogen** replacement, lithium, and corticosteroids adversely affect thyroid functioning.

• Wholistic endocrinologist Dr. William Dean encourages his patients to combine thyroid hormone treatment — either thyroxine or Armour — with alternatives. He checks every few months to be certain the hormones are still needed, and adjusts the dose down when the slower-acting natural remedies kick in.

• Prolonged use of synthetic thyroid replacement hormone is a known risk factor for heart disease and osteoporosis. Once you begin taking synthroid it is very difficult to stop. (See Step 3 for one possible way.) Try all other options before beginning treatment.

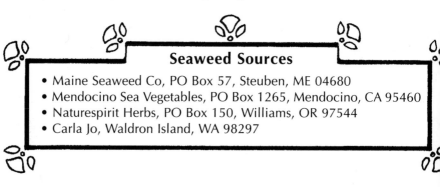

Seaweed Sources

• Maine Seaweed Co, PO Box 57, Steuben, ME 04680
• Mendocino Sea Vegetables, PO Box 1265, Mendocino, CA 95460
• Naturespirit Herbs, PO Box 150, Williams, OR 97544
• Carla Jo, Waldron Island, WA 98297

Fertility After Forty

"Yes, your fertility is changing, dear one. Part of the grief you feel comes from the realization that soon you will no longer be able to conceive, gestate, and give birth to your own children. Your time as a grandmother draws near." Grandmother Growth speaks with the pulse of your blood, her voice deep, reassuring, strong.

"I see your dreams. I know how you long to be a mother. I feel how you push away the idea of yourself as grandmother. I know how much you want to feel the smooth skin of your own baby, to inhale the special smell of the one who came forth from your womb, to hear the cry in the night for your aching breast. I sense your desire, and your doubt, your fear and excitement. Can you do it? Can you have a baby when the authorities urge you to give up or submit to drugs and surgery?

"Yes, you can still do this, dear one. It is harder now than before, and desire alone is not enough to insure success. But everywhere women are commonly surprised with menopausal babies, and in some places, women continue bearing babies until they are in their sixties. What will it take for you to become a mother on the edge of Change? How much chaos can you contain? How strong is your heart? How unflagging your stamina? How secure your sense of self-love? How deep your trust in the universe? Give me your hand. Look into my eyes. I promise you everything, my dear, and nothing."

Step 0. Do Nothing . . .

• Ambivalence about pregnancy and parenthood is normal and natural. But the older a woman gets, the more complicated her emotions about it may be. Add to her emotional soup pot strong opinions from family and friends, confusing information spread by the popular media, and fear-inducing pronouncements from "helpful" medical professionals, and that pot will be in danger of boiling over.

Turn down the heat and increase your chances of conception by meditating. Cultivating a calm attitude, not surprisingly, enhances fertility. Even a quiet five minutes by yourself, free from all responsibilities, can bring big results if done frequently enough.

Step 1. Collect information . . .

The years between 18 and 28 are a woman's most fertile. Even into the mid-thirties, it is usually fairly easy to conceive and carry a pregnancy to term. During these years the hormones that control ovulation, enhance conception, and ensure a healthy pregnancy are usually made easily and in generous quantities. Detrimental life-style choices have not had decades of repetition to create chronic problems.

Is waiting until your late thirties, early forties, even late forties, to have children too late? Are after-forty pregnancies destined to be high-risk? Will these children have more birth defects? The answer to these questions — and others like them — is "No!" Not if you enlist the help of green allies to increase fertility, ensure easy conception, prevent birth defects, and promote a healthy pregnancy and an easy delivery.

Step 2. Engage the energy . . .

• Contrary to current opinion, having children in your forties used to be common. The Bible mentions women having children in their fifties. What is unique to our time is having a *first* child in one's forties. The mothers of our mothers' mothers were having their fifth or eighth or tenth child when they were in their forties, not their first. If people tell you it just isn't done, close your eyes and call upon the spirit of your great-great-great-great-grandmother. Then smile and tell them it seems utterly ordinary to you.

• These Bach Flower Remedies may help. Try:
  ☞ *Aspen* when anxious, apprehensive, or afraid of the unknown.
  ☞ *Mimulus* when dwelling on a specific fear.
  ☞ *Elm* when feeling overwhelmed or inadequate.
  ☞ *Red Chestnut* when you are afraid for or worried about your baby-to-be.
  ☞ *Rock Rose* when you are trembling, shaking, or weeping from anxiety or fear.

★ Regular **gentle massage** or **Reiki treatments** not only help you calm your distress, they also guide you in creating a strong center that's resistant to being pushed around by other people's opinions. Massage prepares your mind/body for a healthy pregnancy and a safe birth.

• Use **lunaception** (explained on page 5) to time your ovulation so you have the best odds of conceiving. It's fine to have sex in the weeks before ovulation, especially if the sex is focused on the woman and her orgasm, but do save your best efforts for those three nights when your "moon" is full and bright and ready to frolic.

★ **Orgasm** on the part of the male is necessary for fertilization. The woman's orgasm does increase the possibility of conception, however. Women who achieve orgasm *after* their partner (up to 40 minutes after his ejaculation) have the very best chance of becoming pregnant.

Step 3. Nourish and tonify . . .

★ **Red clover infusion** is the single best remedy for women over forty who want to conceive but can't — even for those with blocked tubes, diabetes, ovarian cysts, internal scarring, and endometriosis. I know dozens of women with heart-warming success stories starring red clover. Two or more quarts of the *infusion* of the dried blossoms (neither tincture nor tea nor pills will work for this application) per week does wonders for fertility, no matter what your age.

★ Boosting your nutritional status makes birth defects less of a worry. Women who drink 2-4 cups of **stinging nettle infusion** daily and eat cooked leafy greens as well as lettuce salads are getting the abundant folic acid, calcium, magnesium, and other minerals needed to create a healthy baby. (Tinctures, pills, and teas contain little or none of these important nutrients.)

★ **Vitamin E** is an especially critical nutrient for fertility after forty and freedom from birth defects. Freshly ground wheat flour, cold-pressed oils, and nut butters are all good sources of vitamin E, as are stinging nettle infusion and most cooked seaweeds, such as kelp. The man's vitamin E level has as much, if not more, bearing on freedom from birth defects as does the woman's vitamin E level. I avoid supplements.

• Uterine tonics are important for fertility after forty. **Raspberry leaf** infusion helps prepare the uterus for birth and may be drunk freely. **Ginger** root tea is a warming tonic recommended for women who lack vitality, energy, and passion in their uterus. On the other side, cooling tonics, like **chasteberry** or **wild yam** tincture, are a better choice if hot flashes have already begun.

★ Another important herbal ally for women over forty who desire a child is **chasteberry** (*Vitex agnus-castus*). It has been used in Africa and parts of Europe for several thousand years to discourage the male libido. In women, the effects seem to be the opposite! It may also be a fertility enhancer. Most importantly, chaste tree is a strengthening tonic for the pituitary gland, the master control gland for the endocrine system. Daily use of the tincture of the berries (1 dropperful/1 ml 2-3 times daily) increases progesterone (the hormone of pregnancy) and luteinizing hormone (which promotes conception). Because it can lower prolactin levels, chasteberry is best discontinued during the last trimester of pregnancy.

Step 4. Sedate/Stimulate . . .

★ **Avoid heat**, both of you. Hot tubs, even prolonged soaking in a hot bath, can cause temporary (up to several months) sterility in some men. In women, it can endanger the embryo and trigger a miscarriage or birth defects.

★ Feeling tense and distressed about choosing or refusing motherhood? **Motherwort tincture** is my favorite calmative. A dose of 10-20 drops helps clear your mind, eases your tension, and assists you in discerning the best path to follow.

Step 5a. Use supplements . . .

• **Vitamin E** is important for fertility; best consumed in foods. See Step 3.

Step 5b. Use drugs . . .

• Avoid drugs, both of you, including alcohol, tobacco, coffee, as well as over-the-counter drugs and prescription drugs (except those you absolutely need). Your liver needs to be strong, so do your kidneys, so you can conceive and gestate a child. Instead of alcohol, which damages the liver, drink herbal infusions or alcohol-free wine or beer. Instead of tobacco, which may contribute to birth defects and low birth weight, try smoking a little dried peppermint, or, better yet, go for a walk. Instead of coffee, which challenges the kidneys, you may wish to drink green tea or black tea, or try a coffee substitute, especially one made with dandelion roots. Instead of drugs to ease everyday aches and pains, use the gentle herbal remedies collected in *Wise Woman Herbal for the Childbearing Year.*

For Pregnant Women Over Forty

★ The single most important herb for pregnant women over forty is ·**comfrey**. The leaves of the mature plant contain an abundance of constituents beneficial to mother and babe, including generous amounts of minerals, alantoin, proteins, and many vitamins. The minerals in comfrey help insure healthy nervous system growth; the proteins are used by the fetus's developing brain. And the alantoin helps the mother's tissues become stretchy and elastic.

Aging can lead to increased stiffness and brittleness in bones and muscles, making pregnancy more arduous and painful, labor slower and more difficult, and injury more likely during birth. The hormones of pregnancy (which help soften and relax the pelvic tissues) may not be produced in adequate amounts after forty. Comfrey to the rescue!

- Regular use of comfrey leaf infusion, at least a quart a week, promotes a safe delivery by:
  - ☞ strengthening uterine muscles and preparing them to work easily and well.
  - ☞ strengthening perineal tissues so they become resistant to tearing.
  - ☞ strengthening uterine ligaments so the uterus does not prolapse.
  - ☞ strengthening the bladder and increasing resistance to bacterial infection.
  - ☞ strengthening the vagina and helping to promote an environment hostile to infection.
  - ☞ providing easily assimilated minerals to prevent eclampsia and other complications.
  - ☞ helping the bones of the pelvis flex and open during birth.
  - ☞ increasing iron in the blood and thus forestalling post-partum hemorrhage.

★ **Is comfrey safe** for internal use? All parts of wild comfrey, *Symphytum officinale*, contain pyrrolizidine alkaloids which can cause venous liver congestion leading to death. But the leaves of cultivated comfrey, *Symphytum uplandica*, do not contain these alkaloids.[22,23] Four generations of people living at the Henry Doubleday Research Center have eaten cooked comfrey leaves regularly, including during pregnancy and lactation, and no liver problems have been seen in this population. Cultivated comfrey grows up to five feet tall, with purplish, pinkish flowers. Wild comfrey is rarely more than three feet tall with cream-colored, white, or yellowish flowers; it is rarely found in the continental United States. Comfrey leaves sold in bulk are from cultivated plants and are therefore safe to use internally.

Birth Control for Menopausal Women

Step 1. Collect information . . .

Birth control, never simple or easy, is complicated incredibly by the erratic ovulations and unpatterned menses of the premenopausal and menopausal years. Remember your high school chums who unexpectedly had a little baby brother or sister? The biological imperative to reproduce doesn't die without a struggle. This section is for those who don't want to have a(nother) child. If you do, go to page 57.

Step 2. Engage the energy . . .

★ **Barrier methods** (diaphragms, cervical caps, and condoms) are good choices for menopausal women. But the spermicides used with them may provoke vaginal infections, bladder infections, and dryness.

★ Try an erotic **massage** instead of intercourse. Use a special lubricant, like coconut oil. Light candles; buy flowers. Take your time.

Step 3. Nourish and tonify . . .

• Ejaculation control and **withdrawal** won't prevent conception for a woman in the fullness of her fertility, but will for most menopausal women. And it's a wonderful way to nourish intimacy in a relationship.

★ **Self-pleasuring** is safe sex for menopausal women. Guaranteed not to result in pregnancy and promotes health, too! Let Betty Dodson help you with her self-loving books and tapes (page 64.) Your mid-life mate may appreciate learning that sexual pleasure is more than penetration. **Lesbianism** and **celibacy** also work very well.

Step 4. Stimulate/Sedate . . .

★ Get him (and his testicles) in **hot wate**r. Sperm are easily killed at temperatures over 110 F. If he sits in hot water for 15-25 minutes a day for six weeks, he will shoot blanks for at least three months. A **vasectomy** is even safer, and lasts longer.

• Women find a teaspoon of **wild carrot seeds** (*Daucus carota* or Queen Anne's lace) eaten daily in food an effective way to prevent pregnancy.

Step 5b. Use drugs . . .

• Doctors who used to tell menopausal women to stop taking birth control pills, now urge them to start, then switch to "replacement" therapy.

Step 6. Break and enter . . .

• Remove your IUD if it causes heavy menstrual periods/flooding, common menopausal problems which can be serious threats to your health.

• Sterilization and hysterectomy are extreme forms of birth control for menopausal women who will soon need no birth control of any kind.

Sex

"The cycles of fertility pull on you less, my daughter," winks Grandmother Growth. "The urgent cries of your eggs for fertilization are already becoming softer and harder to hear. Do you notice a difference in your desire? You are becoming more than, other than, the woman you were, the woman who was moved to passionate sex when the moon was full and her egg was ripe. You may think your sexual desire is waning, may fear it is leaving you. But observe patiently, my sweet," chuckles Grandmother Growth. "If you will but hold your wise blood inside and stir it in your own cauldron, you will nourish your kundalini, your serpent power, and find yourself, at sixty, passionately sexual with all of life!

"But that is for later; for now, let your focus come in. Bring your focus ever inward, in toward your own wholeness. Do not worry if your desire is not attracted outward, is not sparked by others. This will return in time, transformed to fit your transformed self at the end of your menopausal journey.

"Right now you have a special opportunity to make peace with your children," admonishes Grandmother Growth. "Make peace with the children you have never given birth to. Make peace with the children you have conceived and lost. Make peace with the children you bore and let go of. And then make peace with your own wise child."

Grandmother Growth looks into your eyes and you feel the sparks. "You begin your menopausal years by conceiving your own wise child, your baby Crone. Feel your womb making space to cradle you as a baby Crone, reserving itself to nourish you as growing Crone, gathering strength to birth you to your crowning as Crone. And know that at your emergence as Crone you will hold inside Child self and Mother self. You will be whole. And you will be sexual."

As menopause progresses, ovulation slows and ceases, and the last years of "make-a-baby" lust come to an end, you may feel a distinct lessening of libido, or sexual urges. This can be especially scary if the image in your mirror no longer seems youthful, no longer fits your idealized version of "sexy."

Take heart. Wise crones and old women are very, very sexy . . . when they want to be — not when someone else wants them to be. My R_x for low libido is seven orgasms a week, whether you feel like it or not. You can do one a day or all in one day. Continue for at least three months. Need help even thinking about seven orgasms? See page 64.

References & Resources
Chapter 1: Is This Menopause?

Assilem, Melissa. *Women Ripening Through Menopause.* Idolatry Ink, 1418 Liberty St., El Cerrito, CA 94530, 1994

Beard, Mary. *My Body — My Decision!* HP-Books, 1986

Blum, Jeanne E. *Woman Heal Thyself.* Charles Tuttle Co., 1995

Borysenko, Joan. *A Woman's Book of Life.* Riverhead Books, 1996

Cobb, Jeanine O'Leary. *Understanding Menopause.* Toronto: Key Porter Books, 1996

Cutler, Winnifred. *Hysterectomy: Before & After — A Guide to Preventing, Preparing for, and Maximizing Health After.* Harper & Row, 1988

DeMarco, Carolyn, MD. *Take Charge of Your Body.* The Well Woman Press, 1994

Federation of Feminist Women's Health Centers. *How to Stay Out of the Gynecologist's Office.* Women to Women, 1981

Hobbs, Christopher & Kathi Keville. *Women's Herbs, Women's Health.* Interweave Press, 1998

Hufnagel, Vicki. *No More Hysterectomies.* NAL, 1988

Love, Susan, MD. *Dr. Love's Hormone Book.* Random House, 1997

Madaras, Lynda & Jane Patterson. *Womancare.* Avon, 1981

Our Bodies, Our Selves. Boston Women's Health Book Collective, Simon & Schuster, 1979 (2nd ed.)

Snow, Joanne Marie. *Everything You Need to Know About Menopause.* Prima, 1999

Taking Hormones? National Women's Health Network, 514 10th St. NW, Suite 400, Washington DC 20004

Sex

Chester, Laura (ed.). *Deep Down: New Sensual Writing by Women.* Faber & Faber, 1989

Chia, Mantak. *Cultivating Female Sexual Energy.* Healing Tao, 1986

Corinne, Tee (ed.). *Riding Desire: An Anthology for Erotic Writing.* Banned Books, 1991

Dodson, Betty. *Sex for One: The Joy of Self Loving.* Crown, 1992
  • *Self-loving Video Portrait;* $39.95 + $4 (priority mail); Box 1933, Murray Hill Station, NY, NY 10156. 212-679-4240

Eve's Garden • 119 W. 57th St., Suite 1201, NY, NY 10019

Kensington Ladies. *Ladies' Own Erotica.* Ten Speed Press, 1984

Savage, Linda E. *Reclaiming Goddess Sexuality.* Hay House, 1999

Sex Over Forty Newsletter. 3 Mayflower Lane, Shelton, CT 06484

Mail-Order Books (and Tapes) On Menopause
prices exclude postage

A Book About Menopause. Montreal Health Press, PO Box 1000, Station Place du Parc, Montreal, Quebec, Canada H2W 2N1 ($5)

Bolen, Jean Shinoda. *Menopause as Initiation.* Audio tape from Sounds True, 413 S. Arthur Ave., Louisville, CO 80027 ($12) 800-333-9185

Gladstar, Rosemary. *Herbs for Menopause.* PO Box 420, East Barre, VT 05649 ($6)

Hearts, Bones, Hot Flashes & Hormones ($1) Also, *Taking Hormones and Women's Health: Choices, Risks and Benefits,* expanded ($15) National Women's Health Network, 514 10th St., Suite 400, Washington DC 20004. 202-347-1140

Rouse, Louise. *The Magic of Menopause.* Audio book on tape, 2425 Siskiyou Blvd., Ashland, OR 97520

Weed, Susun S. *Menopause Metamorphosis.* 59 minute video ($29.95) Ash Tree Publishing, PO Box 64, Woodstock, NY 12498 ($13)

Newsletters on Menopause

A Friend Indeed. Newsletter from Box 260 Pembina, ND 58271 or Main floor, 419 Graham Ave., Winnepeg, MB. R3C OM3. Annotated bibliography on menopause. $2 plus SASE. 204-989-8028

Hot Flash. Newsletter of the National Action Forum for Midlife & Older Women, Box 816, Stony Brook, NY, 11790-0609. $25 yearly

Websites for You

- www.tantra.co.nz
- www.sexualhealth.com
- www.bettydodson.com
- www.adta.org
- www.option.org/anxiety.html
- www.womenshealthnetwork.org
- www.soundstrue.com
- www.afriendindeed.ca
- www.thyroid.org
- www.snakeandsnake.com

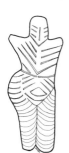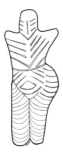

★ www.menopause-metamorphosis.com
★ www.herbshealing.com
★ www.ashtreepublishing.com
★ www.susunweed.com (more links!)

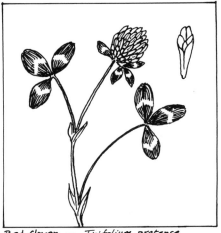

Red Clover — *Trifolium pratense*

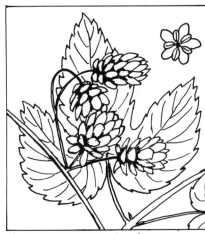

Hops — *Humulus lupulus*

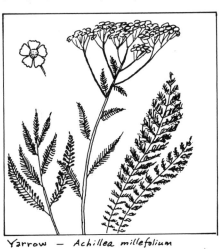

Yarrow — *Achillea millefolium*

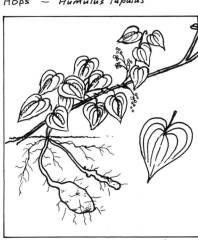

Wild yam — *Dioscorea villosa*

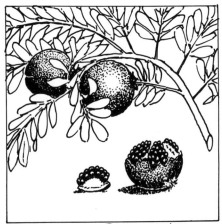

Pomegranate — *Punica granatum*

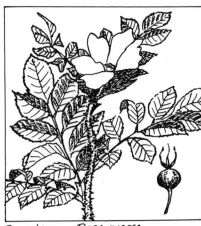

Rose hips — *Rosa rugosa*

Herbal Allies for
Women Beginning Menopause

Modern medicine defines menopause as estrogen loss. So supplementing with phytosterols (plant hormones) and phytoestrogens (plant estrogens) during our menopausal years seems natural. But if we (re)define menopause — as estrogen change accompanied by increased amounts of other hormones — it becomes clear that adding more hormones to our blood during these years involves risk.

During the menopausal years, hormones **Change** throughout the body: not just in the ovaries, but in the uterus, the liver, the fat cells, the adrenals, the pancreas, the thyroid, and the hypothalamus. Hormones trigger each other in feed-back loops. Tampering with one changes how all the rest work, sometimes beneficially and sometimes not.

Phytoestrogenic plants appear to be safe in any amount so long as they are part of the diet, and consumed in their whole form. Eating whole grains, roots, nuts, berries, beans, leafy greens, and drinking nourishing herbal infusions will boost your health tremendously, whether you're menopausal or not. But taking pills and supplements of isolated, concentrated flavonoids entails risks which may equal those associated with pharmaceutical hormones (e.g., cancer and stroke).[24]

Menopausal women have too many hormones, not too few. Luteinizing hormone (LH) and follicle stimulating hormone (FSH) increase dramatically during our menopausal years — and stay increased until well into our postmenopausal years. Progesterone (the baby-making hormone) does decrease, and the monthly production of estradiol (the most active estrogen) stops, but baseline estrogens (the ones that made you a baby girl) remain as strong as ever, so there is a net increase in hormones, not a loss.

Menopausal symptoms are often linked to difficulties in dealing with this increased hormone load: first in making the extra hormones, then, in recycling them through the liver. Food-bound phytoestrogens help us by providing active hormones, and by stimulating sex-hormone-binding globulin synthesis in the liver.[25] Isolated phytoestrogens, such as isoflavone, now found in many formulae for menopausal women, do not act in the same way, though they may reduce symptoms, especially hot flashes, dramatically.

When we consume phytoestrogen-rich plants we allow our individual bodies to create precisely the hormones we need on our unique menopausal journey. The biochemistry of phytosterols and phytoestrogens is an area of intense research. No plant makes human hormones, but almost all contain substances (such as lignans, flavones, daidzein, genistein, and glycitein) that can be converted to hormones. Numerous studies have traced the hormonal effects plants have on animals and people — more than fifteen by-products of phytoestrogen metabolism have been identified in human urine, milk, saliva, and seminal fluids — but only if the intestines are well-colonized with bacteria (e.g. from yogurt). The use of antibiotics completely eliminates the presence of several classes of phytoestrogens in the excretions.[26]

Only after they are fermented (by intestinal bacteria) or altered (by chemical solvents), can phytoestrogens and phytosterols be utilized as human hormones. Diosgenin, found in wild yam roots, is converted in the chemistry lab to pharmaceutical products such as cortisone, birth control pills, and progesterone. "Natural" hormone products (such as progesterone creams) are not natural, and no safer than any other drug.

If you are taking estrogen replacement (ERT) or hormone replacement (HRT), should you avoid phytoestrogens? If you are at high risk of breast cancer, should you worry about phytoestrogens? No, no. The helpful effects of phytoestrogens are especially for you. Numerous studies have shown that the cancer-promoting effects of synthetic estrogens (from ERT, HRT, organochlorines, and plastics) are countered by phytoestrogens in the diet.[27,28,29] In fact, the lower the level of phytoestrogen by-products in the urine, the greater the risk of breast cancer.[30] Phytosterol-rich foods and herbs, with the possible exception of licorice, do not appear to promote breast cancer.[31] Soy isoflavones, when isolated, however, promote rapid growth of breast cancer cells in the laboratory.[32]

Ruth Trickey, herbalist and hormone specialist, believes that phytoestrogenic foodstuffs and herbs rich in sterodial saponins interact with hypothalamic and pituitary hormones and help clear estrogen from the blood, and are thus especially useful for menopausal women with fibroids and endometriosis.[33]

Women who consume phytoestrogenic foods and herbs don't have to adjust their hormone dosages the way women on pills and patches do. Their bodies naturally use the estrogenic glycosides to decrease hormones (by binding them to receptor sites, thus blocking the action of strong estrogens) as well as to increase them (by conversion in the intestines).

Phytosterolic, Phytoestrogenic Plants

Virtually every part of every plant contains some phytosterols or phytoestrogens, but they are most concentrated in **seaweeds** (like kelp, nori), **roots** (like dandelion, carrot, yam), **seeds** (including nuts, whole grains, and beans), **buds** (like artichokes), and **berries** (like blueberries, vitex, and saw palmetto).[34]

Your body's ability to utilize phytosterols is increased when a plant has many different hormonal precursors, and especially when glycosides, saponins, and minerals are present in the same plant. Every herb and whole food offers us a slightly different combination, so more variety is better. Choose from the following three groups:

(1) Unlimited amounts of phytosterolic, phytoestrogenic **foods** (below).

(2) One or more phytoestrogenic **food-like herbs** (page 70) daily. Most are longevity tonics which benefit all women (and men!), before, during, and after menopause.

(3) Only one phytosterolic, phytoestrogenic **herb** (page 72) at a time, and only *when needed*. Most are too powerful to become long-term companions; though a few are used for years. Overuse may be hazardous: Lengthy use of water or alcohol extracts of phytoestrogenic herbs increased uterine weight and changed endometrial cells in lab animals.[35]

And I eat yogurt, because liberation and utilization of phytosterols and phytoestrogens is dependent on healthy intestinal flora.

Eating phytoestrogenic foods, even occasionally, and using phytoestrogenic herbs, even erratically, will mellow your menopause and help you stay healthy. Even small amounts of phytosterols compete with cholesterol for absorption,[36] keeping cholesterol levels healthy and inhibiting the development of colon cancer.[37]

Regular, consistent use will nourish all your endocrine glands (ovaries, adrenals, thyroid, pancreas, thymus, pineal, and pituitary), reward you with vigor, and help prevent diabetes, arthritis, high blood pressure, breast cancer, cardiovascular disease, and osteoporosis during the second fifty years of your life.

Phytosterolic, Phytoestrogenic Foods

★ **Whole grains** and **edible seeds** are superior sources of several quite active phytoestrogens — *lignans* (most concentrated in rye, buckwheat, millet, sesame, flax, and sunflower seeds), *resorcylic acid lactones* (most concentrated in oats, barley, rye, wheat, corn, rice, and sesame seeds), and *isoflavones* (significant amounts in all whole grains) — which are tightly bound into their germ and bran.

★ **Beans** are phytoestrogen champions. Yellow split peas, black turtle beans, baby limas, Anasazi beans, red kidney beans, and red lentils are exceptionally rich sources of the isoflavones genistein and daidzein (more than soy). In fact virtually every edible bean, even green beans, is a rich source of *isoflavones, coumestans,* and/or *lignans.* CAUTION: Beans must be cooked or fermented to remove anti-nutritional substances. Tofu and soy "milk" are not recommended.

★ **Leafy greens** contain isoflavones and other phytoestrogens. Best sources are cooked parsley, nettle, cabbage, broccoli, kale, mustard greens, collards, lamb's quarter, seaweeds, and rhubarb stalks.

• **Fruits** and **berries**, fresh, dried, frozen or cooked are good sources of isoflavones, lignans, and other phytoestrogens. Cherries, grapes, apples, pears, peaches, plums, strawberries, blackberries, raspberries, hawthorn berries, salmonberries, apricots, crab apples, quinces, rosehips, and blueberries are exceptional sources. (See also *citrus* and *pomegranate.*)

★ **Oils** from edible seeds are rich sources of phytosterols, especially corn, rice bran, sesame, and wheatgerm oils. **Olive oil** is even better.

★ **Olives** are an excellent source of phytoestrogenic coumestans.

★ **Roots** such as beetroot, carrots, sweet potatoes, potatoes, burdock, dandelion, sunchokes, and parsnips contain many different phytosterols.

• **Garlic** and its smelly relatives (onions, chives, and leeks) are hormone-rich (and heart-healthy) plants that most women crave.

• **Pomegranate** (*Punica granatum*) is a fruit rich in fertility associations as well as hormones. The seeds of ripe fruits are the exception to the rule that plants do not contain human hormones. (The other exceptions are french beans, rice, apple seeds, and licorice.[38]) There are about 1.7 milligrams of the "weak" estrogen estrone in 100 grams of pomegranate seeds. I eat them right along with the sweet pulp or whir them up in a blender with fruit and yogurt. Olive oil in which ground pomegranate seeds are infused for six weeks and then strained acts as a homemade "estrogen cream" to counter vaginal dryness.

Phytoestrogenic Food-like Herbs

• **Citrus peel** is an exceptional source of estrogenic bioflavonoids. Orange marmalade is a good way to ingest it, as is Peel Power, page 260.

★ **Dandelion**, Löwenzahn, dent-de-lion (*Taraxacum officinale*) is not only exceptionally rich in plant hormones, it is also a supreme nourisher to the liver. Regular use of any part of the plant can ease digestive distress, help prevent diabetes, and really ease hot flashes. The usual dose of the tincture (of fresh or dried roots, or fresh roots and leaves) is 10-25 drops before meals, at least twice a day. To relieve summer hot flashes, I used a dropperful upon arising and another as the day heated up. Drinking dandelion flower wine, a glass with meals, or eating cooked dandelion leaves is also effective. And if you are concerned about your bones, ask calcium- and mineral-rich dandelion vinegar to be your ally.

• **Fenugreek**, bockshornklee, fenugrec (*Trigonella foenum-graecum*) seeds are a rich source of essential fatty acids, lecithin, saponins, and phytosterols. Taken as a tea, or used to season food, they are an inexpensive and tasty way to ease menopausal symptoms, restore blood sugar balance, nourish the glands, improve digestion, and increase libido. Brew a tablespoonful/15 mg of seeds for no more than 15 minutes in a cup/250 ml of hot water. Fenugreek is commonly used in curries. CAUTION: Fenugreek promotes fertility.

• **Flax seeds** (*Linum usitatissimum*) have 75-800 times more *lignans* than other foods and up to five times as much omega-3 fatty acids. No wonder they're a fabulous ally for menopausal women. Daily use of 2-3 tablespoons of ground flax seed has been shown to reduce the risk of breast cancer, shrink tumors, and reverse tumor progression.

• **Green tea** (*Camellia sinensis*) helps block the action of estrogen at tumor sites. Its antioxidant properties recommend it as well. A daily dose is 6-10 cups.

★ **Hops**, Hopfen, Houblon grimpant (*Humulus lupulus*) induces sleep, relieves water retention, and provides abundant phytoestrogens. A strong tea of the dried female flowers (strobiles) is sipped cold throughout the day, or 5-15 drops of fresh strobile tincture is taken just before bed. Drinking home-brew or non-alcoholic beer is another pleasant way to ingest hops.

★ **Nettle**, Brenessel, Ortie (*Urtica dioica* or *Urtica urens*) is one of my dearest friends, a favorite food, and a cherished herbal ally. Her leafy tops are exceptionally rich in hormone-helpful minerals, phytoestrogens, and vitamins. Regular use of nettle infusion helps me keep my bones strong, my heart healthy, my adrenals well-nourished, and my menopausal journey on the high road. (More on page 241.) Avoid nettle in capsules or tinctures; the benefits are slight.

★ **Red clover**, Rotklee, trèfle des prés (*Trifolium pratense*) has ten times more phytoestrogens than soy, as well as lots more bone-building minerals, including calcium and magnesium. The infusion builds energy, eases joint pain, smooths the menopausal passage, prevents (and may reverse) breast cancer, and maintains cardiovascular health. Red clover vinegar is mineral- and hormone-rich; tincture and capsules have little or no effect. (More about red clover on page 161.)

• **Red wine** is an excellent source of phytoestrogens. And heart-healthy, too. Best for postmenopausal women, as those in their menopausal years find alcohol increases the intensity and severity of their hot flashes.

• **Seasoning seeds** such as coriander and cumin, celery and caraway, poppy and sesame, mustard and fenugreek, anise and fennel, all contain phytoestrogens, as do their oils. Use these seeds lavishly when cooking or make tea with a tablespoon/15 mg of any one in a cup of hot water. Drink 3-4 cups a day for best results.

★ **Seaweeds** are second only to flax in concentration of lignans. Seaweed is the real secret of health in the Japanese diet, not soy. I keep a large selection of seaweeds on hand (alaria, dulse, hijiki, kelp, kombu, nori, sea palm fronds, and wakame) and use them as vegetables, not as seasonings. Generous amounts of seaweed can be cooked in with whole grains and beans (kelp and oatmeal is a favorite breakfast) to really boost phytoestrogen levels. For seaweed recipes, see my book *Healing Wise.*

Phytosterolic, Phytoestrogenic Herbs

• **Agave** (*Agave americana*) is a desert plant. In Traditional Chinese Medicine, 1/4-1 teaspoon (1-5 ml) of the fresh juice of the succulent leaves is taken several times a day to relieve uterine prolapse.

• **Alfalfa**, Luzerne, Luzerne cultivée (*Medicago sativa*) is a nourishing source of isoflavones. But menopausal women do well to avoid it, especially in capsules. Alfalfa can thin the blood, increasing the normal tendency of menopausal women to bleed profusely (hemorrhage). If you do wish to use it, for greatest effect, use untreated seeds, not the leaves, to make a cup of tea.

★ **Black cohosh**, Schwarze Schlangenwurzel, Baneberry (*Cimicifuga racemosa*) is a perennial plant of the deep woods. Overuse is making it rare. For many women it is as effective as ERT in relieving menopausal hot flashes, sleeplessness, and irritability. Tincture of the fresh root, 10-60 drops a day, is the preferred preparation. Use caution with dried root products. CAUTION: Do not use black cohosh if you might be (or are) pregnant. (More, page 151.)

• **Black currant**, Schwarze Johannisberre, Cassis (*Ribes nigrum*) nourishes the adrenals and ovaries, and helps prevent urinary tract infections, sore joints, and vascular disturbances (including hot flashes). The dose of a glycerite or alcohol tincture of the fresh leaf buds (or berries); is 10-50 drops.

• **Black haw**, Amerikanischer Schneeball, Viburnum (*Viburnum prunifolium*) is one of the few hormone-rich herbs that can be used by women with a tendency to bleed heavily during menstruation. The astringent action counters cramps and hemorrhage; other constituents ease palpitations. The infusion of the root bark is sipped frequently, as needed, up to a cup/250 ml a day; or use tincture of fresh root bark, 1-25 drops a day.

★ **Chasteberry** (*Vitex agnus castus*) is considered by some as *the* herbal ally for menopausal women. It is especially important for the woman who comes to her menopause through induced means. Consistent use (ok to use for several years) increases the levels of progesterone and luteinizing hormone (LH) in the blood. In the early menopausal years, this can be helpful, but during the "melt-down" years, when too much LH dilates blood vessels, causing hot flashes, panic attacks, and palpitations, vitex can become too much of a good thing. (More, page 153.)

• **Cramp bark** or **Guelder rose**, Schneeball, Biorne obier (*Virburnum opulus*) is similar to black haw, but weaker. Generally considered safe for those who flood. Usual dose is 2-3 cups/500-750 ml of root bark infusion or 20-40 drops of the tincture daily.

★ **Dandelion** is a "Phytoestrogenic Food-like Herb" (page 70).

• **Dong quai** (*Angelica sinensis*) is one of the most frequently used herbs in the world. It is problematic during the menopausal years, however, and needs to be used, if at all, with utmost caution, as the constituents of dong quai promote not only estrogen production, but also hemorrhage. The phytoestrogens in dong quai, like those in soy, promote the growth of cancer cells in petri dishes. (There are no cases of cancer attributed to dong quai.) Premenopausal and postmenopausal women seem to benefit more from the use of dong quai than women in the midst of menopause. The usual dose is 10-40 drops of fresh or dried root tincture (traditionally combined with poria and peony root tinctures) or up to one cup of the dried root infusion. (More, page 172.)

• **Devil's club** (*Oplopanax horridum*) nourishes the pancreas and stabilizes blood sugar levels. Constipation, sore joints, and menopausal flashes give way to the beneficial influences of this spine-covered plant. The usual dose is 5-20 drops of tincture of the fresh or dried root, or a cup/250 ml of the infusion of the dried root bark.

• **False unicorn** (*Chamaelirium luteum*) is a somewhat rare perennial plant whose root has long been considered a profound uterine/ovarian tonic, especially well-suited to women who flood. False unicorn is taken in very small doses: 2-5 drops of tincture of the fresh or dried root, several times a day.

• **Ginseng** (*Panax quinquefolium*) is a heart-healthy herb as well as a hormone helper. It has an enormous reputation as a reliever of menopausal problems, from flashes to indigestion. I prefer to chew on a small piece of the root, but 5-40 drops of tincture is said to work as well. (More, page 169.)

• **Groundsel**, Gemeines Kreuzkraut, Séneçon commun (*Senecio vulgaris*) and her sister Jacob's Groundsel, Jakobskraut, Séneçon Jacobée (*Senecio jacobea*) are closely related to liferoot (page 155). All are important menopausal allies. I tincture fresh flowers and leaves; the roots are considered poisonous. A dose is 10-30 drops per day.

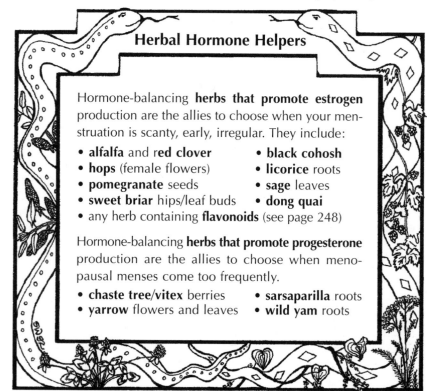

Herbal Hormone Helpers

Hormone-balancing **herbs that promote estrogen** production are the allies to choose when your menstruation is scanty, early, irregular. They include:

- **alfalfa** and **red clover**
- **hops** (female flowers)
- **pomegranate** seeds
- **sweet briar** hips/leaf buds
- **black cohosh**
- **licorice** roots
- **sage** leaves
- **dong quai**
- any herb containing **flavonoids** (see page 248)

Hormone-balancing **herbs that promote progesterone** production are the allies to choose when menopausal menses come too frequently.

- **chaste tree/vitex** berries
- **yarrow** flowers and leaves
- **sarsaparilla** roots
- **wild yam** roots

• **Licorice**, Süssholzwurzel, Réglisse (*Glycyrrhiza glabra*) is a well-known anti-inflammatory. It is one of the richest sources of isoflavones and steroidal saponins. Unfortunately, regular use can elevate blood pressure, aggravate water retention, promote headaches, and possibly encourage reproductive cancers. Maximum dose is a cup/250 ml per day. Or chew on real licorice sticks.

★ **Liferoot** (*Senecio aureus*) promotes menstrual and menopausal ease with its unique blend of liver-strengthening constituents and hormonal components. The usual dose is 5-10 drops of the fresh flower tincture, once a day only. (More, page 155.)

★ **Motherwort**, Herzgespann, Agripaume cardiaque (*Leonurus cardiaca*) is a magnificent ally for women in **Change**: menopause, puberty, menstruation. Almost every woman will benefit from getting to know her. Motherwort moderates hot flashes and night sweats, eases emotional swings and promotes a calm center, strengthens the heart and keeps blood pressure low, and relieves PMS and menstrual cramps. Not only that, motherwort is a tonic, so the more you use it, the less you need it. Tincture of the fresh flowering tops is the usual preparation (tea is very bitter); usual dose is 10-30 drops 1-4 times a day. (More, page 165.)

★ **Nettle** is a "Phytoestrogenic Food-like Herb" (page 71).

• **Peony** (*Paeonia albiflora* or *P. officinalis*) has hormone-rich roots, with poisonous flowers and leaves. Tincture of the fresh or dried roots, 1-25 drops at a time, several times daily, can establish menstrual regularity, ease cramps, and soothe emotional swings. In Traditional Chinese Medicine, peony is usually combined with dong quai.

• **Raspberry**, Himbeere, Framboisier (*Rubus* species) is an important hormonal ally during both the childbearing and menopausal years. The usual preparation is an infusion of the dried leaves and canes of the first-year plants (one ounce of herb steeped for at least four hours in a quart of boiling water), drunk hot or cold, at least a cup a day. The tincture and the glycerin macerate, while not as mineral-rich as the infusion, have the advantage of being tastier; the usual dose is a dropperful twice a day.

★ **Red clover** is a "Phytoestrogenic Food-like Herb" (page 71).

★ The **rose family** contains many members eager to help menopausal women: raspberry, strawberry, sweet briar, and hawthorn. Any part of any rose-family plant can be used — stalks, leaves, leaf buds, flowers, flower-buds, and fruit — to ease headaches, relieve dizziness, nourish the nerves and heart, invigorate the entire being, remedy menstrual cramps, strengthen the bones and prevent osteoporosis, and moderate mood swings and hormonal surges during your **Change**. I put fresh leaf or flower buds, or fresh or dried haws or hips, in alcohol or glycerin or vinegar for six weeks; then use 30 drops/1 ml of the tincture, or a teaspoonful/5 ml of the glycerite, or one or more tablespoonfuls/15 ml of the vinegar daily. I dry and infuse stalks and leaves.

★ **Sage**, Garten-salbei, Sauge officinale (*Salvia officinalis*) relieves night sweats, depression, trembling, and dizziness. It promotes estrogen production, and may lower FSH and LH surges during the meltdown years. I make a full-strength infusion of the dried plant (one ounce brewed for at least four hours in a quart of boiling water) but dilute it by at least a third with water before I drink it, slowly sipping a cup or two throughout the day. Sage vinegar is especially tasty. (More, page 159.)

• **Sarsaparilla**, Sarsaparillawurzel, Salsepareille (*Smilax officinalis* or *S. regelii* or other species) is an old favorite of menopausal women. Confusion reigns when you attempt to purchase sarsaparilla (pronounced sas-prilla). There are not only numerous species — some of which are more effective than others — but also unrelated plants which are commonly called sarsaparilla (most notably *Aralia nudicaulis*). Jamaican *Smilax* is thought to be the most medicinal, Mexican and Honduran the next best. Infusion of the dried root, 1/2-1 cup/125-250 ml a day, or tincture of the fresh or dried root, 10-30 drops several times a day, noticeably supports progesterone production.

★ **Saw palmetto** (*Serenoa serrulata*), best known as a prostate herb, is a respected ally for menopausal women as well. It nourishes and enlivens ovarian, vaginal, breast, and bladder tissues, preventing atrophy and prolapse. Saw palmetto has a long-standing reputation as an aphrodisiac. Those who live along the Gulf Coast or in the deep South will have access to fresh saw palmetto berries and can make vinegars and tinctures; the usual dose is 1 tablespoonful/15 ml of the vinegar or 10-30 drops of tincture, two or three times a day. A cup a day of infusion of the dried berries can be substituted.

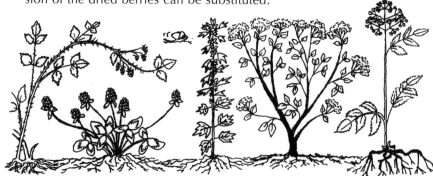

★ **Sweet briar** or dog rose, Haggebutte, Hagrose, Eglantier (*Rosa canina* or *R. pendulina*) is a powerful menopausal ally rarely mentioned in modern herbals. It is a favorite of Swiss herbalists. Glycerin macerate (sold as "non-alcohol tincture") of the leaf buds, or tea, or jam of the fruits/hips, can be used freely, like food.

★ **Wild yam** (*Dioscorea villosa* and 500 related species) is a powerful precursor for LH and FSH, making it an exceptionally poor choice for menopausal women. Infusion (one ounce of the herb brewed for at least 8 hours in 2 cups of boiling water), tincture (10-30 drops several times a day), and tea are used. Wild yam can also promote progesterone and should be avoided postmenopausally. (See page 174.)

• **Yarrow**, Schafgarbe, Millefeuille (*Achillea millefolium*) is especially active in creating progesterone. One herbalist offers the observation that yarrow is excellent for tough, independent women who don't talk about their problems. Given its reputation for sweating out fevers, don't be surprised if yarrow gives you hot flashes or increases the amount you sweat when you flash. The antibacterial, astringent, and tonifying properties of yarrow make it useful for women hoping to get rid of their bladder infections, interstitial cystitis, and incontinence. Tincture of the fresh flowering tops, 5-10 drops several times a day, or a tea of the dried flowers sipped slowly throughout the day is the usual dose. The energy of yarrow is said to revive those who feel drained. Rub some in your hands and inhale the aroma . . . ahhhhh.

How to ingest these herbs? If hot drinks, alcohol tinctures, and spoonfuls of vinegar trigger hot flashes, take your teas and infusions at room temperature, chilled, or with ice. Use your vinegars on salads or add them to soups and marinades. Always put your dose of tincture in at least half a glass of water or juice before taking it. Adding it to hot water is said to drive off the alcohol. A teaspoon/5 ml of herbal vinegar is roughly the same as 10 drops of tincture.

Green Blessings!

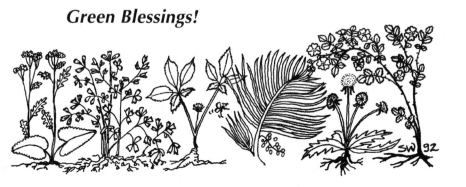

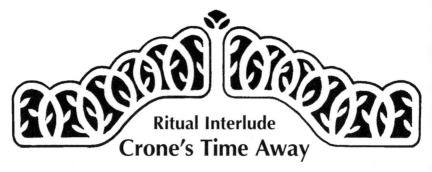

Ritual Interlude
Crone's Time Away

The first stage of metamorphosis is going into a cocoon. The first step of one's self-initiation as Crone is isolation. As you enter menopause, you may feel an urge to let go of the more public parts of your life and retreat.

Just as the menstruating woman naturally seeks to be alone, or has it thrust upon her in the form of painful periods, so the menopausal woman may choose to take time away, or may become the "victim" as her husband leaves her, her children grow up, and her erratic moods alienate her former friends. Chosen or not, manifested subtly or dramatically, isolation stalks the menopausal woman and carries her into her Crone's Time Away.

As menopausal changes increase, our physical processes lead us into ourselves. We want to sleep alone, so the wakings and cover-tossings can be guilt-free. We want to be alone so we can undress and dress as flushes and flashes and sweats and glows of heated energy flow through us. We want to be alone to face our **Change**, to embrace the chaos and our own darkness. We need to be in our cave to sort the experiences of our lives.

This is the first secret of menopause. I want to be alone! (This is not depression.) Don't call me mom! (This is not hysteria.) What do I have to lose by telling the truth? (I am not crazy.)

Deep in our cave we can hear, perhaps for the first time, the voice of our own needs, our own desires. We can take the time, perhaps as never before, to tend to our own needs and our own wants.

Your Crone's Time Away begins with a ritual done by yourself or with others. This is but one possibility. It is designed to tell your family and close friends that your need to be alone is not a rejection of them but a claiming of yourself. It may open into an actual time of isolation, a vacation, a separate room or cabin, or it may create an aura of awe around you that will allow you to feel into your moods and needs without any underlying pressure to tend to others.

*   *   *   *   *

Gather with your family and friends in a public place, the noisier the better, to symbolize the busyness in your life. Walk from this place to a quieter, more isolated area, symbolizing the quiet space you need.

Facing each other, join hands and hum. Don't worry about how you sound. Pay attention to your breath; let the hum vibrate.

Invite the energies of the seven directions to be present with you: east, south, west, north, above, below, and within. Invite your ancestors to be present. Invite your spirit guides and guardian angels to be there with you. Together, bend down to the earth, touching your hands to the earth and breathe out. Then stretch to the sky and breathe in. Bring your hands to your heart, close your eyes, and go inside your self to the place within the within the within.

Using your own words, speak to each of the important people in your life. Stand in front of them and look into their eyes. (Use a photo for those not present.) "You are my lover (daughter, friend, son, sister, mate). I take great joy in pleasing you. I feel great power in making your life easy, beautiful, abundant. For the next few years I will be going through menopause, the great **Change**, the great changer. I will be busy finding my way to my new self, the baby crone, the butterfly. How I will change, I know not now. Of this I am sure, however, my love and affection for you will not change. Together we affirm this bond.

"Yet I must take this journey alone. I ask now for your blessing on me as I begin my **Change**, my journey. I ask you to acknowledge my Crone's Time Away. Let me go with love so my growth will not wrench me from your grasp."

Speak in your own way, in song or dance, in poetry or a prepared script, to each person or to everyone. They need not respond.

When your ceremony is complete, join hands again and begin to hum. Let the hum go on as long as it wants to. Lift your arms to the sky and breathe out. Place your hands on the earth and breathe in. Say goodbye and thank you to the ancestors and angels and guardians. Bring your hands to your heart and feel the vibration in your being.

Drop hands. Leave the circle by yourself. Spend the night alone. In the silence you may hear Grandmother Growth whispering in your ear.

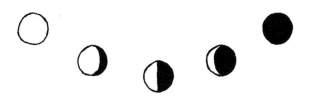

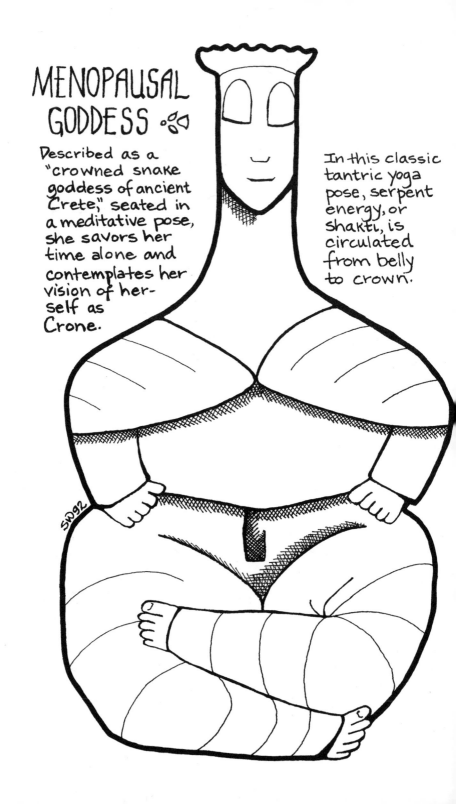

MENOPAUSAL GODDESS

Described as a "crowned snake goddess of ancient Crete," seated in a meditative pose, she savors her time alone and contemplates her vision of herself as Crone.

In this classic tantric yoga pose, serpent energy, or shakti, is circulated from belly to crown.

SW92

This Is Menopause!
Journey Into Change

"Pay attention now," Grandmother Growth says, taking your hand and holding your gaze. "The Change known as menopause deserves your full attention.

"Pay attention now, and relax. Focus, allow, observe, surrender. Your egg basket empties; your memory basket grows heavier.

"Memories are sweeping through you, great granddaughter, like lightning flashes, leaving you shaken and trembling, sweating and panting. Memories too gossamer to catch with words are weaving themselves into your nights and shattering the patterns of your days. Fragments of melodies, half-seen gestures, sketches, muted drifts of color emerge from your memory. All the wild passions of the Maiden are restored to you. All those Maiden things you left behind or pushed aside when you became Mother-woman, return to you now, enriched.

"Do those memories crowd painfully into your head? Do they send your heart racing? Do they make you weep? Sweep you off your feet? Leave you wondering what it would feel like to jump off a high bridge? Take my hand, dear one. Let us walk and talk."

There is no doubt in your mind. Your menstrual cycles are coming to an end. You are in the midst of your menopausal climax years.

During the year or so before the very last period (and the year or so afterward) many women experience some type of menopausal **Change**, such as hot flashes, heart palpitations, sleep disturbances, emotional uproar, anxiety, and/or headaches.

Menopause, like puberty, requires that we give in to **Change** and accept that it is beyond our control. If we arrive at mid-life feeling more in control of our lives than ever before, giving in to menopausal **Change** can be incredibly difficult. The desire to use anything, drugs or herbs or whatever, to avoid disruption of our normal life pattern is strong; it comes from within and is reinforced by society. Why resist?

The Wise Woman Way offers us a new/old story: where hot flashes and wild heartbeats are honored, where menopause is considered woman's greatest transformation — her crowning as Crone — and where old women are vital, flexible, hale-hearted, strong-boned and clear-minded. The Wise Woman Way offers us women's mystery stories and a host of helpful herbal allies that aid the process of menopause instead of attempting to stop it or fix it.

Wise Woman stories say that menopause is an initiation that begins with a period of isolation. The grandmothers say that menopausal women need to draw inward and away from outside responsibilities. From the Wise Woman view, hot flashes, fatigue, headaches, irritability, sleeplessness, and emotional outbursts are allies of wholeness, not problems; they urge me to be alone, to focus on myself and my **Change**, to listen to what I want and to ask for what I need.

Without knowledge of the women's mystery stories, without the help of herbal allies and the reassurance of other women, a woman may feel alone and unsupported in her disturbing and "pointless" changes. She may think the **Change** is only for the worse, or that something is wrong with her. And when she seeks information, she is told (erroneously) that her **Change** will cause heart attacks and crumbling bones, wrinkles and grey hair, and loss of sex appeal and libido. Where is Grandmother Growth to guide her through this immense, frightening metamorphosis, to show her the green gifts of nature that strengthen her heart and bones, soften her skin and sex?

Science defines menopause as lack of estrogen and prescribes the remedy (take estrogen) and tells us that we don't have to mature, or become wise women. We can remain bound to our (and society's) ideas of who we ought to be, instead of exploring who we really are.

If I take hormones will I be able to make room for transformation? take time for solitude? give myself uninterrupted stretches of focused self-loving? encounter, nourish, and sanctify myself as a wise and silly grandmother, a wrinkled wild woman, a lawless fierce crone? My menopausal metamorphosis deserves as much attention as I can give it. And I am not that rare woman who gives herself these gifts without the daily urgings of her body and feelings.

I don't use hormone pills, or patches, or creams. I let the "problems" of my menopause give me the opportunity to claim all parts of myself, even those that are awkward, ugly, old, out of control, and afraid of death. By passing consciously through menopause, by embracing this **Change** in my life, by nourishing myself with green allies, I renew myself. The grandmothers say I make myself complete — reclaiming myself as maiden, redefining myself as mother, and knowing myself as crone. It is so.

"Take my hand, dear one. I will soothe your head, calm your heart, stabilize your grounding, and then teach you to fly. Take my hand, now. You are in the midst of Change."

Flashes and Flushes and Chills

*"Give me your full attention, young Crone," says Grandmother Growth
in a voice deep and resonant. "For you will pay attention, I assure you,
when your menopausal Change lets loose lightning-like hot flashes and
waves of energy that free your feelings and stir your spirit. As you hold
the wise blood inside more and more, menstruating less and less, strong
energies will move in you. The women's mystery teachings of menopause
urge you to take time off to adapt to these energies, to take, symbolically
or actually, your Crone's Time Away and allow those hot flashes and
sleepless nights to guide you into metamorphosis and initiation."*

Hot flashes! The archetypal distress of menopause! After years of
being told to hide my menstrual blood (my womanness), after years of
successfully being in public without anyone suspecting that I was a
menstruating woman, suddenly I am revealed.

The blood that no longer comes so regularly flowing from my
womb now rushes to my face, flushing my skin and covering me in a
damp shimmer. I feel at the mercy of the flash, which takes me when
it decides, and gives little warning. (I am reminded of my labor pains,
and of sexual arousal/release.)

My hot flash tells the world, I am sure, that I am woman (vulnerable and invisible). Not just woman, but old woman (much more
vulnerable and much more invisible). I live in a civilized country
where I am expected to go through a powerful **Change** as though it
were nothing, and where my survival may depend on how I look. I
am urged by both outer and inner voices to do whatever I can to
appear young: dye my hair, have a face lift, and use hormones to
eliminate my hot flashes — the obvious signs of my **Change**.

If I lived in a world safe for women, in a matrifocal culture guided
by the wisdom of the crones, I would cherish my hot flashes. I would
be taught to respect my flashes as part of the gestation of myself in the
fiery womb of menopause metamorphosis. I would learn that my hot
flashes are waves of energy (prana, kundalini, chi, life force). I thrill to
their power, ride them as they rush through me, flashing, flushing, pulsing. I would have guides and role models and stories and herbal and
animal allies to help me. I would be seen as baby Crone. I would be

urged/allowed/supported to take my Crone's Year Away. I would want to be a wise old woman. I wouldn't want to be cured of my hot flashes.

I wonder, did the matrifocal nations, the ancient wise women, have remedies to relieve hot flashes? Even if they respected and valued the transformative power of their flashes and flushes, I'm sure they had wonderful remedies to help the woman distressed by her flashes, for the Wise Woman way seeks both/and solutions. I think they used some of the same herbs and home remedies I do, and you can, too.

Hot Flashes

Step 0. Do nothing . . .

★ My baby Crone friend Marie Summerwood gives herself a "**Crone's Moment Away.**" When she flashes, she closes her eyes and focuses in, taking a moment ("It can seem like a year . . .") away.

Step 1. Collect information . . .

Hot flashes are virtually synonymous with menopause. The vast majority of women will have had at least one hot flash by the age of sixty.

Hot flashes are regarded as a symptom of estrogen deficiency by modern medicine. But women with severe hot flashes have been found to have about the same amount of estrogen in their blood as women who have mild (or nonexistent) flashes. And, while the intensity of the hot flashes is abated in women who take hormones, the overall duration of their hot flashes is more than twice as long as average (five years rather than two).

The far greater hormonal change, and the one more responsible for hot flashes during (and after) the menopausal years, is the elevated levels of luteinizing hormone (LH) and follicle stimulating hormone (FSH). These pituitary hormones are produced in amounts up to 1300 percent greater during the menopausal years than before, and daily (instead of only at mid-cycle as was the case during our menstruating years). LH is a strong vasodilator; that is, it opens the blood vessels and allows body heat to come to the surface. Sounds like a hot flash!

The frequency, intensity, and duration of hot flashes is unique to each woman, but, in general, healthier women have more hot flashes.

During a hot flash, flushes of heat sweep up the body, moving through the upper body and face, reddening the skin, increasing the

"At 56, I've only missed two periods. I've had two rounds of very intense hot flashes—each round lasting six weeks—a year apart."

sensation of heat in the body, and prompting perspiration.

The sensations may be overwhelming or hardly noticeable, the perspiration may be fine or profuse, and the reddening may be even or blotchy. The duration of a single hot flash can be from a few seconds to several minutes. There are reports of flashes going on for fifteen minutes; my experiences lead me to believe that those are analogous to multiple orgasms, that is, not one long release, but many, each one triggering the next.

Hot flashes may occur at irregular intervals, every 60-90 minutes (the adrenal cycle) or only at certain times. Sadja Greenwood, author of *Menopause Naturally*, says flashes are most common between 6 and 9 p.m. My hot flashes came anytime, but most predictably when I laid down to go to sleep and when I got up in the morning. Women have experienced as many as 30 hot flashes an hour, but it is more usual to have only a few a day. The overall average during menopause is less than one a day. Some months I had none, and some days I got an entire month's worth in one day.

Chills may accompany any flash which soaks your clothing with perspiration. Some women say they get cold rushes instead of hot flashes.

While 85 percent of women have hot flashes during menopause, only 5 percent of men experience them firsthand (usually during their forties and fifties). Some of my closest male friends had sympathy flashes with, or instead of, me.

Most women who flash (80 percent) do so for between two months and two years. The other 20 percent have flashes for a decade or more. A small percentage of women continue to flash into their seventies and eighties. (The healthier the woman the more flashes she's likely to have, as she has a stronger life force moving through her.)

Hot flashes often come in groups, appearing and disappearing for no particular reason. This leads women to believe that the remedy they just tried was the one that "eliminated" their flashes, but this is rarely the case, even when the remedy is hormone pills, patches, or creams. And stress can bring them back. Five years after my last period, three after my last flash, a stressful family trip brought on ten days of hot flashes as fierce and frequent as those in my menopausal meltdown year.

When menopause occurs due to surgical removal of the ovaries or other trauma (including chemotherapy, Tamoxifen, radiation, and surgical mistakes), nearly 100 percent of the women experience hot flashes. In women who refuse post-operative hormones, the period of hot flashes is, as with biological menopause, almost always under two

"And at the height of it I was having five hot flashes during the night and one every hour during the day."

years, though the flashes are more frequent and more intense than those of women achieving menopause naturally. In the process of writing this book, I met quite a few women who refused HRT after surgery, or who went off it some years later. All are happy with their decision and all are in good health decades later.

Thinner women experience more rapid changes in their hormone levels during the menopausal years. Fat cells slow the increase of LH and FSH, and moderate swings in estrogen levels.

From an energy standpoint, a hot flash is a release of kundalini energy (see page 96), which "rewires" the nervous system, making it capable of transferring and moving powerful healing and peace-keeping energies for the entire community. (Long-term use of hormones may prevent the emergence of these energies.)

Step 2. Engage the energy . . .

• Judyth Reichenberg-Ullman, a naturopathic physician, finds homeopathic remedies effective 80 percent of the time in relieving menopausal symptoms. One of her favorites for women with hot flashes is **Lachesis**. Try it when the flashes/flushes emanate from the top of your head, are worse just before sleep and immediately upon awakening, and are accompanied by sweating, headaches, or easily irritated skin.

• Other useful homeopathic remedies include:
  ☞ *Belladonna*: the flash centers on your face, which burns and turns bright red; you are restless, agitated, and have palpitations.
  ☞ *Ferrum metallicum*: your flashes include profuse sweating and trembling, are worse in evenings or with exercise.
  ☞ *Pulsatilla*: you flash less outdoors, but your flashes are often followed by intense chills and emotional uproar.
  ☞ *Sanguinaria*: your cheeks are red and burning, feet and hands hot.
  ☞ *Sepia*: flashes make you feel weak, nauseated, exhausted, depressed.
  ☞ *Valeriana*: your face flushes strongly during the flash, and you have intense sweating and sleeplessness.

★ Stay in bed for a day and learn to ride your flashes. Make them your familiar steed. Let go of resistance. Welcome them. Can you feel the kundalini as it surges through each chakra?

"I started having irregular flashes when I was 44. Usually they would come when I was just starting to bleed, which I thought quite unfair. One or the other, isn't that the way it's supposed to be?"

★ **Keep cool.** Drink plenty of water and herbal infusions. Ease off of dehydrating drinks like coffee, black tea, and alcohol. Eat smaller meals more frequently. Walk away from aggravating situations. Soak your feet. Think cool. Sit next to the window so you can lay your cheek against the cold glass. Let your grey hairs blow cool thoughts along your spine. Wear silk. Envision a waterfall. Put ice on your cheeks. Get someone to blow on the nape of your neck. Buy an air conditioner or a fan; or hang out in an air-conditioned store.

★ **Breathe out slowly.** A hot flash is a fire; it will go out faster, and generate less heat, if it gets less oxygen. So blow your breath out, just like when you blow out all the candles on your birthday cake. Slow it down and deprive the fire of its fuel. (Or speed up and make it hotter!)

• Hot flashes are physically comparable to three major experiences: anger, orgasm, and enlightenment. In each case, powerful life-force energies (kundalini) are released. The **Kundalini Meditation** (page 88) helps you become more aware of your sensations and feelings during your flashes. It is best done after you have already had several hot flashes.

• **Baths** are so relaxing. Use menopause as an excuse to jump in. A bath with 3 ounces/80 ml of rubbing alcohol in it can calm fierce flashes. And try the "at-home-ocean-cure": pour 1 cup/250 ml sea salt in a hot bath. Lounge and envision an island paradise.

• Essential oils of **basil** or **thyme or calamus/sweet flag** ease stress from flashes when inhaled or used in a bath or mixed with massage oil.

• **Biofeedback** helps you learn how to consciously dilate and constrict your blood vessels. (This is especially recommended for women who have menopausal migraines.)

Step 3. Nourish and tonify . . .

• Hot flashes deplete vitamin B, vitamin C, magnesium, potassium, calcium, and most trace minerals. Frequent use of **red clover infusion** or **oatstraw infusion** will replace these important nutrients.

"Sometimes there's blip, then a flush whooooshes up to my head; other times it comes on with no warning—flash!—and I'm covered in dampness. Some hover around my neck, some come up my whole torso. Sometimes I get thirsty, sometimes I feel panic. But all of them are HOT."

Kundalini Meditation

Sit or lie down in a private, safe space (bathtub is fine).

Bring all your attention to your breath. As you breathe out, imagine waves flowing out of you with your breath. Breathe out waves of water, of energy, of color, of sound. Allow these waves to flow out of you. Notice where you are tensing, pushing, trying to make the waves happen. And let go, let the waves flow out easily with your breath. Feel the gentle pulsations of the waves deep inside yourself. Feel every cell of your being pulsing peacefully and joyfully with these waves.

When you are ready, begin to draw in red vibrations with your inhalation. Envision yourself filling up with glowing, sparkling, swirling, hot, steaming red. Feel fast spirals of red boiling inside; feel slow vortices of red churning inside. Then breathe out and feel the red flowing out of you in waves. Dissolve into the waves as you breathe out.

With each inhalation, increase the intensity, sharpen the sensation of red: let it be hotter, richer, deeper, more vivid, more consuming. Inhale sun-ripened tomato flesh, sweet cherry juice dribbling down your chin, a sudden flush of menstrual blood blossoming on your clothes. Inhale the seething red sun as it sets into a heaving red sea. Inhale the essence of red roses. Inhale the color of strawberries, the scent of raspberries, the sensation of red satin. Inhale red.

Then breathe it all out. Pause. Feel the emptiness.

Inhale red. Say, out loud or silently: "Sometimes I get upset." Blow out any remaining air as though you were blowing out a candle. Pause. Breathe in red and say again: "Sometimes I get upset." Blow. Pause. Inhale. "Sometimes I get upset."

Blow, pause, inhale, and say, in big red letters: "Sometimes I get angry." Blow. Pause. Inhale. "Sometimes I get angry." Blow. Pause. Inhale. "Sometimes I get angry."

Exhale forcibly. Pause in the emptiness. Inhale red. Say, with passion: "Sometime I feel furious." Again: blow, pause, inhale, and say: "Sometimes I feel furious." Blow. Pause. Inhale. And with intensity say: "Sometimes I feel furious."

Exhale strongly. Make a noise. Pause. Inhale bright red and say or yell: "I." Exhale loudly. Pause. Inhale red; say/yell: "am." Again, exhale with a noise, pause, inhale red. Say/ yell: "enraged." (You can put a pillow or towel on your face and yell into it.)

Breathe out for as long as you can and inhale very slowly. Be intense, be loud if you want to, as you say: "I want to scream." Breathe out, pause, inhale. "I want to kick." Breathe out, pause, inhale. "I want to beat my fists." Breathe out for as long as you can and inhale very slowly. Sigh or moan as you breathe out.

Breathe out with a long sigh. Inhale velvet red, and acknowledge: "Sometimes I only want to think about my pleasure." Breathe out, pause, inhale satin red, and say: "Sometimes I have very sexual thoughts." Sigh fully and pause. Inhale lipstick red and assert: "Sometimes I only want to think about my pleasure."

Breathe out with a long, slow, sound. Inhale blood red and say: "My entire being is nothing but waves of sensation." Sigh, pause, breathe in tropical sunset red and say: "I am nothing but waves of sensation." Sigh and become empty. Wait a moment before inhaling the fresh red of dewy rose petals and say: "I am only waves of sensation." Breathe out with a loud sigh or moan. See how long you can sustain the exhalation.

Breathe slowly and consciously for three breaths. Let the air you breathe be crystalline: clear, sharp, compelling. Let your third inhalation be deeply nourishing, your third exhalation completely freeing. Pay special attention to the energy in your root chakra (lower pelvis).

When you are ready, open your eyes. Get up. Stretch. Record your impressions in words or colors.

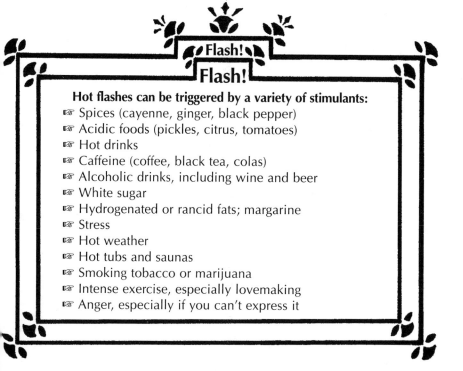

Flash! Flash!

Hot flashes can be triggered by a variety of stimulants:

- ☞ Spices (cayenne, ginger, black pepper)
- ☞ Acidic foods (pickles, citrus, tomatoes)
- ☞ Hot drinks
- ☞ Caffeine (coffee, black tea, colas)
- ☞ Alcoholic drinks, including wine and beer
- ☞ White sugar
- ☞ Hydrogenated or rancid fats; margarine
- ☞ Stress
- ☞ Hot weather
- ☞ Hot tubs and saunas
- ☞ Smoking tobacco or marijuana
- ☞ Intense exercise, especially lovemaking
- ☞ Anger, especially if you can't express it

• **Exercise** affects hot flashes by decreasing the amount of circulating LH and FSH, by nourishing and tonifying the hypothalamus, and by raising endorphin levels (which plummet when you flash). As little as 20 minutes three times a week can reduce flashes significantly.

• Herbal remedies for women with hot flashes include plants that cool the system, such as chickweed; plants that nourish the liver, such as dandelion; and plants rich in phytosterols, such as red clover. Choose one from each group and make your own special blend for your menopausal journey (see boxes pages 92, 93, 94.)

Step 4. Sedate/Stimulate

• Beat the heat of those hot flashes with "personal cool-wear."
☞ Indulge yourself with a beautiful **fan**. If it's old, **fan**tasize about the last menopausal woman who cooled herself with it. Vintage clothing stores have stylish ones; Oriental novelty shops have cheap ones.
☞ **Battery-operated fans** keep you cool with less effort.
☞ **Hydro-headbands** are filled with hydrating gel that stays cool a long time after being soaked and refrigerated. I wear mine around my neck, rather than my head, and keep a spare in the fridge.
☞ The **personal cooling system** is a tiny air-conditioner that you fill with water, turn on, and put around your neck, where it blows a cool breeze over your upper body.
☞ No need for batteries with the **solar ventilator**, a regular baseball cap with a twist: a photovoltaic cell on the top drives a solar-powered fan, causing a breeze to play upon your face.
☞ The **fanteen** combines a canteen, a foam bladed fan, and a spritzer. That's cool!

★ **Witch hazel** extract, sold at the drug store, can help you get cool, cool, cool. Pour some on a hankie; enclose tightly in a plastic bag; off your go. When the flash strikes, you're ready to mop it up, revive yourself, and smell great, especially if you use rose-scented witch hazel.

★ I fill a small plastic mister with water or witch hazel extract and a drop or two of a favorite essential oil, and take it with me on my travels as an **instant refresher** and **cooler**. Passengers around me on airplanes beg me to mist them too!

"It is now four years since menstruation stopped; the flashes are getting lighter, coming less often."

• **What to wear** takes on a whole new significance when you have to cope with being intensely hot or thoroughly chilled, or both, several times a day. Here's advice from the crones:

☞ Dress in **layers** so you can remove and replace clothing easily.

☞ Try **silk** or miracle fibers for the layer next to your skin. Cotton and nylon hold the sweat when you flash and can contribute significantly to the chill that can follow. (Damp, wet cotton: ugh.) Silk and miracle fibers let the moisture evaporate.

☞ Wear **loose clothes**; no turtlenecks or belts. It is not uncommon to feel suffocated during a hot flash. How about a long skirt?

☞ Sweaters and blouses that **button in the front** are a must; pullovers leave you feeling disarrayed when you try to get out of them quickly.

☞ **Elastic waistbands** never looked or felt better. The size of your waist can change several inches in a day during menopause!

Step 5a. Use supplements . . .

Use these remedies only after trying the previous ones. Appendix 1 lists food and herbal sources of nutrients.

★ **Vitamin E** supplements have a well-documented and long-standing reputation as a remedy for hot flashes. Vitamin E supplements may also decrease your risk of dry vaginal tissues and heart disease. The usual dose is 50-200 IU (occasionally as much as 600-800 IU), taken daily for periods ranging from a month to several years. For best utilization, take vitamin E with a meal containing some fat.

The most important thing to look for when buying vitamin E supplements is freshness. Taking rancid vitamin E will increase your risk of heart disease and cancer. Unfortunately, it is almost impossible to buy really fresh vitamin E in capsules.

CAUTIONS: Vitamin E supplements over 100 IU are contraindicated for women with diabetes, high blood pressure, or rheumatic heart conditions; those taking digitalis or anti-coagulants; and anyone who experiences vision disturbances. Vitamin E supplements can promote the growth and spread of breast cancer.[39] If taking vitamin E brings on your period, stop, or reduce your dose.

• Selenium is a synergistic partner of vitamin E. A safe and effective dose of sodium selenite, the most commonly available supplement, is 90 micrograms. CAUTION: Sodium selenite is poisonous in doses over 100 mcg. Elemental selenium is extremely poisonous.

"I love sharing flashes with my 70-year-old mom!"

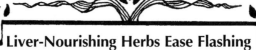

Liver-Nourishing Herbs Ease Flashing

★ **Dandelion** (*Taraxacum officinale*) root is a favorite liver tonic and nourisher wherever it grows, and that's just about everywhere. Regular use of any part, from flowers to roots, helps the liver process the extra hormones generated during your **Change**, thus easing flashes, prickly sensations on the skin, and digestive woes. A dose is 10-30 drops of the root tincture, or a tablespoon/15 ml of the vinegar, taken 1-4 times a day, preferably just before or with meals.

◊ **Ho Shou Wu** (*Polygonatum multiflorum*) roots are nearly as storied as ginseng under their popular name: Fo-ti-tieng. An infusion taken frequently not only nourishes the liver but also restores energy, prevents premature aging and adult onset diabetes, benefits the bones, and strengthens the kidneys.

◊ **Yellow dock** (*Rumex crispus*) root tincture or vinegar and the seeds of the **milk thistle** (*Silybum marianum*) are also liver nourishers of note. Yellow dock is a widespread roadside weed. Try 10-20 drops of root tincture or 1 tablespoon of root vinegar 1-3 times a day. Milk thistle maintains liver health for those going through chemotherapy, alcohol rehabilitation, and menopause. My bottle of milk thistle seed tincture was right at hand when I traveled. If a hot day was in store, I would take a dropperful/1 ml first thing in the morning, and another later as needed.

◊ **Other liver-nourishers**: chicory, oatstraw, burdock.

◊ **Liver-distressers**: coffee, more than an ounce of alcohol in 3 days.

"I'm 48 now; the year I turned 44 I began to have full body sweats on a daily basis, but only in the spring and fall."

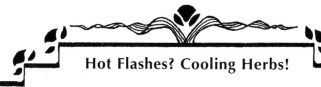

Hot Flashes? Cooling Herbs!

★ Chickweed, Vogelmiere, Stellaire (*Stellaria media*) is often disregarded as a medicinal plant, yet woman after woman has commented to me about the relief she has had during her menopausal years from regular use of chickweed tincture. A dose of 25-40 drops of fresh plant tincture, taken 1-4 times a day, helps reduce the severity and frequency of hot flashes. Results are generally evident within a week or two of regular use. Using chickweed tincture now can help prevent vaginal dryness in your later years. Consistent use shrinks ovarian cysts within a few months.

• **Elder flower**, Holunder, Sureau (*Sambucus* species) tincture is the specific herb for resetting the body's thermostat. When frequent hot flashes or night sweats interrupt your life (and you haven't yet figured out how to take your Crone's Time Away), try using 25-50 drops of fresh elder blossom tincture several times a day. (There is no overdose, so use all you want.) Look for results in a few days.

• **Violet**, Veilchen, Violette (*Viola* species) leaves not only cool the overheated menopausal woman, but also help protect her reproductive tissues from cancer. I use the dried leaves to make an infusion and drink a cup/250 ml a day or more.

• Other cooling herbal allies for menopausal women include oatstraw, mint, seaweeds, all parts of all the mallows (*Malva* species), and the flowers and leaves of any hibiscus (*Hibiscus*).

"I'm 51 and in the past year I had extreme hot flashes for 7 months. I didn't really do anything about them and they've eased up the past couple of months. They did make life more interesting."

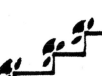

Phytoestrogenic Herbs

★ **Motherwort tincture** has something for every woman, menopausal ones especially. A dose of 5-30 drops, repeated as needed, relieves stress, eases anxiety, cools hot flashes, stops palpitations, increases vaginal lubrication, steadies the mind, and strengthens the heart.

◊ Herbalist Silena Heron's basic menopausal formula (which she adjusts to suit a specific woman's needs) includes ten hormone-rich herbs: two parts chasteberry, one part each motherwort, false unicorn, dong quai, garden sage, and St. Joan's wort, and one-half part each black cohosh, licorice, black haw, alfalfa, and dandelion. If you want to try a formula like this and can't get every one of the herbs, just leave some out, remembering that any *one* of the herbs is sufficient.

◊ Rina Nissim, Swiss herbalist and author of *Natural Healing in Gynecology*, suggests this combination for menopausal women: tincture or glycerine macerate of black currant buds, raspberry leaves, sweet briar (rose) hips and leaf buds. Use one or all, in equal parts, 30-40 drops twice a day.

◊ Georgita Rodriguez, a *curendera* in New Mexico, recommends these herbs to women troubled by hot flashes: yerba de zorillo/wormseed (*Chenopodium ambrosioides*), escoba de la vibora/yellow snakeweed (*Gutierrezia sarothrae*), and yerba mansa/lizard's tail (*Anemopsis californica*). She uses equal parts of the dried leaves or fresh whole plants, boiling them quickly, then allowing the brew to steep for ten or more minutes. The dose is up to three cups/750 mg daily.

★ Make phytosterol-rich **fenugreek** seed tea your wake-up and good-night brew; you'll have easier hot flashes and flushes and, when you do flash your sweat will smell like sweet maple syrup.

◊ Grandfather herbalist Dr. Christopher uses a variety of phytosterol-rich herbs in his formula for the **Change**: ginseng, licorice, sarsaparilla, black cohosh, false unicorn, blessed thistle, and spikenard.

★ Fermented soy products (miso, tamari, tempeh), ground flax seeds, whole grains, red clover infusion, lentils, and cooked dried beans are rich in hormonal precursors and phytoestrogens; daily use eases menopausal symptoms, prevents cancer, lowers risk of heart disease.

• See pages 72-77 for specific dosages of phytoestrogenic herbs.

★ B vitamins, especially B_2, B_6, and B_{12}, are needed in very large quantities during the menopausal years. Many long-time vegetarians suddenly begin to crave (and eat) meat, an excellent source of all B vitamins, during menopause.

• Bioflavonoid supplements, 250 mg 5-6 times daily, may help relieve hot flashes. Hesperidin is the most effective; dosage is 1000 mg daily.

Step 5b. Use drugs . . .

• Estrogen (ERT) is the drug most commonly recommended to menopausal women bothered by hot flashes. In fact, women catapulted into menopause by surgery, radiation, Tamoxifen, or chemotherapy are told that their hot flashes will be "unbearable" without ERT or HRT. Estrogen may alleviate hot flashes, but practitioners and women around the country tell me of women taking ERT and continuing to have intense flashes. Sometimes the only woman in a menopause class who is obviously flashing is the one who is taking hormones. There is little evidence that estrogen relieves hot flashes, so I urge women to try any other alternative.

Happily, fewer then 15 percent of menopausal women in America take prescription hormones. If you are one of these, it is safest to use the lowest dose you find effective, to take it as briefly as possible, to also use liver-nourishing herbs, like dandelion, while on ERT/ HRT, and — after thirteen months — to interface with phytoestrogic herbs and ease off the hormones.

• Other drugs used to control hot flashes include progestins such as Norlutin or Proveramay (side effects include fatigue, depression, weight gain), clonidine (Dixarit), and Bellergal, which contains phenobarbital, ergotamine, and belladonna (a real witches' brew, eh?). For information on other new drugs, see page 225.

Step 6. Break and enter . . .

• Some gynecologists recommend hysterectomy as a cure for hot flashes. This is malpractice, as your uterus doesn't cause hot flashes. Nor is it a benefit that, once your uterus is removed, you can take ERT/HRT without worry of cervical or uterine cancer.

"Experiencing menopause at such an early age (41) is embarrassing. I feel inhibited about discussing it with my peers. Even if menopause is normal, I feel abnormal."

Menopause Is Enlightenment

The energy aspects of menopause are of special interest to me. As a long-time student of yoga, I was struck by the many similarities between menopausal symptoms and the well-known esoteric goal of "awakening of the kundalini." Though the ideas presented in this section may seem strange or difficult to comprehend, they contain powerful messages about menopause which lie at the heart of the Wise Woman approach.

"Kundalini [is] the root [of] all spiritual experiences. . . ."[40] Kundalini is a special kind of energy known in many cultures, including Tibetan, Indian, Sumerian, Chinese, Irish, Aztec, and Greek. Kundalini is said to be hot, fast, powerful, and large. It exists within the earth, within all life, and within each person. Psychoanalyst Carl G. Jung called kundalini *anima*. Kundalini is usually represented as a serpent coiled at the base of the spine, but women's mystery stories locate it in the uterus — or the area where the uterus was, if a woman has had a hysterectomy. During both puberty and menopause, a woman's kundalini is difficult to control and may cause a great number of symptoms.

East Indian yogis spend lifetimes learning to activate, or wake up, their kundalini. This is also called "achieving enlightenment." When they succeed, a surge of super-heated energy goes up the spine, throughout the nerves, dilating blood vessels, and fueling itself with hormones. As kundalini continues to travel up the spine, it changes the functioning of the endocrine, cardiovascular, and nervous systems. Not just in yogis, but in any woman who allows herself to become aware of it. Menopause is a kind of enlightenment. Hot flashes are kundalini training sessions.

To understand the awakening of kundalini during menopause, it is necessary to look at its effects on us throughout our lives. Before puberty, kundalini is primarily outside the body. As puberty commences, a two-valved energy "gate" (imaginary opening) in the "root chakra" (see **Figure 1**) opens, and kundalini circulates up from the earth and into the root chakra. This allows kundalini to build up in the uterus and pelvic tissues until it is released, usually during menstruation. As much as ten days before bleeding commences, the stored kundalini can intensify emotions and sensations, expose powerful feelings, trigger creative outpourings, and generate a house-cleaning frenzy. If pregnancy occurs, kundalini is retained for the duration of the pregnancy and is used in the act of birth.

At menopause, one "valve" of the gate closes. The open valve allows kundalini to enter; the closed one prevents it from leaving. Now kundalini, unable to return to earth, builds up in the pelvic tissues, leading some women to say that menopause is PMS that never stops. If this intense energy collects in the uterus for too many weeks, cramps and flooding may accompany the delayed menses. If it sits in the pelvis for many years, it can dry out the vagina, erode the integrity of the hips, contribute to bladder weakness, and depress sexual desire.

But kundalini naturally, and guided by hot flashes, goes up the spine, conferring enlightenment, not incontinence. But not all at once.

As the kundalini rises, it passes through six energy gates/chakras (see **Figure 2**). If a chakra is resistant to being activated, symptoms relating to the chakra may occur: some painful, distressful, unprecedented, awakening shamanic abilities and perhaps causing the menopausal woman (or her family and friends) to think she's going crazy. She has never been more sane. "After kundalini awakes it becomes impossible to continue believing that external reality is the sole reality."[41] No wonder old women are honored and feared throughout the world![42]

Menstrual pain, bloating, indigestion, heart palpitations, thyroid malfunctions, headaches, and memory loss are all associated with the movement (or resistance to movement) of kundalini through the chakras.

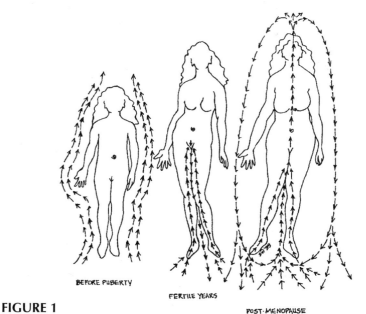

FIGURE 1
Kundalini: maiden, mother, crone

When menopausal symptoms are understood as energy movement a woman feels more at ease. Instead of feeling victimized by her body, the menopausal woman can use her symptoms as a way to pinpoint areas that need special nourishment. Quiet time alone in nature, or sitting in a comfortable chair listening to soothing music allows thoughts and feelings to arise and opens the way for the flow of kundalini. Specific exercises, such as those offered by energy-worker Barbara Brennan,[43] can also be used to help ease into the increased energy flow. After several years of practice, kundalini moves freely up the spine and out the crown, symptoms gradually subside, and overall energy increases.

Handling powerful kundalini energies is easier when the nervous system is strong. Nourishing herbs such as oatstraw infusion, tincture of motherwort, cronewort (mugwort) vinegar, and the many varieties of seaweed, are excellent green allies. Hatha yoga (physical exercise), pranayama (breath exercise), and tai chi (energy exercise) help too.

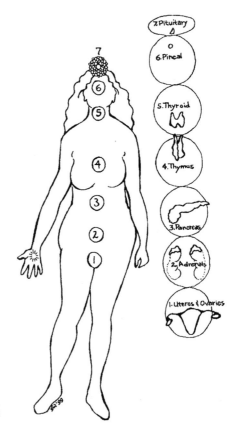

FIGURE 2
The seven chakras

Night Sweats

Step 1. Collect information . . .

A hot flash at night is called a night sweat. While daytime flashes are triggered by many things, night sweats are most often a result of adrenal stress. (Menopausal **Change** requires the adrenals to work hard.) A few hours after you fall asleep, a small sound can trigger an adrenal response, flooding the body with adrenaline (which constricts blood vessels), and awakening you. When you realize there is nothing to fear, you relax, the blood vessels dilate, and zoom! you have a hot flash. Adrenaline-mediated flashes often cause profuse perspiration, sometimes to the point where the bedclothes must be changed before further sleep is possible. Any hot flash, day or night, accompanied or preceded by feelings of anxiety or terror, indicates adrenal stress.

Step 2. Engage the energy . . .

• Try homeopathic *Nux vomica* when night sweats or leg cramps wake you and leave you feeling chilled and irritable.

• Try homeopathic *Sulfur* when whole-body night sweats leave you with a huge thirst and intolerance to heat in any form.

Step 3. Nourish and tonify . . .

★ **Stinging nettle** infusion strengthens, nourishes, and rebuilds the adrenals, thus easing or eliminating night sweats. I found 2-4 cups of iced infusion a day amazingly helpful during periods when I was waking frequently, and the effect was rapid, usually within a few days.

• **Prepare your bed** to help moderate hot flashes in your sleep. Use all-cotton sheets, a mattress of natural fibers (such as a futon), a feather pillow. And perhaps a silk nightgown — or nothing at all? Polyester-blend sheets and nylon sleepwear encourage flashes, and keep you damp and clammy afterward. Foam mattresses and pillows can precipitate volcanic flashes.

• **Oatstraw infusion**, a cup or more a day, strengthens the adrenals, promotes sound sleep, and reduces night sweats.

★ One of my favorite remedies for women disturbed by night sweats is **motherwort**. A dose of 10-25 drops, taken just before bed and each time you awaken, generally brings results within two weeks.

"When I resisted my night sweats, they lasted for several minutes. When I relaxed into them, they were more intense, but only lasted a few seconds."

Step 4. Stimulate/Sedate . . .

★ **Garden sage** (*Salvia officinalis*) is renowned for its ability to reduce and eliminate night sweats. The effect is quite prompt, usually noticeable in a few hours, and long-lived, sometimes up to two days from a single cup of brew. For best results, make an infusion by pouring one quart of boiling water over one ounce of dried sage in a canning jar. Cap tightly and steep for four hours. To use: Put 1-4 tablespoons/20-60 ml sage infusion in a cup of hot or cold water and drink. Undiluted sage infusion stays good for weeks refrigerated. Very antibacterial!

Earthquake Flashes

Step 1. Collect information . . .

"Earthquake" or "volcano" flashes are to a normal flash as a tidal wave is to a normal wave: uncontrollable, huge, devastating. These powerful flashes are more likely to occur in women who achieve menopause by surgery, chemotherapy, or radiation.

Step 2. Engage the energy . . . .

• Try homeopathic *Sulfur* if you have earthquake flashes accompanied by profuse sweating (which may smell strong), especially if the flashes include the torso, hands, and feet, as well as the face.

• Homeopathic *Crotalus* helps the woman with earthquake flashes accompanied by headaches, flooding, restlessness, or/and weakness, worse after sleep.

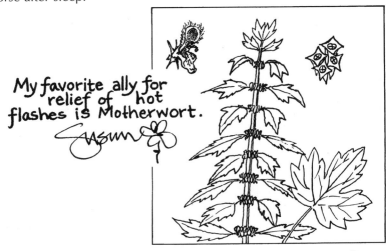

My favorite ally for relief of hot flashes is Motherwort.

Step 3. Nourish and tonify . . .

★ **Motherwort** tincture, 25-40 drops taken every four hours while awake, is a tremendous ally for the woman whose earthquake flashes include emotional uproar, erratic heartbeats, and/or palpitations.

• **Ginseng** (2 grams daily for three months) and lots of jogging put an end to one woman's earthquake flashes following surgery.

Step 4. Sedate/Stimulate . . .

★ Black cohosh root tincture, 30-60 drops taken up to four times daily, effectively reduces and relieves even severe hot flashes.

★ **Breathe out** and out and out. Calm those raging flashes by breathing very, very slowly, with a long, long exhale. Puff out your cheeks and blow like you're playing a trumpet.

• Sucking on a piece of **hard candy** can head off a hot flash or moderate an earthquake flash.

• If I had menopause to do over again, the first thing I would do is **buy an air conditioner** for my bedroom. I spent more than a year dreaming of large refrigerators and trying to crawl into large freezers until I realized I could make my fantasies come true! Visiting air conditioned museums, stores, and theaters also helps. So does putting ice on your cheeks and on the back of your neck.

Steps 5a. and 5b. Use supplements; Use drugs . . .

• Women with earthquake or volcanic flashes take estrogen believing that there is no other remedy, but vitamin E seems equally effective. Very high doses (600-800 IU daily) produce noticeable effects within ten days. (Cautions, page 91.)

Step 6. Break and enter . . .

★ After surgical or chemical menopause, chaste berry tincture, 30-90 drops daily, can moderate the severity and duration of your hot flashes, even if it doesn't eliminate them altogether.

"I started flashing at 47. This peaked the year after my periods stopped, at 54, with hourly flushes waking me in a sweat. They've tapered off in the four years since. I did have a flash this morning, but the last one was three days ago."

Other Overheated Conditions:
Dizziness, Dry Eyes, Burning Mouth, Formication

Step 1. Collect information . . .

As if flushing and flashing and sweating and chilling weren't difficult enough to endure (even enjoy) on our menopausal journey, some women also experience a variety of other difficulties with or apart from their hot flashes: faintness, dizziness, a sick feeling, dry eyes, burning mouth, and formication (from the Latin word for ant, *formica*) — a prickly sensation as if ants were crawling over the skin.

These problems are all related to an overworked and "overheated" liver. In Traditional Chinese Medicine (TCM), the liver controls the smooth flow of energy in the body; if the liver is overworked, as it may well be during the menopausal years, too much energy can go to the head, resulting in dizziness, faintness, and headaches.

That inner "sick" feeling usually centers in the stomach area, just under the ribs, the chakra called the solar plexus, associated with (how did you know?) the liver, and with personal worth/personality.

Lack of vitamin A (produced in the liver from carotenes) results in loss of night vision. In TCM, the eyes are the opening to the liver. Dry eyes are related to an overworked, overheated liver.

Many medical paradigms look to the mouth and tongue as a key to the general state of health of the whole person. A burning mouth and tongue suggests not only a "hot" liver but someone whose whole system is overheated, overloaded. This woman is probably burning to say something, and her thyroid may be overheating as well.

If the nerve endings in your skin seem hypersensitive (even worse than the princess who felt the pea under all those mattresses), that's a sign of liver distress, too.

Note that dizziness may also be from hyperventilation (a by-product of anxiety, fatigue, and stress), dehydration, reduced blood flow to the brain, or inner ear debris (common with age). Regular exercise, especially hatha yoga or tai chi can prevent and relieve these problems.

Step 2. Engage the energy . . .

• *Caladium* is the homeopathic remedy for creepy crawly skin, aggravated by heat and worse at night. So is *Rhus tox.*

• The smell of **lavender oil** is said to relieve dizziness.

• The smell of **cedar** soothes the liver, reduces "touchiness."

• Homeopathic *Thuja* or *Rhus tox.* helps those with a burning mouth.

• Ease **dry eyes**: Place quartz crystals or cucumber slices or steeped chamomile tea bags on the closed eyelids for several minutes. Imagine crying the tears of the earth. Try homeopathic *Berberis vulgaris*.

Step 3. Nourish and tonify . . .

★ Menopausal women with itchy, sensitive skin, light-headedness, hot eyes and mouth find quick relief with 10-20 drops of liver-nourishing **dandelion root** tincture taken 1-3 times daily. **Milk thistle** tincture is another effective liver strengthener, especially used before stress.

• **Lady's mantle** tea, very strong, and lots of it, tones the liver and helps eliminate itchy sensations following hot flashes.

★ Cool and soothe your eyes, mouth, skin, and liver from the inside out with **oatstraw** infusions, and from the outside in with oatstraw baths.

★ A compress of fresh **chickweed** soothes the eyes and restores their moisture. An eyewash of 2-5 drops calendula tincture in a palm full of warm water, used once a day, will also help restore needed moisture to the eyes if used repeatedly for several weeks.

Step 4. Stimulate /Sedate . . .

★ For "instant relief of formication," writes midwife Wonshé, "eat raw **beets**, grated or juiced, three times in one day."

★ If you have crawly, sensitive skin that prevents sleep, reach for the **skullcap** tincture. The dose is 15-25 drops, repeated as needed, up to four times. Tincture of the fresh flowering tops of **St. Joan's wort**, 25-30 drops, can be used with, or instead of, skullcap.

• Relieve burning mouth with a rinse of **calendula** blossom tincture, a dropperful diluted in water, or some **aloe vera** juice, or **plantain seed/oatmeal porridge**.

• When you feel dizzy, breathe into your cupped hands, exhaling as slowly as you can.

• A cup of **primrose** (*Primula*) flower tea can help when you feel nervous and faint, with a sick sensation. (Caution, page 136.)

Step 5b. Use drugs . . .

• Alcohol and prescription medications can dry your eyes, make your skin sensitive, dilate your blood vessels and diminish the blood supply to your brain, making you dizzy, all without a hot flash. (They aren't nice to your liver either.)

Hairy Problems

"Dearest granddaughter, come close and look into my eyes." Grandmother Growth beckons and her voice grows deeper and more resonant. "Look deep into my eyes and acknowledge the beauty there.

"Yes, my skin is wrinkled. My face is the face of age, and to many, that is fearful. But my beauty, like my wise blood, now resides inside of me. Can you see it? Can you feel it? Can you look beyond the hair on my chin?" she says grinning, flicking her fingers under her chin in a most unladylike manner.

"Can you forgive the places where my scalp shines through? Can you find the truth of my beauty, the beauty of age, which is so different from the beauty of youth?" Her eyes grow fierce, but sparkle with amusement. "I know you can, for I know how beautiful I am."

Grandmother Growth takes your chin in her strong hand and looks at you with eyes so intense you fear you may catch on fire. She commands: "When you look into your mirror, I ask you to look deep into your own eyes and to acknowledge your own inner beauty.

"I know, I know, metamorphosis is changing you and you don't like it. Like a teenager, you peer and peer into the looking glass, noting every new wrinkle, every hair on your face (and other new places). Counting each grey hair as it grows. Worrying that your hair seems to fall out by the handful.

"Dear one, my most precious child, take care, but do not fret. And do not tell yourself that you are becoming ugly. I know it is difficult, in fact it may be one of the most difficult tasks of your menopause, but you must recast your own opinion of beauty so that it includes old women who have hairy problems and live well with them — like you!"

Too much hair (on the chin), too little hair (on the scalp), falling hair, thinning hair, greying hair, no matter what the complaint, many women notice something happening to their hair during menopause. As hormone levels shift during the menopausal years, hair responds to the changing hormones by changing texture, falling out, or by growing in "odd" places. Here are remedies for those who want more hair, and for those who want less.

Hair Loss & Grey Hair

Step 1. Collect information . . .

Menopause does not cause grey hair; taking hormones doesn't stop it. Greying, thinning hair is a normal part of aging. Women whose menopause is induced in their twenties and thirties do not suddenly go grey.

Hair loss at mid-life (androgenic alopecia) is more strongly linked to genes than diet or lifestyle. Those of European origins are far more likely to experience it than Asians, Native Americans, Africans, or African-Americans. Hair loss starts earlier and becomes more extreme on men's heads, but just as many women deal with receding hairlines and balding pates. Roughly half of all women experience some hair loss during their menopausal years. Two-thirds of postmenopausal women deal with thinning hair or bald spots. And no one likes it. Americans spend a billion dollars a year trying to regrow their hair!

Normal hair loss (50-100 hairs a day) is gradual. Sudden unexplained loss is not normal. Events which can trigger hair loss include pregnancy, childbirth, menopause, severe emotional stress, thyroid disorders, rapid or profound weight loss, pituitary problems, malnutrition, iron deficiency, lack of protein, chronic illness, scarlet fever, syphilis, large doses of vitamin A, chemotherapy, radiation, general anesthesia, certain medications (see Step 5), and hair abuse including bleaching, permanents, tight braids, tight pony tails, tight wigs, and tight hats.

• The National Alopecia Areata Foundation, 710 "C" St., Suite 11, San Rafael, CA 94901-3853 (415-456-4644) can help you contact a local hair loss support group, and gather more information.

Step 2. Engage the energy . . . .

• Homeopathic remedies for women with hair loss include:
  ☞ *Lycopodium*: loss precipitated by hormonal fluctuations.
  ☞ *Sepia*: especially for menopausal women who have sweaty flushes and heavy bleeding
  ☞ *Phosphoric acid*: loss after grief or extreme emotion, accompanied by exhaustion.

"Hair, hair, everywhere! I have seven cats, and believe me when I say there's a lot of hair in my life. . . . But, I was totally unprepared to find so much of **mine** *lying about. I became obsessed with my hair loss. I imagined life with wigs. Surely I would be bald in months! It didn't happen. I wish I had known that this was common during menopause."*

Step 3. Nourish and tonify . . .

★ Infusion of **stinging nettle**, 2-4 cups a day, strengthens hair and checks falling hair with its superb supplies of protein, B vitamins, vitamin E, iron, and other minerals. Regular use restores thickness, body, shine and sheen to hair. If you have any infusion left over, pour it on your head and rub it into your scalp for faster results.

• "Every grey hair represents a day with too few minerals," a wise woman said to me. Actually, the color of hair is produced by special cells which gradually die as we age. But it is true that hair is loaded with minerals, and getting extra minerals may keep those color cells alive longer. To increase my mineral intake, and keep my hair healthy, I eat more **yogurt**, drink more nourishing **herbal infusions**, prepare more mineral-rich **soups**, use more **herbal vinegars**, and increase the amount of **seaweed** in my diet.

★ Lack of minerals, especially **iron**, can cause hair loss. **Yellow dock** is one of my favorite iron-tonics.

• Natural hair dyes can cure the grey blahs. **Henna** (*Lawsonia inermis*) is a plant that is easily purchased ready-to-use to change the color of your hair temporarily, and you are not limited to carrot-top red. So long as it is not overused (less than four times a year) henna is strengthening to the scalp and hair.

• Other natural hair dyes include **coffee**, **black walnut hulls**, or infusions of **sage** or **rosemary** herb.

• Herbalist Amanda McQuade Crawford suggests using **lemon balm** or **lemon grass** infusion as a hair rinse to prevent hair loss.

• **Burdock seed oil**, one of the best selling hair tonics in Russia, is especially recommended for those with thinning hair or hair loss. Apply to your hair and scalp, leave on overnight and shampoo it out the following day. Repeat as needed.

★ Just plain **olive oil** is also a tremendous hair tonic. So is **jojoba oil**. Apply a handful of either to hair and scalp, wrap well and leave on overnight, washing it out the next morning.

• I know you know, but let me say it again, **exercise**! Yes, it can make your hair healthier too.

Step 4. Sedate/Stimulate . . .

★ While some temporary loss of hair at menopause is considered normal, something worse may be brewing. Thin, dry hair is one of the first signs of an **underactive thyroid**. (See page 52.) Hair loss is also an early sign of **lupus**, an auto-immune disease.

• Chugging down a gulp of **cod liver oil** or wheat germ oil every day for six weeks could help your hair.

• Menopause sends lots of energy to the crown of your head. That can overstimulate the scalp and cause hair loss (and/or headaches). Get your energy moving with a **scalp massage**. Let your head calm down and your hair cool off.

• Blow dryers, dyes, perms, and other harsh treatments damage hair and scalp. **Rosemary** essential oil, a few drops rubbed into the scalp several times a week, repairs the damage, increases hair growth, and improves hair texture.

• Other essential oils which improve hair growth include **lavender, lemon, thyme, sage**, and **carrot seed**. A mixture of 10-20 drops of any of these with 4 ounces of plain olive oil, infused burdock seed oil, or jojoba oil is rubbed into the scalp and left on overnight. Essential oils said to reduce hair loss include **birch, calendula, chamomile, cypress, rose**, and **yarrow**.

• **Avoid** chlorinated water on your hair. A shower filter is more important than a drinking water filter. And cut down on the number of times you wash your hair. Less is more for healthy hair.

• **Avoid cayenne.** Heroic herbalists say it increases hair growth by improving blood circulation to the scalp. But when there is hair loss, says Janet Roberts, MD, specialist in women's hair loss and member of the Oregon Menopause Network, there are inflamed follicles. Cayenne increases inflammation, ultimately increasing hair loss.

Step 5a. Use supplements . . .

• Dry, brittle, thin hair is often due to a deficiency in one or more of these nutrients: protein, vitamin A, vitamin B_{12}, vitamin C, iron, zinc, essential fatty acids. Food and herbal sources of these nutrients (listed in Appendix 1, page 247) are preferable to pills.

• **Avoid hair weaving**, a cosmetic treatment that weaves replacement hair in with the still existing hair; it actually causes more loss (by creating traction alopecia).

Step 5b. Use drugs . . .

• Hair loss can be caused by drugs, including: birth control pills, anti-coagulants, diet pills, thyroid medications; non-steroidal anti-inflammatory drugs including aspirin, ibuprofen, and Aleve; cholesterol-lowering drugs such as clofibrate and gemfibrozil; arthritis medications such as gold salts (auranofin), indomethacin, naproxen, sulindac, and methotrexate; beta-blockers such as atenolol (Tenormin), metoprolol (Lopressor), nadolol (Corgard), propranolol (Inderal), and timolol (Blocadren); and ulcer drugs such as cimetidine (Tagamet), ranitidine (Zantac), and famoridine (Pepcid). And, of course, chemotherapy.

• Minoxidil (Rograine) dilates blood vessels, encouraging baby-fine hair. Only the 2 percent solution is approved for women. Of those who use it only 19 percent achieve even moderate regrowth; 40 percent have minimal regrowth. Meanwhile, 40 percent of the women using the placebo had regrowth! CAUTION: Side effects in women include unwanted hair growth on the face, heart disturbances, and dizziness.

• Fertile women are not allowed to use (or even touch) finasteride (Propecia) for fear of the severe birth defects it causes. This is probably a blessing in disguise, as the side effects (loss of libido, lip swelling, breast engorgement, birth defects) are not pleasant. Finasteride is completely ineffective in reversing hair loss for postmenopausal women.
    Tell your men friends considering using this drug that a dose of .2 mg (one-fifth the normal dose) works just as well, costs less ($10 a month instead of $50), and is gentler on the liver.[44]

• Hormones, including ERT, HRT, birth control pills, and anti-androgens (cypoterone acetate, spironolactone, and fluramide) are used singly or in combination to treat women with androgenic alopecia.

Step 6. Break and enter . . .

• Hair transplants can cover a bald spot but are far less successful on women than on men. Micrografts do a better job of dealing with women's diffuse pattern of hair loss.

• "Scalp lifts" tighten the scalp, making hair appear thicker and fuller.

Hirsutism/Too Much Hair

Step 0. Do nothing . . .

• A few brazen souls just grin and "bare" it. Seriously, does anyone else notice that extra hair? Ask a few people who will tell you the truth. Perhaps you are making a mountain (beard/moustache) out of a molehill (a couple of extra hairs)?

Step 1. Collect information . . .

It is not at all unusual to find extra hairs growing on the chin, upper lip, breasts, and legs during or after menopause. It is thought that menopause makes some hair follicles more sensitive to testosterone's hair-promoting effects. However, sudden hair growth can be caused by a tumor on the ovaries, thyroid, adrenals, or pituitary.

Step 2. Engage the energy . . .

• Visualize a large mirror. Look at yourself in this mirror. When you see something you don't like, ask the mirror how you can change. Finish by telling your image how much you love her. Repeat frequently.

Step 3. Nourish and tonify . . .

• Oatstraw infusion tends to increase the activity of testosterone; increased levels of testosterone contribute to excess hair growth during menopause. It's a long shot, but avoiding oats, oatmeal, and oatstraw infusion may help eliminate or reduce those extra hairs.

Step 4. Sedate/Stimulate . . .

• **Natural bleaches**, like lemon juice or moderate sunlight (or both together), are generally safe even for use on the sensitive skin of the face.

• Shaving, plucking, and waxing are minimally invasive means of removing excess hair. Such means may increase the rate of hair growth, however, or make the texture of the hair coarser, or cause hair follicle inflammation and ingrown hairs.

Step 5b. Use drugs . . .

• Hirsutism may be caused by corticosteroids and medications for high blood pressure. (Rograine was originally a blood pressure drug.)

• Drug treatments — which are 80 percent successful according to one MD — include the corticosteroids prednisone and dexamethasone. Hormones, including birth-control pills and anti-androgens such as spironolactone, are occasionally used.

Step 6. Break and enter . . .

• Electrolysis is expensive, painful, tedious, must be done several times over, and can cause scarring. Most sources advise against home electrolysis.

Emotional Uproar

"Dear woman," sighs Grandmother Growth tenderly. "I see that Change has thinned the protective layers hiding your anger, your fears, your grief. Yes, I see your hidden feelings and secret desires exposed a little more with each hot flash. You may think your feelings are out of proportion, too sharp, quite irrational, possibly insane. But, I assure you, they are only raw from neglect. Receive them without judgment, nourish them, and your 'uncontrollable' feelings during the meno-pausal years will lead you to the deepest heart of your own secrets.

"If you cannot tolerate those about you, leave. Go to the sheltering space of your cave. Claim your Crone's Year Away.

"If you feel called by death, do not mistake this as a call to take your own life. It is a call to embrace your eventual death as fully as possible while living as fully as possible.

"You have given life. You have given life even if you have not had a child, my child; for you have given the gift of potential life to yourself and your people. Giving life is good in your culture.

"Now you leave behind this Mother aspect and take on your identity as Crone. The Crone gives death, knows death, honors the gift of death, feels the truth of death. But death is fearful, bad in your culture. As a baby Crone, you need to acknowledge the facts of life, one of which is that the mate and lover of life is death. Facing one's own death, whether real or symbolic, is an emotionally intense experience. Accepting the death-giving aspect of yourself in the face of your culture's disapproval is an act of great courage.

"Come dear one, and join the dance of feeling, life, and death. Do a crazy Crone step, whirling around the emotional roller coaster; it's part of the journey to 'crazy old lady,' she who can act totally outside the social norms, who can recognize and use the awesome power of her emotions."

We all connect the turbulent hormones of adolescence with the turbulent emotions of young adulthood, and the hormonal changes of pregnancy with the intense emotions of motherhood. Just so, the flashing, flooding hormones of menopause precipitate flashing, flooding emotions in the "pubescent Crone."

With her menstrual moon tides ebbing, then flowing in unpredictable floods, her body sometimes suddenly drenched in sweat, and sleep elusive, how could her emotions remain untouched? Menopause is the classic time in our culture for women to go "crazy." Oversensitivity, irritability, anxiety, fear, extreme nervousness, rage, grief, depression, and crying jags are not uncommon during the menopausal climax years.

The remedies here don't seek to eliminate these emotions, or turn "negative" ones into "positive" ones, but, in the Wise Woman way, to help you incorporate all of your feelings into your wholeness.

"In the midst of a hot flash, I suddenly saw my entire life in a new light. I wanted to rage; I wanted to laugh without stopping. I was afraid I was crazy, but I knew I'd never been more sane."

Depression

"Look here," signals Grandmother Growth, spreading out a story blanket. "See how depression is deeply woven with anger and grief. When our human need for reliable, joyous intimacy is frustrated, and expression of our frustration would endanger us, depression comes and protects us. When there is no way to deal effectively with situations that enrage us, depression comes and helps us quiet our violent impulses.

"Depression is not an easy companion on your journey, but let her go with us for a while. She knows much about life, about your life, and about the give-away of life and death. In her bundle, she carries the anger you have carefully frozen with frigid blasts of fear and kept nourished with your pain. Dare to accept her bundle, to accept your own wholeness. Dare to forgive what hurt you and stop reliving the pain. Dare to thaw your rage. You will need it, daughter, in the days to come."

Step 0. Do nothing . . .

• Welcome the dark. Cherish the deepness. Give yourself over to a day or two of doing nothing.

★ Return to earth. Go into your (metaphorical or real) cave. Lie belly down on the earth. Bury yourself in leaves or sand.

Step 1. Collect information . . .

Depression is very common among women whose menopause is induced. But it is no more common among women achieving menopause naturally than among, say, single mothers. Why is it so associated with menopause in our minds and stories?

Depression can indicate hypothyroidism. Depression can be caused by steroids, high blood pressure drugs, and ERT/HRT. But most often the cause of depression is the belief (valid or not) that nothing you do makes any difference.

Victimization is one of the most significant risk factors in the development of depression; it is estimated that at least 40 percent of all women in the United States have been sexually or physically victimized. Poverty is also a precipitator of depression; women make up more than two-thirds of all Americans who live below poverty level. More than menopause, victimization and poverty put women of all ages at risk for depression and show clearly how depression is a "lid" on rage and pain.

Get help if you are depressed for more than two weeks. Call your local hotline; the number is in the front of your phone book. Or see page 127 for ways to contact feminist therapists.

These remedies are helpful for "ordinary" depression as well as the more severe "clinical" depression.

Step 2. Engage the energy . . .

★ Anger is part of depression. **Find your anger**; cherish it. (See "Rage'" page 117.)

★ Taken together, the **Bach flower remedies** *Wild Rose*, *Larch*, *Mustard*, *Gorse*, and *Gentian* help alleviate feelings of apathy, resignation, despondency, inferiority, despair, hopelessness, discouragement, self-doubt, and intense descending gloom.

• **Homeopathic remedies for women who are depressed:**
   ☞ *Arum metallicum*: with frequent thoughts of suicide, feels cut off from love and joy.
   ☞ *Sepia*: just wants to be left alone, disinterested in sex, and snaps angrily at her family and friends.
   ☞ *Calms Forte* (a blend including calcium): depression with crying.

• Let **sunlight** be your remedy. It's more than idle chatter that we identify depression with grey skies and happiness with sunny ones. Our hormonal/emotional balance is profoundly affected by sunlight. For emotional health (and strong bones) get 15 minutes of sunlight on your uncovered eyelids (take contacts out) daily. If you can't get out (or if the sun doesn't cooperate) try sitting next to special lights for thirty minutes each day upon waking. (See page 127.)

★ **Sing the blues**; dance 'em too. Women have depended on songs and dances to carry them out of depression for centuries. If you don't know how, sing along with Rosetta Records, page 127.

• **Dance therapy** or **massage therapy** is more effective than talk therapy for reaching and healing hidden traumas and relieving depression. Even a single session may have a dramatic effect.

• Aromatherapists suggest the smell of **lemon balm** (*Melissa*) tea or oil to lift spirits and ease depression.

• Menopause is an ideal time to renew your relationship with your **inner child**. As we embrace our past and bless it, depression lifts and the future smiles. (See Cathryn Taylor's *Inner Child Workbook*.)

• Write in a journal. Talk to a friend.

Step 3. Nourish and tonify . . .

★ **St. Joan's wor**t, Johannaskraut, Herbe de la St. Jean (*Hypericum perforatum*) lives in the sunniest locations and blooms when the sun is at its maximum. The bright red tincture is a dependable reliever of the blues. I call it bottled sunshine. A dropperful/1 ml, taken 1-3 times daily for months (years if need be) has helped many women relieve SAD (seasonal affective disorder), move through grief, ease the physical pain of depression, and walk on the sunny side! CAUTION: *Hypericum* in capsules is associated with sensitivity to the sun. This is not true of the tincture, even at high doses.

★ Adrenal exhaustion gives rise to depression, fatigue, irritability, and unpredictable mood swings. Your adrenals expend a lot of extra energy making hormones during your menopausal years. Give them tender loving care with **nettle** infusion, up to 4 cups/1 liter daily.

★ **Oatstraw** infusion has been an ally for hysterical and depressed women since earliest times. Gentle *Avena* nourishes the nerves and helps you remember why life is worth living. Drink as many cups a day as you wish. Or try an oatstraw bath.

• **Garden sage** (*Salvia*) is an ancient ally for emotionally distressed midlife women. In some societies, only crones were allowed to drink the brew made from the nubbly leaves (at least partly because it delays menses and dries up breast milk). I make a full quart of infusion, steeping an ounce of dried sage overnight. I dilute this strong brew, mixing a few spoonfuls into hot water or warm milk and honey when I want to consume it. The undiluted infusion keeps for weeks refrigerated, unlike most infusions which spoil quickly. It's a great hair rinse, too.

★ **Walk and sing!**

★ Short-term cognitive behavioral therapy or interpersonal therapy has been clinically verified to be as effective as drugs in relieving depression. Not only that, two-thirds of those who simply read about therapy improved significantly.

★ **Thirty minutes of aerobic exercise**, especially soon after awakening, has been shown to relieve depressions resistant to all other treatments, including drugs.

Step 4. Stimulate/Sedate . . .

★ **Sleep less**. While we sleep, a depression-causing substance is produced. We usually awaken when we've used all we produced that night. Depressed women overproduce this substance while asleep and find it difficult to wake up. Going back to sleep compounds the problem. Staying up all night once a week can cure you of depression. If you can't cope with no sleep, even mild sleep deprivation (such as sleeping five hours or less for two nights in a row) dramatically decreases depressive symptoms in some people.

★ **Imitate joy**. Stand tall, smile with your whole face (mouth, cheeks, eyes), and breathe deeply. You will either actually start feeling happier or make your rage/grief more visible and more easily accessed.

★ To **energize** yourself when depressed: 1) lift your sternum and sigh deeply many times, 2) hold your arms out in front of you for several minutes, 3) bounce up and down on the balls of your feet.

Step 5a. Use supplements . . .

• Increasing the amount of **vitamin B complex** in your diet with whole grains and supplements of up to 50 mg daily can ease depression.

• Low levels of **calcium** and **zinc** in the blood are associated with depression. Eating more cheese and yogurt, garlic and mushrooms will help, as will supplements of up to 20 mg zinc and 1500 mg calcium.

• Lack of **vitamin B$_{12}$** doubles the risk of severe depression for older women,[45] and is vital for good vision. This critical nutrient, found only in animal products, is difficult to assimilate. Tofu and soy beverages interfere with its absorption.[46] Supplements (25 mcg daily) are recommended for women 65 and older, and required for those who eat little (or no) meat or dairy.

• **SAM-e** is short for A-adenosylmethionine, a biochemical found in every cell of your body. It helps form vital compounds like DNA and neurotransmitters. Well-nourished people make SAM-e from the amino acid methionine. As a supplement, 1600 mg of SAM-e relieved the symptoms of moderate depression as did imipramine (Tofranil, Janimine), but no better than *Hypericum*. CAUTION: Half the brands tested by Consumer Reports failed one or more tests. Only Natrol,

Nature Made, TwinLab, and GNC passed all tests. (Cost of a daily dose — four 400 mg capsules — ranges from $8-$13.)

Step 5b. Use drugs . . .

• Depression can be a side effect of estrogen/progestin therapy (HRT) as well as estrogen therapy (ERT). It is wise to avoid hormonal replacements if you already feel depressed during your menopausal years. Two studies assessing the effectiveness of ERT on menopausal depression found ERT ineffective in improving women's mental states, but strongly associated with an increase in suicide attempts.

• Antidepressant drugs are used frequently to relieve (control) menopausal women's feelings. But adverse reactions to antidepressant drugs are quite frequent in women (much more so than in men). CAUTION: Fatal interactions can occur if you take Prozac (fluoxetine) with any of these: lithium, tricyclic antidepressants (Tofranil/imipramine, Elavil/amitriptyline, Norpramin/desipramine) or monoamine oxidase inhibitors (Nardil/phenelzine, Parnate/tranylcypromine).

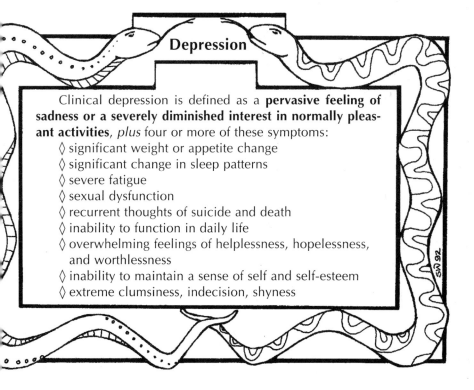

Depression

Clinical depression is defined as a **pervasive feeling of sadness or a severely diminished interest in normally pleasant activities**, *plus* four or more of these symptoms:
◊ significant weight or appetite change
◊ significant change in sleep patterns
◊ severe fatigue
◊ sexual dysfunction
◊ recurrent thoughts of suicide and death
◊ inability to function in daily life
◊ overwhelming feelings of helplessness, hopelessness, and worthlessness
◊ inability to maintain a sense of self and self-esteem
◊ extreme clumsiness, indecision, shyness

Thoughts of Suicide

Like uncontrollable emotions, thoughts of suicide are normal for menopausal women. Remember that the death phase of menopausal initiation does not imply actual physical death. Yet it would be foolish to deny that the feeling of dying can be as real emotionally as if it were actually happening.

There is a physical/emotional logic to thoughts of suicide. These rightly disturbing thoughts can show the menopausal woman the next steps on her journey. Real suicide is an act of desperate self-empowerment. But thoughts of suicide can be pathways to wholeness, health, and self-realization. Like depression, suicidal thoughts during menopause are potent guides to truth and joy.

Explore the logic of your suicide thought. What is its gift? How can you receive it without harming yourself? Suppose you want to take a flying leap. Jumping off a high place gives an intense experience of falling, flying, being free of restraint, unsupported, giving in to gravity. What other means are available to achieve these feelings? The answer may be as simple as learning to stand on your head, or as complex as doing something you've never done, never thought you could do: something exciting, terrifying, such as going on vacation totally on your own, alone, taking flying lessons, learning to ski, or trekking in the Himalayas.

If you feel like taking a gun to your head, you may need to learn to open the crown chakra. If you'd like to end it all by taking pills and passing out, you may need to admit to your exhaustion and take a rest. If you were to cut your wrists (cut off your hands, symbolically), what would you no longer have to handle?

If you feel compelled to actually hurt yourself, do call the local crisis hot line in the front of your phone book. As with any decision about health, a wise woman seeks a second opinion.

"When a woman wakes up suddenly in the middle of the night feeling suicidal, estrogen-enhancing herbs such as sage or black cohosh offer relief. It's important to let women know this is common and other women experience it."
— Holly Eagle

• Women taking lithium say they have gradually switched over to skullcap (*Scutellaria lateriflora*) with similar results. A dose of infusion is one cup/250 ml or more per day; of fresh plant tincture is 5-8 drops twice a day; of the dried plant tincture is a dropperful/1 ml several times a day.

Step 6. Break and enter . . .

• Electro-convulsive treatments (ECT), previously known as shock treatments, have been updated for the new century with special care taken to minimize harm to the recipients. ECT has been effective for women whose depression resists all other therapies.

• Medicine is not so quick these days to take menopausal women from their homes and lock them up. Now women are locked away in their own minds and not allowed to come out until they can think "straight." The crazy Crone breaks all the rules; she jimmies all the locks.

Rage

With a great grin, Grandmother Growth winks and confides: "The self-initiated Crone is an outrageous hag. In order to be outrageous, you must contact and own your rage. Focused anger is the same energy as the uterine contractions of birth and menstruation: it pushes; it is hard. Give your anger a sturdy obstacle to push against; let it move outward. Anger focused outward with Crone wisdom has changed, and will continue to change, the courses of nations. Beware of hiding your anger, of focusing it inward; this brings resentment, spite, sulkiness, depression, death of the community, and fantasies of self-destruction."

Step 1. Collect information . . .

Anger makes your heart pound, your palms sweat, and your blood pressure rise, for a short time if you express it, for a long time if you don't. Anger doesn't cause disease. Repressing it does, especially in women.

Menopausal women are described as irrational, ill-tempered, out of control, and insane when we speak the angry truth about our individual and collective lives in women-hating societies. To maintain the current social order, the rage of mature women must be disparaged and silenced. Unheard, unseen, unable to create the **Change** we envision, we turn our rage inward, we internalize social hatred toward women and naturally think of suicide. Why not, instead, be mad enough to live?

Step 2. Engage the energy . . .

★ *Cherry plum* is the **Bach flower remedy** for menopausal women about to do something desperate. Use it when you're afraid your anger is almost out of control, when you're on the verge of mental collapse, or when you're obsessed with thoughts of doing terrible things. The dose is 1-4 drops, under the tongue, frequently, while considering: Is there some way to achieve my vision other than this desperate action? "I want to kill my mate. Then I would be alone. Hmmmm . . . How about a vacation? Alone!" If you don't have *cherry plum* put some water in a special glass and use that as your remedy.

• Homeopathic *Lachesis* is suggested for the menopausal woman whose rage is evidenced by outbursts of irrational jealousy.

• Read *The Dance of Anger* (Harriett Lerner). Read *Kali: The Feminine Force* (Ajit Mookerjee). (See "References and Resources," page 127.)

• Do the Kundalini Meditation (page 88).

Step 3. Nourish and tonify . . .

• Try the "**NO!**" remedy on page 190.

• **Twist** a towel and growl; you can bite it, too. GGGRRRR . . .

• **Hit** a hard object (like a wooden chair) with a rolled up newspaper or use Elisabeth Kübler-Ross's favorite, a length of rubber radiator hose and a big city phone directory or two. Start with inarticulate sounds. Gradually add short, simple phrases such as "No!" or "I'm furious!" IMPORTANT: Stay in the present and prevent dizziness while doing this by keeping your eyes open and focused. Pick a point on the floor or wall and concentrate on it, stare at it. Let the fire in your eyes come through. See if you can burn a hole in the wall with your gaze.

• Take time to be gentle with yourself after feeling rage, especially if rage is a new ally for you. Go for a walk, rearrange the bookshelf, listen to music, draw, eat chocolate.

Step 4. Stimulate/Sedate . . .

★ With thanks to my teacher Gay Luce, I offer you the **temper tantrum** in a small space, for those times when you must have a raging fit but it just won't do to have it in public. To start, find a toilet stall, closet, or other small private space; you will need a little room to move. Then disorient yourself by shaking everything energetically: arms, legs, lips, eyes, fingers, head, toes, shoulders, all at once and without rhythm. Continue for at least a minute. Then inhale massively and hold your breath while you stamp you feet and strike out with your hands. You can sit on the toilet and kick with your feet, instead of stamping. If you can make some noise, let a sound come out when you finally stop and exhale. If I really put energy into the disorientation, one tantrum is usually enough; you may need to do it 2 or 3 times at first. And one more hint: practice this before you really need to use it.

• The color **pink** relaxes muscles in seconds. Pink rooms are currently used quite successfully in prisons to calm hostile, aggressive inmates.

Step 5b. Use drugs . . .

• **Tranquilizers** end that terrible feeling of wanting to destroy everything. So does alcohol. But it only *seems* easier to drown sorrow than to be angry. The Crone's rage keeps her community alive with conscience, truth, and beauty.

Step 6. Break and enter . . .

• Go ahead and break something. The sound of shattering glass sings the truth of rage. Go to your local recycling center and see if you can safely break glass there. One friend has a special set of dishes and a special (safe) place to break them when she's "uncontrollably enraged."

Grief/Crying Jags

"Gone are the days when you wept uncontrollably one day and found yourself bleeding the next. Now you cry and there's no blood the next day. So you cry; and cry. Love your tears, Crone-to-be," croons Grandmother Growth. "Feel the grief of life, the grief of death. Let these tears flood your heart with compassion.

"Grieve all that is lost to you, dear one. Grieve all potential that never thrived. Grieve the beauty extinguished too soon. Grieve the wounds of all women, all souls.

"Grief is an important part of your self-initiation as Crone, great granddaughter. As a menopausal woman you are watching the death of yourself as fertile Mother-woman. So it is fair to cry, to weep, and to grieve. Come, cry here on my shoulder."

Step 0. Do nothing . . .

• When the grief is deep and mourning is fully engaged, sobbing will sound hysterical (that is, as though coming from the womb/belly). This will stop when exhaustion sets in, rarely before. Go to bed. Be patient. Love yourself.

Step 1. Collect information . . .

Denied and restricted, grief contracts the muscles, especially those of the throat and chest. Allowed, grief can throb through your body and soul in deep, loose, primal sobs; then tenderly and eagerly push you, birth you, into vital and vibrant new life.

Step 2. Engage the energy . . .

★ Grief historian Marie Summerwood says: "In traditional cultures grief is considered sacred, a vital aspect of wholeness and health. It is the women who wail and lament and **sing the songs** of death and dying."

• Grief likes to cling, so hold on; hold on to something soft and plush. And if it is a small pillow stuffed with **hops** (soothing) or **lavender** (sweetening) or **sage** (transforming), all the better.

• What rituals of mourning have you participated in? What rituals of mourning have you read about? **Create a ritual of mourning** for yourself, just exactly as you would like it.

Step 3. Nourish and tonify . . .

★ **Motherwort**, tincture of the fresh plant in flower, 10-15 drops, 2-3 times a day for several weeks, mellows the sharpness of grief.

★ **Passion flower** (*Passiflora*) relieves hysteria. (Hysteria, by the way, refers to feelings from the womb, which is *hystera* in Greek.) Try it if your crying brings on a headache or leaves you twitchy and restless. A dose of the tincture of the fresh plant in flower is 10-25 drops as needed.

• **Lemon balm** (*Melissa*) is a soothing friend to a crying woman. Brew a tea of the fresh leaves and drink freely, seasoning with honey.

★ **Hawthorn berry** (*Crataegus*) tincture (or a tea of the flowers) helps the heart heal from deep grief. A dose is 20-30 drops, as needed.

Step 4. Stimulate/Sedate . . .

• **Hops** tea offers lots of B vitamins (depleted when you cry or sweat), a calming touch, and phytoestrogens to ease your **Change**. Over-indulgence may put you to sleep—and that may be just what you need.

★ When sobbing continues for days, muscles can get very sore. **St. Joan's wort** to the rescue. A dose of 25 drops/1 ml of the tincture (not capsules), taken up to 6 times a day, helps eliminate lactic acid build-up in the muscles, deepens sleep, eases depression, and strengthens the nerves.

Step 5a. Use supplements . . .

★ Large doses of B vitamin complex for several days can dramatically improve your ability to handle the stress of grief.

Step 5b. Use drugs . . .

• Tranquilizers, again? See pages 119.

Anxiety/Fear/Extreme Nervousness

"Have you noticed?" whispers Grandmother Growth. "Your hot flashes and menstrual irregularities disrupt your normal patterns, make openings for your buried fears to emerge. Welcome these fears; they bring memories. Memories of childhood, memories of other lives. Often these memories find easiest access to your consciousness through fear. If you reject your fear, it will immobilize you, shorten your breath, leave you speechless, and dim your full delight in life. Approach with curiosity; let your fear bring you gifts of self-awareness. (Note how dilated the pupils become in fear. Anxious eyes take in everything.) Hold my hand. Say 'I'm afraid.' And take a step forward."

Step 1. Collect information . . .

Adrenaline, made by the adrenal glands, is the "fight or flight" hormone. During menopause, when the adrenals take on the extra task of contributing estrogen/estrone to the hormonal dance, they can easily become depleted. Depleted adrenals often over-react, giving rise to sudden sensations of anxiety, fear, and nervousness. For example, the need to make a minor decision can cause a surge of adrenaline, triggering a hot flash and leaving you feeling mentally blank, physically wiped out, anxious, and fearful. Use these Wise Woman ways to ease the tension.

Step 2. Engage the energy . . .

★ Try these Bach flower remedies, 1-4 drops at a time, as needed:
  ☞ *Aspen*: fear of the unknown, apprehension, and anxiety.
  ☞ *Mimulus*: fear of the known.
  ☞ *Red Chestnut*: anxious and fearful for others' safety.
  ☞ *Elm*: overwhelmed and inadequate.
  ☞ *Rock Rose*: renowned for easing terror and panic.

★ Even one session of **massage** can cause a marked decrease in anxiety and fearfulness. Fear and anxiety give rise to hard, contracted muscles and shallow breathing. To unfreeze yourself, curl up in a fetal position (on your side with knees drawn up), breathe deeply, and hum. It's fine to rock back and forth. What feeling wants to emerge? Grief is soft, but still contracted. Rage is hard and will make you uncurl.

• If you are overcome with unfocused anxiety, **focus** your eyes. Look at anything, steadily, concentratedly, and breathe deeply. Feel a warmth in your upper abdomen; breathe, focus.

★ With the assistance of a friend, use **gentle touch** to restore your sense of calm. Lie on your stomach. Have your friend rest their right hand on your sacrum, fingers touching and pointing toward your head; their left hand is at your neck, fingers together and pointed toward the head. In silence let the hands rest comfortably for 1-5 minutes.

• Allow your fear to speak (in a safe space, with or without help). Pay close attention to what it says. **Become friends with your fear**. Care for it.

• Aromatherapists use **rose** to ease anxiety and fear. Put the essential oil on the seam of your sleeve and wrap yourself in its calming scent.

★ **Claim your boundaries**. Anxiety arises when we feel unsafe. Where can you be safe? Who supports you in the full expression of your self/selves? Identify and create the physical, psychic, emotional boundaries and rules you need in order to feel really safe.

• If your anxiety/nervousness is specifically focused, take all your worrying energy and use it to create a huge **image of safety** (like a cowrie shell, Buddha's or Christ's palm, a giant mother's lap, pink light). Surround the object of your anxiety with this image as often as necessary. Fear locks up movement and speech; a clear visualization can unfreeze you.

Step 3. Nourish and tonify . . .

• How about a class in **self-defense**? There really are things to be afraid of; best to know how to deal with them.

★ Sister stinging **nettle** is the remedy of choice to nourish the adrenals and relieve anxiety. Brew a rich infusion and drink freely.

• When the worries go 'round and 'round in your brain, **talk** to someone who will listen in silence. No matter how stupid or silly your fears seem, express them out loud with a witness.

• **Nourish your fear. Fear and desire are not opposites; they're the same.** When I don't want to admit to myself what I want, I turn my desire into a fear so I can hold it close and keep it at a distance at the same time. What would your life be like if your fears came true?

• **Yoga** postures, yoga breathing, and quiet, focused meditation tonify (and soothe) the sympathetic nervous system. Regular practice alleviates anxiety, often permanently.

• I use a dropperful (or two) of **St. Joan's wort** (*Hypericum*) tincture when I'm on the edge and feel like anything will push me over it. The dose can be repeated safely several times an hour if needed. This nerve-nourishing and nerve-strengthening herb relieves the immediate anxiety and helps prevent future distress as well.

Step 4. Sedate/Stimulate . . .

• Fear wants to pull in, contract; let the muscles relax in a **hot tub** or **sauna**. Ahhhh. . . . Or try a **lemon balm** or **oatstraw bath**; both are ancient remedies for bad cases of the "nerves."

★ **Exercise** of any kind is often a ready remedy for overwhelming anxiety. Movement and fear don't coexist easily. If you feel like running away from it all, running might be the very thing to do. Fifteen to twenty minutes of heart-pounding exercise will use up your excess adrenaline and "eat up" your stress.

★ If you feel so anxious you think you might burst and do crazy things, try the **lion pose**. Open your mouth very wide; even wider! Stick your tongue out; even further. Open your eyes really wide; bigger. Rotate eyes left, then right. Breathe deeply and exhale audibly, expelling breath through mouth. Relax. Do this up to ten times. Keep the shoulders and the forehead relaxed. This pose unblocks the throat, releases facial tension, relaxes the breathing muscles, and relieves anxiety.

• Extreme fear or anxiety may lead to hyperventilation. If you are breathing rapidly and shallowly and feel spaced out you can 1) breathe into a paper bag until normal breathing resumes or 2) hold your breath (you can actually put your hand over your nose and mouth) for a count of 20; then breathe out as slowly as you can.

• Reach for **skullcap** or **motherwort**, 10-20 drops of fresh plant tincture (1-2 dropperfuls of dried plant tincture), to calm your thoughts.

• **Valerian** is the herbal tranquilizer. Try tiny five-drop doses of the fresh root tincture, but repeat every 10-15 minutes until you are calm. Use for no more than three weeks at a time to avoid addiction.

Step 5a. Use supplements . . .

★ Calcium supplements, up to 1500 mg a day, help relieve anxiety. (See page 30.)

Step 5b. Use drugs . . .

★ **Tranquilizers**, more commonly prescribed for menopausal women than estrogen, are dangerous.

☞ Prescription tranquilizers are addictive. Sudden withdrawal causes severe symptoms, including seizures. Slower withdrawal causes the very distresses the tranquilizer was supposed to relieve: anxiety, restlessness, sleep disturbance, headaches, shaking, visual disturbances, and a generally "yucky" feeling.

☞ The majority of women taking tranquilizers feel drowsy all day. Many also have side effects such as dizziness, decreased coordination, slowed reaction times, inability to concentrate or read a book, and decreased mental functioning, including memory loss, learning blocks, and confusion. One MD states: "Three-quarters of my patients on Librium or Valium have impaired intellectual functions."

☞ The risk of breaking a bone is five times greater among those taking tranquilizers; and the effect continues for three or more months after taking the last one. Most people on tranquilizers don't realize how shaky on their feet and slow to react they've become.

★ If a chemical tranquilizer/sleeping pill is chosen, the advice of Sidney Wolfe, MD, is to use 7.5 milligrams (1/2 of a tablet) of oxazepam (Serax) for no more than seven days. Have the doctor write NO REFILL on the scrip. Do not drink any alcohol. Do try at least one remedy from Step 2 and one from Step 3 at the same time.

Step 6. Break and enter . . .

★ Suicide has been linked to regular use of tranquilizers, as have nightmares, sleep disturbances, and depression.

★ In an ironic twist, some women seem to discover their rage when dosed with tranquilizers.

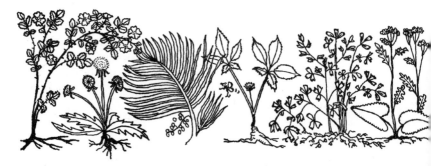

Oversensitivity/Irritability

"If you would be Crone, dear woman, you will be as sensitive as I am," says Grandmother Growth from the shadows. *"My skin is sensitive; I feel the tiniest crinkle in my bed. My ears are sensitive; I seem to hear and understand the conversations of all life. My eyes are sensitive; I see exceptionally well at night. My nose and mouth are sensitive; I can find water by smelling, identify the uses of a plant by tasting. My emotional body is sensitive; I feel untruths as physical discomfort.*

"Do not think of this sensitivity as a problem, a disability. Experience it as expansion, not limitation. Sensitivity isn't easy to live with; like nature, it doesn't tolerate sloppiness. In your civilized world, sensitivity may be a detriment, but in the natural world, sensitivity keeps you alive.

"Let us honor the heightened sensitivities of the Crones. Our communities depend on the Crones' irritability for their very survival. In their sensitivity, the Crones are irritated first by that which has the ability to poison all of us, whether it is a food, a feeling, or a rule."

Step 0. Do nothing . . .

• Is your oversensitivity a way to create some space around yourself? Is this Grandmother Growth's way of reminding you to take some time alone? It is OK to be antisocial. Dance by yourself. Stay home and read: *Reinventing Eve* (Kim Chernin) or *Circle of Stones* (Judith Duerk).

Step 1. Collect information . . .

PMS-like emotional sensitivity is aggravated during the menopausal years by sleepless nights, embarrassing hot flashes, and short-term memory loss. Nourishing the adrenals offers smoother emotional responses. Nourishing the nerves allows more energy to move with less friction. Nourishing the self-image encourages the emergence of the wise Crone.

Step 2. Engage the energy . . .

★ The Bach flower remedy *Walnut* offers protection from outside influences. Use it as a buffer during the height of your menopausal sensitivity and as a guide when you encounter (or call up) symbolic death states. A whole walnut in the shell carried with you also works.

• The Bach flower remedy *Impatiens* helps when you feel irritable and impatient. Buy it or make a similar remedy by floating the flowers from cultivated Impatiens or wild jewel weed (*Impatiens capensis*) in a bowl of spring or rain water for several hours in the sun. Add vodka to your remedy to preserve it. A dose is 1-4 drops as desired.

Step 3. Nourish and tonify . . .

★ **Oatstraw** gives the emerging crone amazing endurance and eases irritability by soothing nerves. Drink infusion freely. (The Bach flower *Wild oat* is for those seeking the true goal of their life.)

★ **Yoga** — not just the postures, but the breathing and focusing exercises as well — helps create strength in the nerves, adrenals, and heart, making sensitivity and irritability an ally rather than a liability.

• Traditional healers of India and Asia say oversensitivity is connected to the **liver**. What's your local liver-loving weed? Dandelion, yellow dock, thistle? Find out. Make friends; invite her to dinner — often.

Step 4. Stimulate/Sedate . . .

★ Treat yourself to a full-body **massage**. It will relax your muscles so you can be at ease with your heightened sensitivity, and it may awaken deadened places in your emotional body, as well.

★ **Skullcap** tincture strengthens the nerves and eases oversensitivity. I take 4-8 drops in water in the morning if I want to be a little "tougher" emotionally; I take the same at night if I need to sleep deeply.

• Television, alcohol, and drugs are common ways of numbing sensitivities. Substitute volunteer work, gardening, and exercise; they keep you just as occupied in the short run and improve health in the long run.

★ If you suddenly stop drinking coffee, you may feel hypersensitive. Lots of **water** (a glass every hour) helps calm the sensory overload.

Step 5a. Use supplements . . .

★ Calcium supplements, 250-500 mg a day, help calm the most jangled nerves. So does a cup of warm milk. Ahhhh. . . .

Step 5b. Use drugs . . .

• Tranquilizers are frequently prescribed for menopausal women who are too "uppity." See pages 119.

Step 6. Break and enter . . .

★ Being **buried** for 8-24 hours in sand or earth (with face exposed) and left alone is a dramatic way to transform your feelings of extreme sensitivity. I have found this "primitive psychotherapy" — which involves a real, yet symbolic, statement of the underlying desire ("I don't want to feel anything") — to be incredibly effective in helping the individual integrate and contact a rich wholeness/healthiness.

Emotional Uproar
References & Resources

American Dance Therapy Association, 2000 Century Plaza, Suite 108, Columbia, MD 21044 (410-997-4040)

American Environmental Products, 625 Mathews St., Fort Collins, CO 80524 (800-339-9572) • 10,000 lux light fixtures

Association for Women in Psychology, Ellyn Kaschak, Dept. of Psychology, San Jose State, CA 95192 • List of feminist therapists

Bailey, Linda. *How to Get Going When You Can Barely Get Out of Bed.* Prentice Hall, 1984 • Practical advice and exercises

Burn, DD. *Feeling Good: The New Mood Therapy.* NAL, 1990

Chernin, Kim. *Reinventing Eve.* Harper, 1994

Depression: What Can Be Done? Health Facts, Vol. XV, #128, Jan. 1990

Drinker, Sophie. *Music and Women.* Zenger, 1977

Duerk, Judith. *Circle of Stones: Woman's Journey to Herself.* Lura Media, 1989

Feminist Therapy Institute, Polly Taylor. 128 Moffitt St., San Francisco, CA 94131 (415-586-9061)

Haldane, Sean. *Emotional First Aid.* Station Hill, 1989

How Anger Affects Your Health. University of California at Berkeley Wellness Letter, Jan. 1992

Lerner, Harriett. *Dance of Anger: A Woman's Guide,* Harper & Row, 1990

Levine, Stephen. *Healing Into Life and Death.* Anchor/Doubleday, 1987

Lewisohn, P. *Control Your Depression.* Prentice Hall, 1991

Mookerjee, Ajit. *Kali: The Feminine Force.* Destiny, 1988

Option Institute, 2080 S. Undermountain Rd., Sheffield, MA 01257 (413-229-2100) • Feeling workshops

Pierrakos, Eva. *Pathwork of Self Transformation.* Bantam, 1990 • Highly recommended

Rosetta Reitz, 115 W. 16th St., Apt. 267, NY, NY 10011 • Women's jazz

Sewell, Marilyn (editor). *Cries of the Spirit: A Celebration of Women's Spirituality.* Beacon, 1991

Stone, Thomas A. *Cure by Crying.* Cure by Crying, Inc., 1995

Taylor, Cathryn. *Inner Child Workbook.* Tarcher, 1991

Wise Woman Center, PO Box 64, Woodstock, NY 12498 • Workshops exploring grief, anger, spirit healing, more

Zweig, Connie & J. Abrams, (eds.). *Meeting the Shadow: The Hidden Power of the Dark Side of Human Nature.* Tarcher, 1991

Sleep Disturbances

"Do you know the way to your dream time?" The voice of Grandmother Growth comes inside your ear, just as you thought you were falling asleep. "When you claim the transformation of menopause, you can enter dream time any time. When you hold your wise blood inside, dreams comes at your bidding. So does sleep.

"But not just yet. Not until after you've journeyed with me into seeming chaos, into the sleepless, timeless, visionary place of the Crone. Much that has bound you, young Crone, will unravel in the nights to come. Your wisdom is waking. And so will you.

"You won't sleep well during the short part of your menopause when you may be swept by waves of volcanic heat, shiver through arctic chills, have sweat rivering through your bedclothes, and feel powerful surges of emotion. There may be times when your mind and hormones and memories make a crazy quilt of your dreams and days. Surely you wouldn't expect to sleep peacefully through that.

"Inspiration may shake you awake before dawn. Be ready to receive the gifts of this Change, whether awake or asleep. Be ready; what you thought were walls are veils," comes her voice, like the breeze, soft.

Step 0. Do nothing . . .

• Relieve yourself of all responsibility for even a day or two (better a week or two) so you can be free to sleep whenever the mood strikes.

• Free yourself from the rule of time so you can catnap and tap into your creativity at any hour of the day or night. Put away all clocks and watches for a few days. Don't listen to the radio or ask for the time. Let the earth and moon and sun provide your timing.

Step 1. Collect information . . .

Sleep disturbances are a short-lived, but recurring, part of menopausal **Change**. Most menopausal women are so exhausted they can fall asleep with their clothes on, but wake after a few hours. A few menopausal women wake so frequently, for so many nights, that they acquire the dazed look of a new mother of twins. Some catch up with a nap later. Others stay tense all night and are achy and irritated all day.

"I was 40; my tubal ligation accidentally fried my ovaries. I'd go to sleep and wake up in a terrible sweat. I'd throw the covers off and open the window and go back to sleep. In 15 minutes I was frozen, awake again, covering up, dropping off to sleep, only to awaken 20 minutes later in a terrible sweat. I'd throw the covers off and open the window and go back to sleep. In 15 minutes I was frozen, awake again, and again, and again all night."

Step 2. Engage the energy . . .

• Create a **bedtime routine**: Go to bed at the same time each night, read or listen to taped music for thirty minutes, then turn out the light. If not asleep in thirty minutes, read or listen to more music for another half hour. Turn out the lights again. (This is behavior modification; see Step 5.)

★ **Keep a journal** by your bed. Creative juices flow wildly during menopause; if you're up when they are, grab 'em.

★ **Lavender blossoms** and their essential oil are crone classics; didn't your granny smell of lavender (at least in your imagination)? The strong but agreeable odor brings sleep at night, relieves dizziness and faintness during the day. Sleep with a little pillow of lavender blossoms; slip it into your pocket when you dress. Or use a few drops of the essential oil on a handkerchief tucked into your pillow or purse. A lavender bath before bed (use a handful of dried flowers or a few drops of oil) eases the mind and body, and evokes soothing dreams.

★ No matter how little sleep you get, you can feel energetic and refreshed if you **relax** deeply and completely instead of struggling to sleep. Visualizing or fantasizing is an ideal way to relax, often leading to sleep. (If other thoughts intrude, just return to your fantasy.) My favorite relaxation is on the next page.

Step 3. Nourish and tonify . . .

★ Let **oatstraw** strengthen your nervous system, smooth your energy flow, and give you more restful sleep. Her cooling nourishing ways ease night sweats, anxiety, and headaches. Oatstraw is renowned for her antidepressant effect. Try a cup of infusion before bed, warm, with milk. Ahhhh. And another at breakfast. Ummmm. Or try sleeping on an oat hull pillow. You can't overdose on bone-strengthening, gland-nourishing oatstraw; drink freely.

• **Hops** tea is a powerful sleep inducer and wonderful hormonal ally to the woman awakened frequently by night sweats. Keep a cup on the night stand to slip you back to sleep. A small pillow of dried hops blossoms under your head also helps entice sleep into your bed.

★ **Nettle**, astonishing nourisher of the energy circuits and the adrenals, isn't usually considered a sleep inducer. But it might be if your adrenals are waking you up. They work hard during your menopausal years and can become over-reactive. If a small noise triggers an adrenaline rush, you awaken, heart pounding, anxious. Then, you have to urinate — a sure sign of an adrenaline-mediated flash. Every time you go through this cycle, the adrenals are stressed a little more, making it ever more likely that your sleep will be disturbed. Remedy? Nourish the adrenals. Ally? Stinging nettle infusion, one cup at least, four times a week.

• Try **ear plugs** (the little foam cylinder ones are inexpensive and highly effective). Soon you'll sleep, sleep, sleep.

• Nerve-nourishing **St. Joan's wort** (*Hypericum*) tincture is also a gentle beckoner of sleep. Use a dropperful in a cup of fresh hops or lemon balm tea for a double dose of slumber.

Susun's Favorite Relaxation

I am peacefully and happily lolling on a sandy beach listening to the waves. The wind and the sun and the shade touch me in just the right proportions.

The sound of the waves gets gradually louder as the tide comes in. The flowing waves lap over my toes and then recede. Slowly. I smell the tang of the brine as the waves cover my ankles, then pull down to my toes. Slowly, caressingly, the waves rise up to my knees, slide down my calves.

I hear and feel the waves as they reach up to my mid-thighs and pull back down to behind my knees. The waves rise and fall rhythmically; up to my hips, down my thighs. Content, at ease, I settle deeper into the sand as the warm water curls up and around me and pulls the sand away from underneath my back and buttocks.

The waves continue to spread over me, then pull away. The water covers my hips, my fingertips, my waist, my lower arms, my breasts, my shoulders.

I feel safe and secure as the moving water rocks me. I let the water come as high as I like. Sometimes it covers my face as I breathe out and slips away just before I breathe in. Sometimes I float. (Actually, I usually fall asleep before the water gets past my knees.)

Step 4. Sedate/Stimulate . . .

★ Delicious, aromatic **skullcap** tincture is my favorite pain-killer and sleep-inducer when made from the fresh flowering plant. (Dried plant tinctures are less effective; use 30-60 drops as a dose.) *Scutellaria lateriflora* even brings sleep to those addicted to sleeping pills. Though powerful, skullcap rarely leaves a muggy feeling next morning. Long-term use is not addictive, but rarely needed. I use 3-8 drops in water ten minutes or so before lights out. And another dose just as I lie down. (And once again in ten minutes if need be.)

★ **Passion flower** herb, Passionskraut, Passiflore (*Passiflora incarnata*) is an old wives' remedy for women with nervous insomnia, hysteria, restlessness, and headaches. With its unique, purple-crowned flowers, it visually says "crone." A dose of 15-60 drops of the fresh flowering plant tincture before bed each evening can relieve ongoing sleeplessness. (Passion fruits are a rich source of estrogenic bioflavonoids.)

• Tincture of the fresh root of **valerian**, Baldrian, Valériane (*Valeriana officinalis*) is a powerful plant sedative. It is a special ally for menopausal women desperate for a night's sleep. Valerian also helps resolve chronic headaches (even migraines), decrease anxiety, and reduce fatigue. A dose is 20-30 drops just before bed, repeated in thirty minutes if needed. CAUTION: Valerian can be as habit-forming as some drugs if used nightly. Some people are stimulated by valerian.

• Coffee, black tea, or alcohol contribute to night sweats and unrestful, agitated sleep. For some menopausal women, these stimulants prevent sleep altogether and trigger intense hot flashes.

Step 5a. Use supplements . . .

• A bedtime dose of 500 mg **calcium** can bring a sound night's sleep.

• CAUTION: Amino acids in pill form are synthetic drugs, not natural substances. Yes, L-tryptophan helps induce sleep, but it is different than the naturally occurring tryptophan found in foods.

Step 5b. Use drugs . . .

• *Sleep-inducing drugs are habit-forming.* The ones most commonly prescribed are benzodiazepines such as Valium, Xanax, Dalmane, Doral, Halcion, ProSom, and Restoril. Side effects of benzodiazepines include next-day memory loss, confusion, anxiety, and excitability. Considering their stressful effects on the nervous system, these drugs seem totally inappropriate for the sleep-deprived menopausal woman.

To avoid the worst side effects of these drugs, take them for no more than 2-3 weeks and at half the usual dose.

★ **Behavior modification** therapy has been shown to be four times more effective than drugs in reducing the time needed to fall asleep and in increasing the actual span of restful sleep. (See Step 2.)

"Sleep deprivation has been a very powerful tool for me in breaking down my control barriers and making way for the information that the universe wants me to have. In my opinion, sleep deprivation is more powerful than most psychoactive drugs."

Fatigue

"Fall into my arms and sleep," offers Grandmother Growth. "You don't have to make this change happen; it will happen on its own. Let me hold you. Let go. Don't resist. Rest. You are in the midst of the labor of giving birth to yourself as Crone. Of course you are tired. This is hard work.

"Let the pushing energy of your uterus move your energy up to your crown, rather than down and out, as with menstrual blood and babies. This birthing of your wholeness is something you'll retain, not something you'll birth and give away. Rest in my strong arms. Take courage."

Step 0. Do nothing . . .

• Extreme fatigue during menopause indicates a profound need to do nothing. Take a Crone's Time Away or at least arrange a short time-out.

• Give yourself a "well day" before you have to take a sick day. Ask family and friends to give you a day totally off . . . and take it! Barricade yourself in your room if need be (or, like the cartoon character Sylvia, in the bathroom).

Step 1. Collect information . . .

Internal processes occurring during menopause demand tremendous amounts of energy, leaving a deficit for your external life unless you provide yourself with very high quality nutrients (especially minerals and fats) and use your energy wisely.

Women whose menopause is induced generally experience more extreme fatigue than women who achieve menopause naturally. And women whose sleep is disrupted with frequent night sweats frequently feel worn out and tired all day. Even if you achieve menopause naturally and are resting well, you may have less energy for things outside yourself during the most intense part of your **Change**.

Step 2. Engage the energy . . .

• *Olive* is the Bach flower remedy for exhaustion.

• For every hour you work, take a 60-second break. Breathe deeply; stand up and stretch; change your view; drink some herbal infusion.

★ List ten good things about fatigue, laziness, lethargy, and procrastination. I've found laziness to be my best guide to efficiency; lethargy has stopped me from taking foolish risks; and procrastination helps me find more efficient ways to proceed. Love and honor your fatigue for helping you conserve energy and giving you the time to find creative *new ways to do the same old things.*

Step 3. Nourish and tonify . . .

• **Seaweeds** of all kinds help restore energy by nourishing nervous, immune, and hormonal systems. Make it a habit to eat some every day.

★ When you feel bone-tired, get grounded energy with **ginseng, black cohosh, yellow dock,** or **dandelion roots**. Use 5-10 drops of the tincture of any one of these with each meal for several weeks.

• **Stir** up your wise blood so it doesn't just sit there making you feel exhausted. Stand up, feet shoulder-width, knees relaxed. Swing your arms toward one side, then the other. Let the shoulders and hips move as you twist your upper body. The arms move freely. After a minute or two, stop. Rock the tail bone and pelvis forward and back, forward and back for at least a minute. Repeat several times a day.

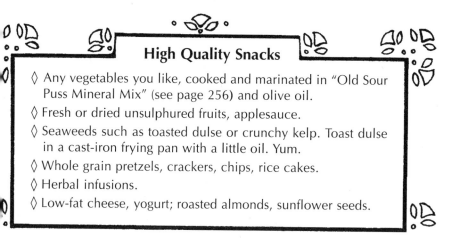

High Quality Snacks

◊ Any vegetables you like, cooked and marinated in "Old Sour Puss Mineral Mix" (see page 256) and olive oil.

◊ Fresh or dried unsulphured fruits, applesauce.

◊ Seaweeds such as toasted dulse or crunchy kelp. Toast dulse in a cast-iron frying pan with a little oil. Yum.

◊ Whole grain pretzels, crackers, chips, rice cakes.

◊ Herbal infusions.

◊ Low-fat cheese, yogurt; roasted almonds, sunflower seeds.

★ **Green** is the color of plant energy. The plants with the deepest green give you the most energy. A daily cup of **nettle** infusion increases energy without wiring your nerves.

• An evening cup of **oatstraw** infusion builds deep energy for the next day, especially when you have been riding an emotional roller coaster.

• **Eat more**. When you're too tired to eat, you get more tired. (If this sounds like an old wive's tale, remember that old wives were the wise women. But, actually, it's the latest scientific thinking.) In addition to at least one really good meal a day, eat high quality snacks hourly.

Step 4. Stimulate/Sedate . . .

★ Though it seems contrary, **St. Joan's wort** (*Hypericum*) tincture relaxes the nerves yet increases energy. Take 25-30 drops several times a day, including before bed. You'll sleep better, ache less, and wake up with more energy and a brighter outlook on life.

• Warming herbs such as **cayenne**, **ginger**, and **cinnamon** increase energy (but may increase hot flashes, too). Make a tea with 1 cup/250 ml boiling water and $1/2$ -1 teaspoon (1-2 grams) of the powder of any one of these.

• Does raw food make you tired? Traditional Chinese Medicine thinks so. Uncooked food and chilled foods, especially cold drinks, use up your internal energy to cook and warm the food. Use a stove instead.

• **Wheat grass** juice, **green barley** powder, **spirulina**, and **blue green algae** are stimulants, not nutritional supplements. I don't use any of them, as my diet supplies me with plenty of energy.

Step 5a. Use supplements . . .

• **Vitamin E**, up to 1,300 IU daily, and **vitamin B** complex, up to 50 mg daily, are suggested to remedy fatigue.

• Low levels of **potassium**, **iron**, and **iodine** contribute to fatigue. Supplemental levels as high as 6000 mg potassium, 100 mg iron, and 100 micrograms iodine have been recommended.

Step 5b. Use drugs . . .

• "Energy-producing" foods/drugs such as coffee and candy are not recommended for menopausal women.

• Pharmaceutical drugs that increase energy are not recommended either.

Headaches/Migraine

"Oh, how densely packed your head is, my sweet," sighs Grandmother Growth. "I'm afraid there's no room for new growth. If you could empty your mind, leave off worrying and planning for a while, and give in to the chaos and its random pleasures, just for a short time, I think you'd feel less pressure and your head would hurt less. The energy of your womb now circulates inside you and throbs in your head. Sit quietly; breathe out through the top of your head and imagine the breath falling gently down to earth. Rest your forehead against the earth. Place this cool stone on your third eye. Your Crone's Crowning comes closer. This is the work of your body; let your mind rest."

Step 0. Do nothing . . .

★ Follow your natural instinct: Lie in total silence, in complete darkness, and sleep, if possible, until the headache is gone.

★ Like fatigue, a headache, especially a migraine, is a way to get some **time alone**. Is finding time for yourself usually a headache?

Step 1. Collect information . . .

Menopause often brings relief to the woman who has had migraine headaches since adolescence. Other women experience headaches for the first time during menopause, usually the result of fatigue, stress, rapidly changing hormone levels racing through the liver, and rushes of kundalini moving into the crown area.

Menopausal headaches may also be triggered by sudden (and usually short-lived) allergies to certain foods.

Headaches and migraines are a common side effect of ERT/HRT.

Step 2. Engage the energy . . .

• Rub a drop of lavender or chamomile oil briskly between your hands. When palms are warm and tingly, place them on the part of your head that aches. (It's also wonderful to have someone do this for you.)

• If it's tolerable for someone to hold your head, try this: Sit in a chair or lie down. Lean your head back into your friend's hands and allow them to support your head in their palms (fingers pointing down, thumbs above the ears) for up to five minutes. Breathe fully.

★ Blinking **red lights** can relieve extreme or severe migraines, within an hour, 72 percent of the time. Wear goggles that restrict side vision for maximum effect.

★ Women with chronic migraines often benefit greatly from the help of a skilled feminist therapist.

Step 3. Nourish and tonify . . .

★ Tea, infusion, or tincture of **garden sage** leaves offers immediate relief from a headache and helps prevent future ones.

★ **Black cohosh** root tincture or a vinegar of fresh **willow leaves** will ease a headache with pain-killing methyl salicylate. Ten drops of the tincture or one teaspoon/15 ml of the vinegar is equivalent to two aspirin.

★ **Vervain** (*Verbena officinalis*) was a sacred herb in ancient matriarchal cultures. Menopausal women use the tincture of fresh vervain flowers, 20-40 drops in water, before bed and as needed, to strengthen the nerves, relieve insomnia, dispel depression, treat nervous exhaustion, and moderate headaches, including migraines. (Vervain was a favored plant for the Maiden's altar and the moon lodge, where she was used to promote the onset of the menstrual flow, ease cramps, reduce flooding, and quicken desire.)

• **Lady's mantle**, another ancient sacred plant, has many magical attributes, including an ability to aid women who are taking on or leaving the role of mother. What a wonderful friend for an emerging crone! Try 10-25 drops of the tincture of the fresh herb several times a day to relieve headaches.

• The beautiful spring **primrose** (*Primula veris*) offers relief from menopausal headaches if taken regularly. The golden carpet of Schlesselblume on Bavarian pastures and roadsides is one of my favorite memories of Germany. If you don't visit or live in Bavaria, you can grow and gather the blossoms of *Primula officinalis* instead; they're also a good source of pain-killing salicyn. Make a tea of the dried flowers and drink several cups a day for some months. CAUTION: Sip your first cup mindfully and slowly, as some folks are allergic to primrose. NOTE: The roots of most primroses contain oil-soluble estrogenic factors and cell-softening saponins, suggesting use as an ointment for tender, dry vaginal tissue.

• Connections between foods and headaches are sketchy. There is little evidence that plants indigenous to the Americas, such as chocolate and nightshades (tomatoes, potatoes, eggplant, peppers, tobacco) contribute to headaches. I do suspect that chemicals in processed foods (such as aspartame, MSG, and nitrates) and in some natural ones (aged cheeses, miso, red wine) can trigger headaches. With other foods, you're the best judge.

Step 4. Stimulate/Sedate . . .

• **Avoid alcohol**. It is a known headache trigger.

• **Keep cool.** Being hot, from hot baths, saunas, hot flashes, exertion, or air temperature, is the second most common headache trigger. Stay cool. Stay in the shade. And just say "no" to hot tubs.

• Sedate headache pain with tinctures of **skullcap**, 3-5 drops, and **St. Joan's wort**, 25-30 drops. I take them together, as frequently as needed, up to half a dozen times a day. Migraine sufferers take them as soon as the aura begins, before there is pain, and repeat every ten minutes for 3-6 doses.

• Anti-inflammatory, hormone-rich **wild yam** eases the aching heads of menopausal women. A dose of wild yam root tincture is 10-30 drops up to 6 times a day, or infused, 1-2 teacupsful a day. The lower dose, taken daily, relieves chronic headaches. In acute situations, use the higher dose.

• **Soak your feet** in cool water scented with a few drops of rosemary oil. Breathe deeply.

• Migraines are most frequent between 6 a.m. and noon. Take headache remedies before bed and on awakening to insure maximum effect.

• To banish simple headaches, soak a handful of fresh **lemon balm** (*Melissa*) leaves in a glass of wine for an hour and sip it, or drink a tea of dried leaves. If you want sleep as part of your headache cure, substitute catnip (*Nepeta cataria*) for the melissa.

• **Feverfew** (*Chrysanthemum parthenium*) is a much publicized remedy for migraine. It is most effective as a preventative measure: eat a sprig of the fresh plant daily. For acute headache, 2-4 fresh leaves or a cup of strong tea may help. CAUTION: May irritate mouth.

Step 5b. Use drugs . . .

• Painkillers are many women's first thought for a headache remedy. But habitual use increases the duration and frequency of headaches.

• Taking ERT/HRT? Ease off and see if your headaches ease up.

Step 6. Break and enter . . .

• Some women say their headaches are so bad that they want to blow their brains out. Perhaps menopausal headaches, like sleeplessness, are part of the physical "mind-altering" process of becoming a crone.

Heart Palpitations

"All of your energies are changing, dear one," affirms Grandmother Growth. "Your heart is changing. It is expanding into the broad heart of the self-initiated Crone, who honors excitement and thrills, as well as calm and subtlety. This part of the journey may make your heart pound.

"Do your heart palpitations bring up thrilling memories and quivering fears, which are also your secret desires?

"Listen to your heart. Let the energy of your uterus spiral strongly into your heart. Nourish your heart, young Crone, so she can beat strongly for many more years and carry you into very old age."

Step 1. Collect information . . .

Heart palpitations (a pounding, racing pulse of up to 200 beats a minute) may accompany flashes during menopausal years. Palpitations are not indicative of heart disease. They may be caused by electrolyte imbalances from fluid loss if you sweat frequently or heavily. They may also be triggered by strenuous exercise and strong emotions.

It is not surprising that menopausal **Change** affects the heart as well as the uterus, for they are very similar organs: both are smooth muscle tissue and both produce some hormones. The uterus is the strongest muscle in a woman's body; the heart, a man's strongest muscle.

Herbs that treat the uterus treat the heart as well. The healing color for the uterus is red; for the heart, green. Plants that strengthen heart/uterus are often green/red: for instance, hawthorn, rose, strawberry, raspberry, and motherwort.

NOTE: If you have a minor heart valve prolapse (10 percent of the population does), it may suddenly be noticeable at menopause, when the prolapse allows palpitations. Seek expert help if your palpitations leave you extremely breathless, very dizzy, or in great pain.

Step 2. Engage the energy . . .

★ **Rose** flower essence calms and steadies the heart.

★ Close your eyes. Put one hand on your heart, the other on your belly. Breathe slowly until your heartbeat is even and quiet.

Step 3. Nourish and tonify . . .

★ **Hawthorn** (*Crataegus*) is a slow-acting but very reliable heart tonic. (It also remedies insomnia.) Try berry tincture (25-40 drops, 2-4 times a day) but don't expect results for over a month.

★ Prevent palpitations by maintaining a good mineral balance. Drink lots of mineral-rich herbal infusions. Keep some by your bed to drink when you wake up in the night and first thing in the morning.

★ **Motherwort tincture**, 10-20 drops with meals and before bed, tones the heart and helps prevent palpitations. Try 25-50 drops for immediate relief when your heart is pounding crazily.

"My mother is astonished, and relieved, that motherwort dependably stops her irregular, wild heartbeats, a frightening experience for her. And there it is, growing right outside her bedroom window, planted by the Great Creator."

★ **Black Haw** (*Viburnum*) root bark exerts an antispasmodic effect on the heart and uterus and supplies phytosterols as well. It's all a menopausal woman with a racing heart could want. Sip the infusion frequently or try 25 drops of tincture. NOTE: Although black haw contains some blood-thinning coumarins, experience has shown it unlikely to promote flooding during menopause (or while giving birth).

Step 4. Stimulate/Sedate . . .

★ **Valerian** root tea by the mouthful, or tincture by the dropperful, promptly slows and eases racing hearts.

• **Ginger** root tea, hot or cold, warms, soothes, and calms the heart. It may, however, increase sweating and flooding.

• Try real **licorice** (the root, not the candy) when your heart starts to race. CAUTION: Prolonged use may elevate blood pressure, increase fluid retention, and upset bowels.

• Heavy smoking, large intake of caffeine, or regular use of alcohol increase the severity and incidence of palpitations.

Step 5a. Use supplements . . .

★ **Vitamin E** (200-400 IU daily) may remedy menopausal palpitations but increase cancer risk. (CAUTIONS: page 91.)

★ **Magnesium** glyconate relaxes the chest, heart, and lungs. Daily use of 500 mg helps prevent palpitations and deepens sleep.

Step 5b. Use drugs . . .

• Antihistamines (like Benadryl, Nyquil, Dimetapp) can cause palpitations.

Step 6. Break and enter . . .

• Invasive diagnostic tests are contraindicated for those with palpitations.

For Women Taking Hormones

"When you turn off the radio and the CD-player, can you hear me? When you turn away from the television and stare out the window do you see me? Do I live behind your eyelids? Am I in your dreams? Do you know me? Do you want me? Do you love me?" The words of Grandmother Growth are tinged with grief.

"I want to guide you through the mystery of menopause. But you cringe away. You look for ways to prevent your Change. You believe that staying young forever will make you happy forever. But, you are not happy now. You fear change, and there is wisdom in that, yet you are wise enough to know that Change will come, no matter how you resist it, and this kills your happiness.

"Only those who feel secure in their own bodies experience happiness. Controlling your hormones so they mimic fertility prevents the growth of your body's wisdom and the flowering of your power as a Wise Crone.

"Menopause is about Change, not about clinging to the past," says Grandmother Growth emphatically. "I love you. I want you. I see you."

Step 0. Do nothing . . .

• The National Women's Health Network advises women to resist pressure from doctors to accept a prescription for hormones and try alternative remedies first. **Take your time** and make up your own mind. Separate the claims from the realities of hormone replacement. Investigate the real risks.

• Taking hormones does not cure menopause, it only delays it.

Step 1. Collect information . . .

There was a time, in the 1960s, when most menopausal women took hormones. But today, at the beginning of the twenty-first century, a mere thirteen percent of women over the age of fifty do so. In 1998, more than half of the women who started on HRT quit within a year; two-thirds quit within two years. The promise of hormones has been hollow. It becomes ever more undeniable that a healthy diet and daily exercise go further toward preventing heart attacks and broken hips than hormone therapies.

Susan Love turned me on to the best reason for taking hormones: to have time to prepare for a Crone's Year Away. Whatever your reason, if you take hormones there are special things you can do to protect your health from the effects of those hormones. And there are special problems you may encounter if you take hormones. Most commonly: water retention (remedies: page 40), nausea, breast tenderness (p. 42), spotting (p. 19), migraines and headaches (p. 135); also, dizziness (p. 102), depression (p. 111), severe mood swings (p. 125), discoloration and wrinkling of facial skin, increased facial hair (p. 108), and loss of libido (liferoot, 155; ginseng, 169; oatstraw, 239; fenugreek, 71).

Step 2. Engage the energy . . .

• **Collect butterflies.** What's a butterfly? Any woman older than you, whom you want to grow up to be, who doesn't take hormones. Caterpillars who eat hormones rarely become butterflies, alas.

• Did you know your grandmothers? Your great-grandmothers? Whether they lived to ripe old ages or not, they didn't take hormones to get through menopause. Perhaps one of them will come to you (in your dreams?) and guide you through your **Change**.

Step 3. Nourish and tonify . . .

★ Drink at least a quart of **red clover infusion** every week. And eat more **lentils**. Both of these bean-family members fight cancer three ways. First: They contain large amounts of phytoestrogens which prevent cancer cells from utilizing the cancer-stimulating estrogens you take. Second: They contain a "repair kit" for damaged DNA, stopping cancer before it starts. Third: They improve the mineral balance in the body and strengthen the immune system.

• Nourishing herbal infusions, a whole foods diet, enough exercise, and yogurt — every day — will protect you from most of the detrimental effects of ERT/HRT.

• Protect against blood clots by using herbs with a mild blood-thinning effect, like red clover (others, page 213).

• Taking ERT increases your risk of losing your gallbladder. Protect yours (and your liver) with **milk thistle seed** or **dandelion root**. Try a dropperful/1 ml of tincture in the morning, or a glass of dandelion flower wine with supper.

"I've been taking HRT since I was 38. Every time I try to taper off, my symptoms — night sweats, mood swings, and bone aches — return rapidly. I'm 53 now."

Step 4. Stimulate/Sedate . . .

- Use of ERT/HRT for as little as five years can:
  - ☞ Double your risk of breast cancer
  - ☞ Double your risk of lung cancer
  - ☞ Double your risk of ovarian cancer
  - ☞ Increase your risk of gall bladder surgery
  - ☞ Increase your risk of endometrial cancer
  - ☞ Increase your risk of blood clots and stroke
  - ☞ Increase blood levels of sodium, which increases blood pressure

★ **Coming off hormones** is best done by reducing the dose. Some women use a pill cutter to make their daily dose smaller and smaller. Some take a whole pill but skip more and more days until they take none. Some cut their patches in half. (Check to see if the kind you use can be cut; some can't.) Be prepared to have menopausal symptoms — which may be worse than the ones you had before you took hormones.

Step 5a. Use supplements . . .

- Use of hormone supplements degrades your nutritional status by interfering with or depleting **folic acid**, **magnesium**, and vitamin **B₆**.

Step 5b. Use drugs . . .

- Wait a decade — or two — before you take hormones. Women who begin taking ERT/HRT in their 60s or 70s maintain bone density as well as women who begin during menopause.[47]

- There are now dozens of designer hormones available for women. Determining the right ones in the right dose is not easy. Go slow; start with the lowest possible dose; adjust, adjust. And read *Dr. Susan Love's Hormone Book.*

- Taking Hormones? Claims — and Realities:
  - ☞ Prevents fractures — if taken past the age of 80
  - ☞ Prevents bone loss — but doesn't increase bone mass
  - ☞ Prevents Alzheimer's — in retrospective studies only
  - ☞ Prevents heart disease — but increases mortality by increasing risk of stroke (see page 207)
  - ☞ Keeps you looking young — if pimples, blotchy patches, and easily sun-damaged skin is your idea of young.

- Hormone creams are billed as a "natural" alternative to ERT, and pushed by NDs and pharmacists. It's hard to resist something that's "uniquely crafted for you, adjusted to fit you exactly." Gynecologist Carol Shaak, MD, says she individualizes a combination of estradiol, progesterone, and testosterone to bring a woman's hormone levels to Day 17 of a (mythical) menstrual cycle.

While there are some benefits to using creams instead of pills — the dosage is more easily adjusted, and the load on the liver is lighter — Wise Women use neither. We trust our bodies, our good diets, and our green allies to provide us with all the hormones we need.

Step 6. Break and enter . . .

• Women who have their uterus (and breasts) and use hormones are advised to have an endometrial biopsy yearly to watch for endometrial cancer, and a yearly mammogram to watch for breast cancer.

"You are not a brain running a body by switching on hormones. Nor are you a body running a genome by switching on hormone receptors. Nor are you a genome running a brain by switching on genes that switch on hormones. You are all of these at once. . . ."
— Matt Ridley

Progesterone Creams

"Overblown claims for natural progesterone have been made by people with financial interests in the product."   — National Women's Health Network

Step 0. Do nothing . . .

★ Be at peace with your menopausal metamorphosis. Like puberty, like birth, menopause is a process not aided by hormonal manipulation. Extra progesterone is for pregnant women, not emerging crones.

• *Lancet* reported: twenty women who used 2-4 times the amount of ProGest suggested on the label absorbed virtually no progesterone.[48]

Step 1. Collect information . . .

★ Women who use progesterone creams are participating in one of the largest unsupervised trials of hormone use ever conducted. Is it safe?

• A chemical process "completely unrelated to biochemical process-es"[49] turns wild yam roots into natural progesterone. Dr. John Lee says: "In the laboratory diosgenin is chemically synthesized into real human progesterone."[50] Since when does "real," "natural" come out of a lab?

• Progesterone is for (pro) pregnancy (gestation). Postmenopausal women no longer get pregnant. Do they need progesterone?

• Progesterone promotes the rapid growth of cells, especially in the breasts. Can progesterone creams promote cancer?

Carolyn De Marco, MD, says low progesterone correlates with increased breast cancer.[51] But in mice, increasing both progesterone *and estradiol* slows breast cancer, while increasing progesterone alone spurs it.[52] At least two-thirds of the women in Dr. John Lee's ProGest trials used oral estrogen as well as progesterone cream.[53]

Since "natural" *progesterone* and "unnatural" *progestin* are both made from diosgenin, studies confuse them. Proponents of the creams claim only progestin has detrimental effects, not progesterone. I don't agree. Hormones are strong players with adverse as well as beneficial effects.[54]

Healthy menopausal women are sometimes low in progesterone (at certain times in their cycles). If this is you, go to Step 3.

Step 2. Engage the energy . . .

• Bless your belly. Rub it with olive oil infused with aromatic herbs.

Step 3. Nourish and tonify . . .

★ **Chasteberry** and wild yam are well known for increasing progesterone, only maybe they don't. Wild yam seems to nourish the hypothalamus, and chasteberry nourishes the pineal, thus improving health by increasing the responsiveness of the body's own feedback systems.

Step 4. Sedate/Stimulate . . .

• Progesterone creams sedate hot flashes four times better than a placebo.[55]

• Twenty percent of the women who used progesterone creams in studies spotted or bled erratically — a sign of increased uterine cancer risk.[56]

• Progesterone creams have not lived up to their promise of improving bone density. Most studies show no gain. In several studies, women using progesterone cream lost more bone than those using a placebo.[57] Only a few studies, with small numbers of women (all of whom no longer have their ovaries) show improvement in bone mass.

The women in Dr. Lee's study ate leafy greens daily, took vitamin D and calcium supplements, drank no sodas and little alcohol, smoked no cigarettes, had red meat less than four times a week, and excercised regularly. Do the same and you won't need a cream for strong bones.

Step 5b. Use drugs . . .

• Progesterone creams are sold without regulations, as cosmetics, not medicines. None are approved by the FDA for continuous long term use. The dose suggested is 50-100 times the FDA recommended dose.[58]

Preventing Breast Cancer

Hot flashes won't kill you, but breast cancer could. Three-quarters of all breast cancers occur in women over 50.

While it is beyond the scope of this book to deal with all the ways to prevent breast cancer, I can give you a few strong recommendations. For more information, see my book *Breast Cancer? Breast Health! The Wise Woman Way.*

☞ **Reduce use of seed oils.**

Conflicting evidence about the role of fat in the diet arises because some fats protect against breast cancer, and some seem to promote it. The largest study to date followed 61,000 Swedish women and found that: "For each 10 grams of monounsaturated fat [from dairy products and meat in the daily diet, breast cancer] risk fell by 55 percent."[59] Greek women consume lavish amounts of olive oil, goat cheese, and animal fats (up to 60 percent of total calories), yet have some of the lowest rates of heart disease and breast cancer in the world.[60] In fact, the more olive oil a Greek woman eats, the lower her risk of breast cancer.[61]

But regular use of "vegetable" oils (soy, corn, cottonseed, sesame, sunflower, canola) increases risk of breast cancer. "For each 5 grams of polyunsaturated fat [from vegetable oil], the risk [of breast cancer] rose by 70 percent."[62] Vegetable oils alter prostaglandin production, flooding the body with inflammation-promoting omega-6 fatty acids.

☞ **Don't take supplemental hormones of any kind.**

The January 2000 *Journal of the American Medical Association* reported: five years of hormone use can increase breast cancer risk by 40 percent. A recent study of 46,355 women found breast cancer risk increased by 8 percent for every year of HRT use. (ERT increased risk by 1 percent per year of use.)

And the longer taken, the greater the risk.

Other studies showed women who took ERT for 2-5 years had 38 percent more breast cancer than those who didn't; after 5-9 years breast cancers increased by 55 percent; and after 10 years of ERT, by 70 percent. To be effective in controlling osteoporosis, ERT must be taken for at least 15 years, or from the last menses until roughly the age of seventy. Some doctors advise taking ERT for life.

The use of "natural" hormones may not be safer for the breasts; the jury is still out on the risks incurred by women who use progesterone creams.

☞ **Don't have mammograms; do examine your breasts regularly.**
A mammogram may help *find* cancer but it cannot *prevent* it. Repeated mammograms may even cause it. (A mammogram, with 250-300 millirads of radiation per dose, is one of the three highest-dose X-ray procedures currently done.) It is a given that damage from radiation includes cancerous changes in cells. *Of all the body tissues, breast cells are among those most easily damaged by radiation.*

☞ **Eat more beans.**
High dietary intake of phytoestrogen-rich beans protects breast tissue from cancer. Lentils are exceptionally strong protectors. So are red clover and astragalus. What about soy? There is a relationship between the large amounts of *fermented* soy products (miso and tamari) in the Japanese diet and low incidence of breast cancer. But no relationship has ever been shown between the consumption of processed, fake, imitation soy foods, and breast cancer reduction. Soy beverage is used moderately, or not at all, depending on the specific Asian country.

☞ **Eat more fruits and vegetables.**
Whether you eat them fresh, canned, cooked, dried, boiled, baked, frozen, or fried, fruits and vegetables have many more anti-cancer compounds than any other foods. Eat at least five servings a day, including something from the cabbage family, something dark green, orange, or red, and some garlic and onions, too.

Male Menopause/Andropause

"My children, your attention is precious to me," says Grandmother Growth in the tenderest, yet fiercest of voices. "The brightness of your faces as you consider the wisdom of the Ancients is a balm to my soul and a joy to my heart. Know that we are all together. We are always all together in this dance of life, this dance of death.

"I see your faces and they are not the faces of children, no matter how much younger than me you are. I see your grey hair, your balding patches, your wrinkles. I see the thick waists you swore you'd never have, the changes in your sex lives, your indigestion and your night terrors. I see it all. I know it all. I understand it all.

"Mid-life brings far-reaching changes throughout the entire body/ psyche/mind for all of you: women and men. Men and women alike must embrace (or resist) the task of aging and ponder (or deny) the reality of dying. Approach yourselves with loving kindness during the process of

your menopause, your andropause. Let go of how you are accustomed to seeing yourself. Allow yourself to act in new ways. Then, as those very strong hormones that have ruled your behavior since puberty wane, you will find yourself open to greater peace, deeper satisfaction, and a more fundamental abundance than ever before.

"Nourish yourselves. Love yourselves. Simple remedies are the best for those who would be the Ancients. Grow older with me my children, so you may take my place as the Wise Ones."

Step 0. Do nothing . . .

• Doing nothing is not about denial. But most men I talked to were deeply into denying their mid-life change. One man put it like this: "Male menopause? I have no language to talk about it. I never heard my uncles or my dad talk about it. And I don't want to talk about it. I don't even want to think about it. I don't want to admit I am getting older and changing. I don't want to change."

Step 1. Collect information . . .

Technically, men can't have menopause — since they never started men(struating). But that begs the real question. Some authors argue that testosterone levels drop in men after the age of forty and that this is analogous to the drop in estrogen that women experience. And they suggest — surprise! — that men take supplemental testosterone.

Wise women say supplementation of hormones is not necessary for either women or men who wish to live long, healthy, happy lives. Wise dietary choices, including nourishing herbal infusions and vinegars, are. So is regular exertion.

The analogy between andropause and menopause is rather thin. Men reach their testosterone peak in their teens; women reach their estradiol peak in their mid-twenties. Men make less and less testosterone as they age, but never stop making it; women make less and less estradiol as they age, and finally stop producing it. The decline of testosterone is subtle and easy for most men to ignore; the cessation of estradiol production causes difficult-to-ignore symptoms for most women.

But the results may be the same. Lower levels of hormones reduce cancer risk; supplementation increases cancer risk. Lower levels of hormones conserve chi (life force) and nurture old age according to Taoist sages; supplementation leaves one exhausted of core chi.

Men's symptoms during andropause are similar to women's during menopause: disturbances of self-image triggered by weight gain, hair loss, and wrinkles; memory problems; lessening of sexual urgency;

emotional sensitivity and anxiety; even hot flashes. Additionally, men experience more visual problems during andropause, and lose some strength and endurance. The herbs suggested in this book for these (and other) problems work as well for men as they do for women.

• To learn more about andropause, read *Male Menopause* by Jed Diamond; and *No, It's Not Hot in Here* by Dick Roth (Ant Hill, 1999).

Step 2. Engage the energy . . .

• Envision yourself ten years older . . . twenty . . . thirty. Who will you be? What will you be doing? What are you doing now that helps you get there? What are you doing that hinders your vision?

Step 3. Nourish and tonify . . .

★ **Oatstraw infusion** is the herbalist's choice to raise testosterone levels in men (and women). I use one oz. of dried herb in a quart canning jar, filling it to the top with boiling water and lidding it tightly. After 4-8 hours, I strain the herb out and drink the resulting liquid.

★ Hormones are specialized forms of fats. Get more **essential fatty acids** from fatty fish, olive oil, cod liver oil, purslane (*Portulacca oleracea*).

Step 4. Sedate/Stimulate . . .

• "I didn't know I had a drinking problem until menopause," is a statement I have heard from more than one woman, so I asked men if they experienced changes in their ability to drink in their forties or fifties. Many did. A glass of red wine with dinner is heart healthy, but two may be too many for your liver to handle during andropause.

Step 5. Use drugs . . .

• European doctors view oral ethyl testosterone as a potential liver antagonist and carcinogen; it is still for sale in the USA, however.

• For those who (wisely, I think) avoid needles, the FDA has approved a transdermal patch of testosterone (applied to the scrotum).

Step 6. Break and enter . . .

• Testosterone is commonly injected intramuscularly in one of two forms: testosterone propionate (wears off after 2-3 days) and testosterone cypionate (lasts for 7-21 days). An abundance of testosterone is known to promote prostate cancer, however.

References & Resources
Chapter 2: This Is Menopause!

Airola, Paavo. "Menopause: Dreadful Affliction or Glorious Experience?" *Let's Live,* July 1976

Andrews, Lynn. *Woman at the Edge of Two Worlds.* Harper, 1993

Anonymous. *A Book About Menopause.* Montreal Health Press, 1988

Anonymous. *The Gift of Menopause.* (No Imprint), 1981

Appleton, Nancy. *Healthy Bones.* Avery, 1991

Batten, C. "Menopause: A Journey Homeward." *Woman of Power* #14, 1989

Boylan, Kristi M. *The Seven Sacred Rites of Menopause.* Santa Monica Press, 2000

Brody, Jane. "Can Drugs Treat Menopause?" *The New York Times,* May 19, 1992 (Front page, Science Times)

Cobb, Janine O'Leary. *Understanding Menopause.* Key Porter Books Limited, 1993

Costlow, Judy, M. C. Lopez & M. Taub. *Menopause, A SelfCare Manual.* Santa Fe Health Education Project, 1991

Crawford, Amanda McQuade. *The Herbal Menopause Book.* Crossing, 1996

Dickson, Anne & N. Henriques. *Women on Menopause.* Healing Arts, 1988

Greer, Germaine. *The Change.* Knopf Canada, 1991 • Recommended

Greenwood, Sadja. *Menopause, Naturally.* Volcano Press, 1984

Hasselbring, Bobbie; Sadja Greenwood & Michael Castleman. *Medical SelfCare Book of Women's Health.* Doubleday, 1987

Heron, Silena. "Botanical Treatment of Chronic Gynecological Conditions, Including Symptoms of Menopause." 1988 (unpublished paper)

Hudson, Tori. *Women's Encyclopedia of Natural Medicine.* Keats, 1999

Ito, Dee. *Without Estrogen—Natural Remedies for Menopause and Beyond.* Random House, 1994

Kenton, Leslie. *Passage to Power—Natural Menopause Revolution.* Random House, 1995. • Highly recommended

Lark, Susan. *The Menopause Self-help Book.* Celestial Arts, 1990

Lichtman, Ronnie. "Perimenopausal and Postmenopausal Hormone Replacement Therapy" and (Part 2) "Hormonal Regimens and Complementary and Alternative Therapies." *Journal of Nurse Midwifery,* 41:3-28 and 41:195-210, 1996

Love, Susan M., MD, with Karen Lindsey. *Dr. Susan Love's Hormone Book.* Random House, 1997

Maleskey, Gale. *Take This Book to the Gynecologist with You: A Consumer's Guide to Women's Health.* Addison-Wesley, 1991

"New Directions in Menopause." *HealthFacts,* Vol. XIV, #126, Nov. 1989

Nissim, Rina. *Natural Healing in Gynecology.* Pandora, 1986

Northrup, Christiane. *The Wisdom of Menopause.* Bantam Books, 2001

Ojeda, Linda. *Menopause Without Medicine.* Hunter House, 1989

Orrick, Phyllis. *The Menopause Rag.* New York Press, Vol. 5/4, June 1992

Page, Lafern. *Menopause & Emotions — Making Sense of Your Feelings when Your Feelings Make No Sense.* Primavera Press, 1993

Perry, Susan & Kate O'Hanlan, MD. *Natural Menopause — The Complete Guide.* Perseus Books, 1997

Raymond, C. "Good News About Menopause." *American Health,* Nov. 1988

Reichenberg-Ullman, Judyth. "Menopause Naturally." *Natural Health,* March 1992

Reitz, Rosetta. *Menopause, A Positive Approach.* Penguin, 1979

Roth, Dick. *"No It's Not Hot In Here"—A Husband's Guide to Understanding Menopause.* Ant Hill Press, 1999

Saline, Carol. "A Change of Thought on Change of Life." *Philadelphia Magazine,* January 1992

Sander, Pela. "Natural Health Remedies." *Women of the 14th Moon,* Crossing Press, 1991

Saul, D. "Menopause: A Dance Between Delight and Regret." *ANIMA,* Vol. 18/1, Fall 1991

Sheehy, Gail. *Silent Passage: Menopause.* Random House, 1992 • See excellent critique in "The Menopause Rag"

Showler, Linda. "Menopause: If It Isn't Broken, Don't Fix It." Letter to *Townsend Letter for Doctors,* May 1990

Siegal, Diana. "Menopause Changed My Life." *Sojourner,* March 1991

Smith, T. *Homeopathic Medicine For Women.* Healing Arts, 1989

Taylor, Dena, & Amber Sumrall (eds.) *Women of the 14th Moon: Writing on Menopause.* Crossing Press,1991 • Recommended

"The Estrogen Question." *Consumer Reports,* September 1991

Tree Farm Communications, 23703 NE 4th Street, Redmond, WA 98053. • Audio tapes of various women herbalists (including Susun Weed) speaking on menopause

Trickey, Ruth. *Women, Hormones & the Menstrual Cycle: Herbal and Medical Solutions.* Allen & Unwin (Australia), 1998. • Recommended

VanNostrand, Jillian & Christie V. Sarles. *Wild Woman's Garden — 7 Radical Weeds for Women Over 40.* Radical Weeds, 1998

Voda, Ann & M. Eliasson. "Menopause: The Closure of Menstrual Life." From *Lifting the Curse of Menstruation.* Haworth, 1983

Warga, Claire. *Menopause and the Mind.* The Free Press, 1999

Weideger, Paula, et al. *Menopause.* Health Right, 1975

Wolfs, Honora Lee. *Second Spring: A Guide to Healthy Menopause Through Chinese Medicine.* Blue Poppy, 1990

Herbal Allies for Women in the Midst of Menopause

Here, without further ado, are ten herbal allies for women in the midst of **Change**: black cohosh, chasteberry, liferoot, kava kava, sage, red clover, motherwort, ginseng, dong quai, and wild yam.

Black Cohosh
Cimicifuga racemosa
Schwartze Schlangewurzel, Cimicifuga
Chinese herbalists use Sheng Ma: *C. foetida, C. dahurica,* and others

This stately and striking perennial plant of the hardwood forest has been so overharvested that I can now walk for an entire day in its prime habitat and see only a few small groups of it. (Most of the harvest is shipped to Germany and formulated into Remifemin.) Native Americans have long considered it a powerful ally for women — especially during menopause — and science agrees.

Numerous studies show black cohosh tincture to be as effective as ERT in relieving common menopausal problems such as hot flashes, headaches, joint pain, water retention, and fatigue. Recent analysis finds black cohosh does not suppress luteinizing hormone, has no estrogenic effect, and contains no compounds related to estrogen, thus making it safe, perhaps even helpful, for women with a history of breast cancer.[63]

Use black cohosh during your menopausal years to:

• *Calm hot flashes, reduce night sweats*
Black cohosh supplies an amazing array of micronutrients that help you produce and use all kinds of hormones. Try 10-15 drops once or twice a day for 2-6 months.

• *Counter menstrual pain, regulate menses*
• *Relieve headaches*
• *Ease joint pain, fibromyalgia, arthritis, and rheumatism*
Black cohosh contains antispasmodic factors and aspirin-like salicylates that dilate the blood vessels (constricted blood vessels are a common reason for headaches) as well as con-

stituents that slightly depress the central nervous system. A dose is 15-25 drops as needed.

• *Increase energy, calm the nerves, ease agitation, bring sleep*
Black cohosh invigorates chi and helps balance the nerves. It has long been praised as a remedy for hysterical women. Try 5-10 drops a day for 1-3 months as a long-term tonic; use a dropperful/1 ml as a sedative.

• *Alleviate water retention and breast tenderness*
• *Treat incontinence*
Black cohosh tonifies the kidneys and adrenals, eliminating fluid buildup. It treats incontinence by stopping spasms in the urinary system. Use 15-25 drops as needed.

• *Relieve heart palpitations and angina pain*
Black cohosh lowers blood pressure, improves circulation, causes dilation of blood vessels, and thins the blood. For acute use, try 25-30 drops as needed. As a cardiotonic, use 10 drops daily for 3-6 months.

• *Increase vaginal lubrication, counteract prolapses*
Black cohosh is the herbalists' favorite for helping women with weak pelvic muscles, uterine and bladder prolapses. Try a dropperful/1 ml a day for 1-3 months.

• *Improve digestion*
A 3-5 drop dose of bitter black cohosh tincture with meals improves digestion and increases digestive juices. Use of the powder, in capsules, may do the opposite.

Pungent, bittersweet, fall-dug black cohosh roots are so popular the wild population cannot keep up with the current demand. Please buy only cultivated roots/products.

Dosage: Infusion of dried root, up to a teacup a day, by the spoonful. Tincture of the fresh rhizome/roots, 10-60 drops, daily.

CAUTIONS: Do not use black cohosh if you have menstrual flooding, suspect pregnancy, or are breast feeding. Large doses can cause flushing, low blood pressure and depressed heartbeat. Side effects — headache, dizziness, visual disturbance, nausea — are more common, and more severe, with preparations made from dried roots.

Chasteberry or Vitex
Vitex agnus-castus
Chinese herbalists use Man Jing Zi: *Vitex rotundifolia* or *V. trifolia*

The dried berry-like fruits of this small tree have been used by menopausal women since antiquity. Today's woman, whether she achieves menopause naturally or through surgery, radiation, or drugs, agrees: chasteberry helps smooth the way.

Taken during the early menopausal years vitex keeps cycles more regular. Daily use enhances progesterone, luteinizing hormone (LH), dopamine, and luteotropic hormone, but inhibits follicle stimulating hormone (FSH) and prolactin. (Approximately 62 percent of the women suffering with PMS have very high levels of prolactin.)

Vitex is a legendary anti-aphrodisiac to men; hence "chasteberry" and "monk's pepper." It can be a powerful aphrodisiac for some women, however. Whether it makes him droop or you horny, vitex does affect your glands. But not quickly. Chasteberry contains tonifying flavonoids, glycosides, and micronutrients, but no fast-acting phytosterols. Two or three months of daily use may be required for noticeable benefits.

If you have the patience, chasteberry can:

• *Calm down severe hot flashes, counter dizziness*
Chasteberry is especially useful for the woman who flashes due to high levels of estrogen and FSH.

• *Improve your chances of having a baby in your 40s*
• *Reestablish menstruation that has stopped prematurely*
• *Reduce and eliminate menstrual cramps, endometriosis, or fibroids*
Vitex berry tincture has a pronounced anti-inflammatory effect on the endometrium. Large doses taken persistently for several years slowly but steadily relieve endometriosis and fibroids. Moderate doses improve fertility, increase the likelihood of ovulation, and provide sufficient progesterone for successful implantation of the embryo.

• *Stop flooding, spotting, oozing, and irregular cycles*
Chasteberry is an incredible nourisher to the pituitary gland,[64] which controls and coordinates the menstrual cycle. Especially beneficial to women in the early years of menopause when progesterone levels may need a boost to keep cycles even.

• *Redirect hysteria into focused action and emotional calm*
Chasteberry provides slow, steady grounding so you can use your hysteria (literally: "wild womb energy") wisely. For acute care, try motherwort.

• *Clear hormone-related skin problems*
If those pimples and spots of puberty have returned to haunt you, or new skin disturbances have cropped up, reach for the vitex. Change for the better is often evident after even a few weeks of use.

• *Relieve hormone-related constipation and digestive distresses*
Chasteberry helps prevent, or improve, sluggish action of the digestive tract during menopause.

• *Lessen tenderness and lumps in the breasts*
• *Relieve water retention, edema, bloat*
• *Eliminate headaches, migraines, and depression*
These are three of the main complaints of women with PMS. Those who took chasteberry, in a double-blind study of 350 women, reduced the severity and amount of their PMS symptoms by 50 percent in three months.[65] For best effect, continue use for at least a year.

• *Protect against reproductive cancers and reverse early cancers*
• *Lubricate vaginal tissues*
Vitex gently alters hormone levels to protect reproductive tissues from cancers and keep vaginal walls strong and flexible.

Though not native to North America, chasteberry bushes are easily grown here. Fresh or dried berries may be infused in water or tinctured. If vitex doesn't grow near you, buy a quarter pound of dried berries and make your own tincture: Fill a bottle one-third full of chasteberries, then fill it to the top with 100 proof vodka. Wait six weeks, then use.

•**Dosage: Tincture of berries, 1 dropperful/1 ml, 1-4 times daily.**
　　　　Tea of freshly powdered berries, 1 cup/250 ml, 1-4 times daily.
　　　　Freshly powdered berries, 20 mg daily.

CAUTIONS: In use for over 2000 years in North Africa, vitex has a reputation for being free of side effects; however, physician herbalist Tioronna Low Dog says she has seen capsules trigger a rash in a few women.

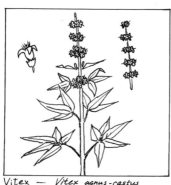

Vitex — *Vitex agnus-castus*

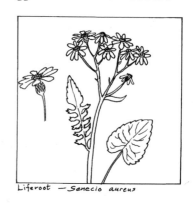

Liferoot — *Senecio aureus*

Liferoot
Senecio aureus
Groundsel
Senecio vulgaris
Gemeines Kreuzkraut, Séneçon Commun
Jacob's Groundsel
Senecio jacobaea
Jacobskraut, Séneçon Jacobée

The *Senecios* have a bad reputation for poisoning livestock, but a great reputation for helping women during menopause, birth, and menstrual distress.

These glycoside-rich "troublesome perennial weeds" are good sources of phytosterols. Many authors warn against their use, but I have seen nothing but favorable results with small doses of tincture made from fresh blossom. Liferoot and groundsel are classic tonics, having far greater effect over a long time than as quick-acting remedies. Commit to daily use for two weeks out of each month for at least two months before expecting to see results.

Use any one of the *Senecios* during your menopausal years to:

• *Completely eliminate severe menstrual pain, nausea, debility*
Liferoot is an ally without peer for women incapacitated by chronic severe menstrual distress. For best effect, take 5-8 drops daily for two weeks before your bleeding begins. Continue for 3-9 months.

• *Help you ride your hot flashes*
• *Tonify your uterine muscle*
• *Regulate your menstrual cycle, slow flooding, cure anemia*
Powerful plant hormones and an ability to increase circulating iron are the gifts of liferoot. Senecio is considered safe to use even if you flood.

• *Soothe the nerves, moderate emotional swings*
• *Relieve PMS symptoms, especially breast tenderness*
• *Reduce gravel and other urinary tract problems*
• *Increase libido*
Senecios choose to grow where they can collect a wide spectrum of trace elements and micronutrients, which slowly accumulate in your body as you consume them, balancing and nourishing the nerves,

endocrine system (including adrenals), and kidneys. Once all of these are in top shape, the libido kicks in. I've seen it happen many times. Don't discount this effect or you may be in for a surprise.

Out of respect for the alkaloids concentrated in the roots, I use only the flowering tops and leaves of liferoot. The lively yellow flowers turn into dandelion-like fluff balls and blow away if dried, so I tincture them in vodka when they bloom in the spring.

Dosage: Tincture of fresh flowers, 5-15 drops per day. Best if taken during luteal phase only.

CAUTIONS: *Senecio* can cause temporary (but distressing) changes in your menstrual and premenstrual patterns during the first few months of use.

Barbara didn't have hot flashes at menopause, she had cold sweats. "First I'd be cold, then hollow in my gut, and I'd think I was going to wet my pants I had to pee so bad. Then my heart would pound and I'd be wet from scalp to toe, and really chilled. I'd have to bring changes of clothes with me wherever I went, I'd get so wet so unexpectedly. If I was stressed, I'd get very dizzy, too." She read about Ginseng, bought some whole roots and chewed them "as much as I could for the past three moon cycles." She even cooked them for hours in her soups. "And I just realized I haven't had a chilling sweat in over a week."

Alex had taken estrogen for three years to control her severe hot flashes, and she was ready to try something else. Since she had always gotten chilled after her flashes, had been anemic off and on, and really liked celery and cilantro, she decided to ally with dong quai. "For the first few weeks, I took a little dong quai with my whole dose of ERT. Then I gradually withdrew from the estrogen by cutting my pills to smaller and smaller sizes and eating more dong quai."

A year later, Alex is still free of sweats, chills, and flashes, and is considering cutting out the dong quai as well.

Kava Kava
Piper methysticum

This beautiful shrub with heart-shaped leaves has powerful effects on alertness, memory, and emotional balance. Kava kava easily induces tranquility, with no sedation and no addiction, and brings deep restful sleep. But it can also be used to focus energy.

Traditionally used as a social lubricant and a spiritual connector, kava kava is a sacred plant whose consumption is surrounded by ritual and myth. It produces a gentle joy that allows one to feel at ease in almost any situation.

South Sea Islanders chew the juicy fresh rhizomes and roots (to activate the hypnotic lactones), mix this mass with water, ferment it for a few hours, strain it, and ingest it as a community event. Uri Lloyd comments: "This is the 'Intoxicating Long Pepper,' from which a disgusting drink is prepared by the natives, and even by the whites, of those islands." Everyone participates in the kava kava ceremony, including individuals who conservative modern herbalists believe should avoid it: pregnant and lactating women, children, infants, and elders.

Menopausal women love kava kava because it helps them:

- *Relieve anxiety, ward off depression*
- *Loosen up, chill out*
- *Remember, focus*

Kava kava acts on the amygdala region of the brain to modulate fear and anxiety, while increasing mental alertness. Noticeable results occur within a week of using tea or tincture daily. Those taking prescription antidepressants or sedatives, and those with a tendency toward thoughts of suicide, do best with very small doses or none at all.

- *Cool hot flashes*

Kava kava has a reputation for being an antipyretic, that is, an herb that puts out fires. A small (20 women) double-blind study found significant improvement in patients' well-being and reduction of hot flashes when 100 mg of dried root was taken three times a day.[66]

- *Sleep deeply*

After the gentle warm bubbly feeling and mental stimulation of kava kava wear off, one is left pleasantly tired, free of thought, worry, doubt, or stressful memories. Yaaaaaawn . . . time for bed, or a nice nap.

• *Be free of muscle and joint pain, relieve menstrual cramps*
Kava kava is one of the most powerful muscle relaxers known. The Herbal PDR lists it as antispasmodic and anticonvulsive. The infusion or tincture (as needed) helps those with problems like fibromyalgia, whiplash, muscle spasms, and restless legs syndrome. Regular moderate use (3-5 times a week) releases soft tissue tension and increases flexibility. For strongest effect, **let the infusion ferment** at room temperature in a loosely capped jar until bubbly. A cup, sipped slowly, begins to work in fifteen minutes and continues to relieve pain for 6-10 hours.

• *Stay unbothered by urinary and vaginal infections*
• *Counter bloat (water retention)*
• *Avoid (or correct) incontinence*
• *Increase sexual interest*
Kava kava soothes, tones, cools, and clears infection from mucus tissues, easing bladder infections, urethritis, UTIs, gout, vaginitis, and interstitial cystitis. By cooling inflammation in the neck of the bladder, it eliminates incontinence. Twice daily use brings results in a day or two.

Kava kava is not native to North America, nor is it grown here. Dried rhizomes may be infused in water or alcohol (tinctured). To test for activity, chew the dried herb and note how quickly the mouth becomes numb. Daily use is best restricted to 3-4 months. Irregular use can continue indefinitely.

Dosage: Tincture of rhizomes, one dropperful/1 ml , 1-4 times daily.
Infusion of dried rhizomes, 1-4 cups/250-1000 ml, daily.

CAUTIONS: Side effects from normal use of kava kava are restricted to mild gastrointestinal disturbances. Prolonged ingestion of excessive amounts can lead to skin discoloration, a dry scaly rash (even lesions), dizziness, muscle weakness, and vision impairment.

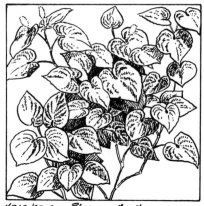

Kava kava - *Piper methysticum*

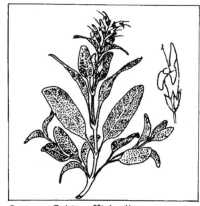

Sage - *Salvia officinalis*

Garden Sage
Salvia officinalis
Garten-salbei, Sauge officinale, Shu Wei T'sao

DO NOT USE sagebrush/desert sage (Artemisia tridentata).

"Where sage doth grow well and vigorous, therein rules a strong woman."   — Old wives' saying

The ancients called sage sacred. *Salvia* means "s/he saves." Since earliest memory, sage has dried breast milk and stopped menopausal sweating, eased the minds and wombs and bellies of women everywhere. There is no herb as effective as sage at drying up the flowing springs of perspiration that gush with some women's hot flashes. But that's not all.

Use garden sage during your menopausal years to:

• *Dry up night sweats, cold sweats, and hot flash sweats*
Sage's effect is generally noticeable within two hours and can continue for a day or more from a single dose. In Traditional Chinese Medicine (a Wise Woman tradition), sweat is regarded as a precious pure fluid of life and a cooling substance.

• *Regulate hormonal* **Change**
• *Improve chances of pregnancy after 40*
Sage's hormonal effects have long been noted; our foremothers used it to increase fertility. Sage contains flavonoids and phytosterols.

• *Ease irritated nerves, banish depression*
Mineral-consolidating sage is rich in mellow calcium, calming magnesium, peppy potassium, sexy zinc, and anti-stress thiamine.

• *Relieve dizziness, trembling, and emotional swings*
Sweating doesn't remove toxins from the body, but it does remove minerals. When you sweat profusely, the mineral loss can cause dizziness, trembling and emotional swings, and even joint pain. Sage not only stops sweating and the resulting mineral loss, its rich mineral reserves help you make up for previous depletion.

• *Eliminate headaches*
Sage contains headache-easing saponins, which keep the blood flowing freely; carotenes, which nourish the liver (in TCM, headaches are related to liver weakness); and essential fatty acids, which keep the blood vessels flexible.

• *Strengthen the liver, aid digestion, decrease excess gas*
Like its sister mints — peppermint, rosemary, thyme, spearmint and savory — sage is rich in essential oils that help the stomach and liver produce more digestive enzymes and acids, thus easing indigestion, nausea, and gas.

• *Relieve menstrual cramps and flooding*
Sage's antispasmodic oils and sweat-stopping tannins exert their influence all the way to the uterus, giving you prompt relief from pain and excessive bleeding.

• *Reduce bladder infections*
Sage contains highly disinfectant oils that concentrate in the urine, discouraging bacterial growth.

• *Prevent joint aches, improve circulation*
Sage's essential fatty acids and minerals are boons to those suffering from aching joints. When you receive optimum minerals from herbs, mineral deposits at your joints are more likely to dissolve into the blood. Sage's saponins also grease your joints and ease inflammation.

• *Gain mental clarity, a strong memory, and a calm "craziness."*
One who is wise is a sage. To burn sage is to clear the air. In legend, to rub a person with sage kept them safe in a transformed state. Breathe in the deep scent of sage and welcome the crazy old crone you are becoming.

• *Slow the aging process*
Sage lives up to its seemingly absurd claim of bestowing extra decades of life on its users: it is antiseptic to most bacteria inside (and on) your body, filled with anti-oxidants that retard wrinkles and grey hair and help prevent cancer, blessed with heart-healthy oils, abundant with much-needed minerals, and easy to grow, even in a pot. Why not make a cup of sage tea, right now?

Powerful-tasting sage is a welcome addition to whole grain dishes (and, yes, turkey stuffing). Try fresh sage finely chopped and sprinkled on salads, potatoes, carrots, parsnips, beans. Use dried sage in soups; or as a condiment at the table. Infused, sage makes a dye-like rinse to keep hair dark, an antiseptic rinse for infected gums, and a tasty drink.

Dosage: Infusion of dried leaf, 1-2 spoonfuls, 1-8 times daily.
Tincture of fresh leaf, 15-40 drops, 1-3 times a week.

CAUTIONS: Avoid sage if you have dry mouth or very dry vaginal tissues. If used daily, its essential oils accumulate in the kidneys and liver.

Red Clover

Trifolium pratense
Rotklee, Trèfle rose, Triphyllon

Even finding a four-leaf clover isn't as lucky as finding out about red clover. It's everything you thought soy would be, with none of soy's drawbacks. Instead of leaching minerals from the bones, red clover contributes generously to bone health. Instead of disturbing the thyroid, red clover helps normalize it. And red clover has an iron-clad reputation for preventing and countering breast cancer. So do miso and tamari, but not other soy foods.

Red clover contains more active phytoestrogens in greater quantity than soy. Strong infusions of the blossoms are thoroughly safe to use and highly effective. Countless women who have wanted to become pregnant have succeeded after drinking red clover infusion for 3-18 months.

Whether you are still longing to be a mother, or yearning to be done with your childbearing years, red clover is an ally you will lean on for the rest of your life. It is a subtle, complex herb, mild yet deep, superbly nourishing and wonderfully grounding.

Use red clover before and during your menopausal years to:

• *Keep yourself hormonally fit*
• *Reverse premature menopause*
• *Improve your chances of having a child after the age of 40*
Red clover flower heads contain many hormone-like flavonoids, including isoflavone, daidzein, genistein, formononetin, biochanin, sitosterol, and coumestrol, a particularly strong phytoestrogen (six times more active than the one in soy).[67] Red clover contains all four major estrogenic isoflavones; soy has only two of them. A cup of red clover infusion (not tea) contains ten times more phytoestrogens than a cup of soy beverage, is richer in calcium, has less calories, and contains no added sugars.

• *Moderate the intensity of your hot flashes*
Women who took powdered dried red clover in capsules had as many hot flashes as those taking a placebo. Not surprising, but misleading. Red clover blossoms need to be infused in water to liberate their minerals and phytoestrogens. Women who drink red clover infusion have high urinary excretion of phytoestrogens, and that correlates strongly with easier hot flashes — and less breast cancer.

• *Prevent and reverse breast cancer*
Red clover strengthens the immune system, improves lymphatic functioning, repairs damaged DNA, turns off oncogenes, reverses pre-cancers and in situ cancers, and has been used for hundreds of years by those who wish to become very old women. To promote breast health, I drink a 1-2 quarts of infusion a week.

• *Improve memory, clear confusion, increase energy*
Red clover infusion is rich in iron, chromium, B vitamins and other trace nutrients necessary for good mental and physical functioning.

• *Ease your anxiety*
• *Relieve muscle and joint pain, diminish headaches*
The tincture of red clover is a profound relaxer and soothing calmative. Its salicylic acid content (similar to aspirin) makes it an excellent pain reliever, too.

• *Keep your skin supple and healthy*
• *Increase vaginal lubrication*
• *Ease incontinence, relieve cystitis*
Red clover infusion nourishes and soothes the mucous surfaces of the lungs, throat, bladder, and vagina, countering inflammation and relieving dryness. Regular use relieves skin rashes and may reduce wrinkles.

• *Prevent osteoporosis*
• *Prevent strokes*
Red clover's minerals build strong bones twenty ways. And its blood-thinning coumarins help prevent strokes.

Sweet, bland red clover blossoms are welcome in salads, a nice addition to a pot of rice, and tasty steeped in vinegar. I like to add a pinch of mint to my red clover infusion to counter its black-tea taste.

Dosage: Infusion of dried flowers, 1-4 cups/250-1000 ml per day.
Tincture of fresh blossoms, 15-25 drops, 1-4 times a day.

CAUTIONS: Overconsumption of red clover's coumarins can lead to a breakdown of red blood cells and increased risk of hemorrhage. Excessive use might increase uterine weight in females who no longer have their ovaries; at least, that's what happens to sheep.

Soy
Glycine max

"The highly processed soy foods of today are perpetuating . . . nutrient deficiencies all over the world." — Sally Fallon

Like red clover, soy is a member of the bean family. All beans contain generous amounts of phytoestrogens, those wonderful substances that help menopausal women take heart, stand tall, and stay gutsy. Since I wrote the first edition of *Menopausal Years*, the world seems to have become saturated with articles and ads advising all menopausal women to eat soy.

Is there something wrong with this picture? I think so. Soy has a dark side. It all has to do with how seeds protect themselves.

All seeds (beans are seeds) contain substances — such as phytates and trypsin inhibitors — that interfere with our ability to liberate, utilize, or create key nutrients, such as calcium, zinc, vitamin B_{12}, and thyroid hormone. These substances are known collectively as anti-nutritional factors.

In most instances, soaking and cooking are sufficient to remove the anti-nutritional factors, making beans generally safe to eat. But not always. Some types of beans retain their anti-nutritional factors unless treated in severe ways. Soy is one such bean.

Fermentation destroys soy's anti-nutritional factors and increases its mineral availability. **Miso, tamari, tempeh, and natto are fermented.** Tofu, soy beverage, soy nuts, soy granules, and fake soy foods (soy-burgers, soy dogs, soy cheese, and so on) are not. Tofu is the only unfermented soy used consistently in Asian cultures.

Traditionally, tofu is eaten with seaweed (to offset its thyroid-damaging effects), and miso (to offset its B_{12}-disrupting effects), and, whenever possible, fish/meat (to offset its mineral-depleting effects). When unfermented soy is eaten frequently in a diet low or lacking in animal protein (as is the case for many vegetarian and all vegan women) the anti-nutritional factors can create havoc: brittle bones, thyroid problems, memory loss, vision impairment, irregular heartbeat, depression, and vulnerability to infections.

Unfermented soy is high in hemoglutin, which causes clumping of red blood cells and may increase risk of stroke. It is also impressively rich in aluminum (up to 100 times more than is found in the same amount of real milk).

"Soy did me in." — Michael Moore, PhD herbalist

What can soy do during your menopausal years?

• *Reduce hot flashes?*
So true, so true. Up your intake of plant hormones and you will have fewer hot flashes. Study after study has looked at this effect and it is quite strong.

• *Protect against breast cancer?*
Fermented soy foods (such as miso and tamari) clearly protect against breast cancer. But tofu, soy "milk," and other soy products expose breast tissues to extra estrogens which may increase breast cancer risk especially during and after menopause. And when women take hormones isolated from soy, the risk increases even more.

Eating soy all your life is vastly different than eating a normal American diet for fifty years and then supplementing with isolated isoflavones. *To protect your breasts, use miso and tamari, both proven anti-cancer champions, lavishly.*

• *Prevent heart disease?*
Soy lowers total cholesterol and increases HDL. In monkeys without ovaries, soy isoflavones dilated blood vessels as much as estrogen did. While we know that lower cholesterol and more relaxed blood vessels are signs of health, we don't know that soy actually prevents heart attacks or stroke.

• *Help your bones?*
Rats without ovaries who eat soy have thicker bones. Real-life women with their ovaries find the opposite to be true. Soy is not a good source of calcium. Tofu and soy beverages are supplemented with calcium, true: calcium carbonate. That's chalk, and chalk is brittle.

• *Improve your memory?*
Soy is deficient in fats needed for healthy brain/memory functioning.

Soy protein isolate, texturized vegetable protein, isolated isoflavones — processed soy foods come in more forms than I can list. I eat miso and tamari freely, tofu and tempeh occasionally, and other soy products not at all.

Dosage: 50-200 grams of isoflavones per day, preferably from food.

CAUTIONS: Excess soy can cause liver damage and is said to feminize men. Soy may be difficult to digest, may cause allergic reactions.

Soy bean – Glycine max

Motherwort
Leonurus cardiaca
Herzgespann, Agripaume cardiaque, Yi Mu Cao

"Everyone ought to have a little Mother around the house," Grandmother Edith would frequently say. The Mother she meant is motherwort, a locally common weed and a treasured ally to women stressed by menopausal problems. Grandmother Edith's love affair with motherwort began when her hot flashes knocked her out in the supermarket, continued as it mended her husband's heart, and grew and grew as her five daughters found relief from PMS and menstrual cramps, constipation and the crazies with the help of the little Mother, motherwort.

Use motherwort regularly during your menopausal years to:

• *Lessen the severity, frequency, and duration of hot flashes*
Motherwort regulates and tonifies the functioning of the thyroid, blood vessels, liver, heart, and uterus. For best results use 5-25 drops of tincture daily for 3 months. But don't neglect to try a dropperful (in a splash of water) even after a flash has begun.

• *Relieve faintness with flashes*
Motherwort is traditionally used to relieve shortness of breath and congestion in the respiratory passages. She invigorates the circulation and increases oxygen in the blood. Use 15-25 drops of tincture as soon as you feel faint or dizzy.

• *Ease stressed nerves, relieve anxiety*
Motherwort calms, supports, and strengthens you the way the smell of your mother did when you were very young. Used regularly, motherwort feeds your nerves and your good common sense, relaxing and unclenching any held tension. Motherwort is not sedating, but calming, leaving you ready for action, not flying off the handle or bouncing off the walls. Ask motherwort to be your ally in tough times, in shaky times, in enraging times, in scary times, in depressed times, in grief-filled times. Try 10-20 drops as soon as you feel your nerves starting to fray or just before a stressful event. Repeat every five minutes if needed.

• *Relieve insomnia and sleep disturbances*
Use motherwort's high-calcium calming effect when you are awakened by night sweats and have difficulty getting back to sleep. Keep a glass of water and a bottle of motherwort tincture by your bed and take 10-15 drops and a swallow of water as soon as you wake, even if it's three times an hour. Motherwort eliminates the nightmares some women experience with their menopausal **Change**.

• *Strengthen the heart, reduce palpitations and tachycardia*
Motherwort calms a rapidly beating heart with readily usable minerals, trace elements, and an alkaloid exceptionally tonifying to the heart (and uterus). Rudolf Fritz Weiss, a German herbal doctor, uses motherwort tincture for those with functional heart complaints. The botanical name translates as "lion-hearted." A dropperful/1 ml of motherwort tincture acts quickly to ease palpitations and tachycardia. Regular use lowers hypertension, and sets you up to be a hale-hearted crone.

• *Eliminate menstrual cramps*
• *Relieve uterine pain*
Motherwort tincture is my favorite remedy for women with uncomplicated menstrual cramps. I find 5-10 drops usually eases cramps in five to ten minutes. Repeat every ten minutes as needed. Motherwort encourages strong (but not crampy) uterine contractions, which strengthen the uterine muscle. So the more you take motherwort to ease your cramps, the more toned your uterus becomes, and the less likely cramps are in the future.

• *Restore thickness and elasticity to vaginal walls*
Motherwort brings blood to the pelvis and thickens all tissues there (bladder, uterus, vagina). Noticeable results occur within a month of taking 10-15 drops daily.

Eva told me she was having 24-30 powerful hot flashes daily, and had been for the past two years. She had tried ERT, but it made her feel "miserable, premenstrual." When I visited her, I wasn't surprised to find a motherwort "weed" growing in the flower bed beside her front door. It was in full flower; the perfect time to harvest and tincture it.

Six months later, Eva called to tell me that she was now having only one or two flashes a day. She'd been taking a dropperful of motherwort tincture 2-4 times a day, and she was involved in the Pathwork (see page 127), which supported her wholeness in very new ways.

"I was always the perfect wife and mother, friend and community member. I never got mad, or even very upset. Last year I had a flash every time someone was rude to me. Motherwort and Pathwork have given me permission to be rude back. I thought you said motherwort would make me calm. Instead, it helped me find my anger."

• *Lift depression*
A dose of motherwort first thing in the morning is far kinder to your system than coffee and helps you ease into the day with a renewed sense of life.

• *Reduce water retention, edema*
Small, frequent doses of motherwort will reduce bloat in a few hours. For chronic care, use a dropperful/1 ml a day for 3-6 weeks.

• *Relieve constipation and extend life*
There is a Japanese saying about the heirs of those who take motherwort: they are grumpy because they must wait so long for their inheritance. But does it really work? A small dose (5-10 drops as needed) does ease gas pain, encourage regular elimination, and improve digestion. That alone would make anyone want to live longer.

Bitter with minerals and alkaloids, motherwort is unwelcome in salads and nasty as an infusion, so it is used as a tincture, vinegar, or syrup. In Oriental herbalism, Yi Mu Cao is cooling, pungent, bitter.

Dosage: Tincture of fresh flowering plant, 15-25 drops, 1-6 times a day. Vinegar of fresh plant, 1-2 tablespoons/15-30 ml, as desired.

CAUTIONS: Motherwort can aggravate a tendency toward flooding. Do not use daily if you bleed heavily or are easily habituated to substances that make you feel really good. Motherwort is so soothing, so calming, that you may begin to lose some of your own standing and lean too heavily on your Mom.

Ginseng & Dong Quai
Adaptogenic Roots

Panax Ginseng is one of the best known of all herbal medicines. It is more frequently associated with relief from severe menopausal problems, especially hot flashes, than any other plant in Western herbalism.

Dong quai is the East's most frequently recommended herbal ally for the mid-life woman. It is considered by many to be the finest woman's tonic in the world.

Both of these roots specifically support transformation by helping us adapt to **Change**. Unfortunately, they are expensive, difficult or impossible for an amateur to grow, and rare in the wild. Fortunately, they are effective even in very small doses.

Ginseng is yang; it is a chi (energy) tonic. Dong quai is yin; it is a blood (substance) nourisher. If yang and yin are mistakenly identified as male and female, then we arrive at the common (mistaken) notion that ginseng is for men and dong quai is for women.

Native Americans made no such mistake. Among the Iroquois Nations, ginseng was well-known as a woman's remedy. The Penobscot Indians also considered it a woman's herb, and advised women wishing to conceive to cook it and eat it.

In fact, both men and women benefit from ginseng's yang chi tonifying and from dong quai's yin blood nourishing, the more so as we age. Blood is the mother of chi; chi is the promoter of blood. Oriental medicine says menopause is the yang (energized) manifestation of yin (wise blood). And we can all benefit from ginseng's and dong quai's rich stores of minerals, plant hormones, and B vitamins.

Menopausal women may want to take ginseng (alone) for two weeks and then dong quai (with other roots) for four weeks, alternating in this fashion for up to two years or until your menopausal transformation is complete. This alternation is highly recommended for women experiencing premature menopause, naturally or through surgery or drugs.

While I generally use one herb at a time, Chinese herbalists insist that dong quai must be moderated by other herbs. One of the most ancient and beloved combinations is equal parts of dong quai, rehmannia, ligusticum, and peony roots. (See page 259: Four Roots Tonic.)

Ginseng can be combined with other roots, too. That's the way Native Americans used it. (See "Menopausal Root Brew," page 257.)

Sweet, smoky, warm, spicy, exotic, and interesting, the tastes of ginseng and dong quai are intriguing in soups, remarkable in teas, powerful in tinctures, and quite pleasant to chew. The most enjoyable way to purchase ginseng and dong quai is to stroll through Chinatown, stopping at herb stores until you find the roots you want to savor on your journey through menopause.

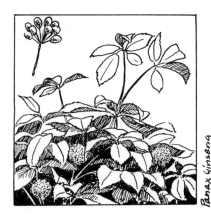

Panax ginseng   Codonopsis tangshen

Ginseng
Oriental Ginseng/Ren Shen *Panax ginseng*
American Ginseng *Panax quinquefolius*
Tienchi Ginseng *Panax pseudoginseng*
Not "true" ginseng, but used interchangeably:
Dang Shen *Codonopsis pilosula*
Siberian Ginseng *Eleutherococcus senticosus*

All varieties of ginseng are roughly interchangeable in effectiveness. I prefer wild American ginseng, which is less stimulating, less heating, and perhaps less strongly hormonal than the ginseng grown in Korea and China.

During the past fifty years, ginsengs have been the subject of intense scientific scrutiny. For centuries, the indigenous peoples of the lands where the different ginsengs grow — wild mountainous areas of North America, China, and Russia — have considered them fountains of youth and cure-alls. Science validates their native wisdom: all varieties of ginseng are energizing, rejuvenating (especially to the hormonal system), immuno-protective, and adaptogenic.

Although the benefits of taking ginseng are cumulative, you'll note improvement in 2-3 weeks if ginseng is your menopausal ally. The lore of the Catskills (where ginseng, or 'seng, still grows wild) tells me to chew on a little 'seng spring and fall, and whenever I'm under stress. Since ginseng is rare in the wild, and expensive to buy, I use it quite sparingly. The pint of tincture I put up with two large wild roots a decade ago will last me the rest of my life.

Wild *Panax* roots, whether American or Chinese, are the most effective of the ginsengs. They are the most desired, and most expensive as well. The least effective ginseng is powdered, in capsules or foil packages. Well-handled commercially grown roots of any ginseng, dried or tinctured, offer maximum effect at the lowest price.

Ginseng's effects are neutralized by vitamin C supplements (if taken within three hours). Ginseng's effects are doubled when combined with 200 IU vitamin E or a spoonful of fresh wheat germ oil.

Take ginseng, especially *Panax*, during your menopausal years to:

• *Reduce the intensity and frequency of hot flashes*
With eleven hormone-like saponins, several phytosterols, and a ready supply of hormone building blocks such as essential fatty acids, min-

erals (especially manganese), and glycosides, ginseng is amply prepared to help ease your menopausal flashes.

• *Improve nervous functions, ease depression and anxiety*
By nourishing the nerves, moderating blood sugar swings, and regulating the hormones, ginseng helps you use your powerful menopausal emotions instead of being swept away by them. Ginseng is at its best when you are under the most stress.

• *Reduce the effects of stress*
• *Boost your brain*
Of all ginseng's benefits, this is the most demonstrated. When you're burned out, exhausted, numb, clumsy, and feeling dull, make a ginseng soup, or take the tincture twice a day. Ginseng nourishes and strengthens the energy centers — adrenal cortex, pituitary, thyroid, and hypothalamus. Taken with ginkgo, it promotes fast, accurate thinking and improves both short- and long-term memory in healthy adults.[68]

• *Stop menstrual flooding, regulate endocrine activity*
Ginseng contains a rich supply of plant hormones and micronutrients that nourish your ability to create the estrogen and progesterone you need to continue menstruating regularly, without flooding, until the final period.

• *Improve energy level, reduce fatigue, increase stamina*
Not to be confused with herbal "speeds," which give one a false sense of energy, ginseng rebuilds energy and stamina from the inside out by nourishing, regulating, and tonifying virtually all systems. It also lessens fatigue by diminishing night sweats and promoting deeper, more restful sleep.

• *Improve memory, concentration, mental acuity, and clarity*
Ginseng improves all mental functioning, especially during stress.

• *Improve cardiovascular health*
Ginseng's scientifically validated cardiotonic properties nourish heart and blood vessels, improve blood flow to the heart, lower elevated blood pressure (without reducing normal blood pressure), reduce cholesterol, increase HDL (good fats) and reduce LDL (bad fats). Animals on high-fat diets which included ginseng did not gain weight nor develop atherosclerosis.[69]

• *Reduce mild hyperglycemia, prevent diabetes*
Ginseng is particularly valuable for stabilizing blood sugar swings, since it affects the metabolic processes of the liver and sugar utilization within the muscles. Regular use lowers the levels of sugar in the urine and blood, reduces thirst, and increases sexual desire.

• *Eliminate menopausal headaches*

• *Improve digestion*

Ginseng helps the liver that is so busy during menopause it can't tend to digestion. In Traditional Chinese Medicine, a weak liver allows energy to fly to the head, causing a headache. Chewing on a ginseng root before or after you eat can help.

• *Enhance libido*

Ginseng may not make you feel like a young doe in estrus, but you might find yourself having some very "adult" thoughts.

The taste of ginseng is sweet, aromatic, and warming, to a greater or lesser degree depending on individual plants and the species. Ginseng roots lend themselves to savory soups, satisfying teas, and robust tinctures, but the classic way to consume ginseng is to put a piece in your mouth and "just worry it around for an hour or so, until it's all gone."

Dosage: Tincture of fresh or dried root, 5-40 drops, 1-3 times daily. Infusion or tea of dried root, 4-8 oz/25-50 ml, per day. Piece of dried root as big as a third of your little finger daily for 6-8 weeks.

Note: Dosage varies more among individual plants than among species.

CAUTIONS: Ginseng is contraindicated if you have a fever, feel jittery or have sleep difficulties. Some women report overstimulation from ginseng. There are documented cases of ginseng causing hot flashes and menstrual-like bleeding long after menopause has culminated. (If this happens to you, discontinue use.) Do not use ginseng if you are taking insulin, stimulants, or blood pressure drugs.

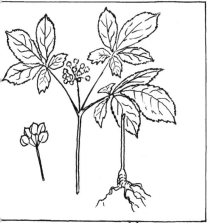

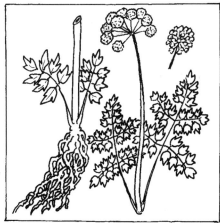

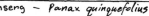

ʌseng — *Panax quinquefolius*

Dong Quai — *Angelica sinensis*

Dong Quai
Angelica sinensis
also spelled Dang Gui, Tang Kwei, Tang Kuei, Dong Gway

Cherished all over the Orient as a supreme ally for women with reproductive/uterine/hormonal distresses, dong quai roots are now readily available in North America. Traditional Chinese Medicine always uses dong quai with other roots. Scientific studies of dong quai alone consistently find it ineffective.

Use dong quai combinations as nourishing menopausal allies to:

• *Regulate menses, reduce spotting and flooding caused by anemia*
Dong quai's stores of iron, folic acid, and phytosterols help diminish bleeding in pale, undernourished women. Vital, feisty, hot-blooded women may have the opposite reaction. Dong quai is tricky to use during menopause. It relaxes the uterine muscle and excites contractions (both actions increase the likelihood of heavy bleeding). In addition, it appears to increase the blood flow to the uterus. For this use, combine with yellow dock root and burdock or white peony root. A dropperful/1 ml of the tincture is taken twice a day. Discontinue immediately if bleeding increases.

• *Revivify thin, dry vaginal tissues*
Dong quai has long been noted for its ability to nourish and thicken vaginal and bladder walls. Consistent use brings a soothing flow of moisture into the pelvis, hydrating the bowels and easing constipation as well as increasing vaginal secretions. A mixture of half dong quai roots and half wild yam roots, tinctured together and taken (a dropperful twice a day) for 6-12 weeks should do it.

• *Restore a youthful face and complexion*
Dong quai stirs and heats the blood, and the effect is often immediately obvious in the face, where it gradually plumps out facial wrinkles, and quickly brings a rosy glow to the cheeks. I once saw a tall, thin man drink a cup of dong quai tea. As he set the cup down, he flushed from the chest up to his crown (just like a hot flash!) and fainted. We're after a less dramatic effect, however. (See Four Roots Tonic, page 259.)

• *Relieve hot flashes for cold women*
Dong quai's sterols and minerals work promptly to modify hormonal chaos; they accumulate in the body, offering continuing benefits with repeated use. However, in several double-blind studies, women taking dong quai had as many hot flashes as women taking a placebo. In fact, if you feel hot much of the time anyway, dong quai may make you flash all the more.

• *Relieve menstrual cramps, uterine pain*
• *Eliminate incontinence*
• *Reduce headaches, relieve water retention*

Dong quai's warming, relaxing qualities bring ease to the entire pelvis, relieving aches and spasms in the uterus, vagina, bladder, ligaments, and muscles. As its healing energy moves to the head, it throws off headaches. And it stirs the kidneys to eliminate excess fluid, ending swollen ankles and bloated bellies. In this instance, combine dong quai with dandelion root, licorice, elecampane root, and/or burdock root. A dose of the combined tincture is one dropperful/1 ml, taken as needed, up to four times in an hour.

• *Eliminate palpitations, decrease heart disease*

Dong quai reduces high blood pressure, counters atherosclerosis, promotes healthy blood circulation, and markedly increases coronary blood flow. Its coumarins thin the blood much as aspirin does. Combine with motherwort and/or hawthorn tincture, half and half, and take up to a dropperful as needed.

• *Ease menopausal insomnia*
• *Restore emotional calm*

Nerve-mellowing magnesium (depleted by frequent night sweats) and rare elements such as cobalt help stabilize emotional upheavals and improve the quality of your sleep when dong quai and valerian pair up.

• *Relieve menopausal rheumatism*
• *Tonify the liver*

Dong quai soothes achy joints during (and after) menopause and is a grand ally of the liver during the menopausal years.

Dong quai smells and tastes a little like its family members: celery, lovage, carrot, parsnip, parsley, cilantro, anise, cumin. Dried sliced roots are wonderful to chew on. Garden angelica is related to dong quai and is a tolerable substitute, as are wild varieties of angelica, including osha (*Ligusticum porteri*).

Dosage: Combination tincture, 30-60 drops (1-2 ml), 1-3 times daily. Infusion or tea of dried root, 4-8 oz/125-250 ml daily.

CAUTIONS: Dong quai may increase bleeding from fibroids. Do not use during menstruation if bleeding is heavy. Do not use if you regularly take aspirin or blood-thinning drugs. Do not use if you are bloated. Do not use if you have diarrhea. Discontinue use of dong quai if it causes breast tenderness or soreness. Dong quai may cause spontaneous miscarriage in susceptible women.

Wild Yam
Dioscorea villosa (and other species)
Wilde Yamwurtzle, Shan yao

Also known as colic root or rheumatism root, wild yam has very large roots (some weigh a hundred pounds or more). All the most commonly prescribed synthetic hormones — including progesterone, progestin, testosterone, estrogens, and cortisone — are made from wild yam.

Human gut bacteria can cleave a sugar molecule from wild yam's steroidal saponin, producing diosgenin. Labs make progesterone from diosgenin, but our bodies can't. Diosgenin has a weak estrogenic effect. According to Australian herbalist Ruth Trickey: "A more probable explanation . . . is that [diosgenin] interacts with hypothalamic and pituitary hormones and . . . initiates ovulation."

Anecdotal evidence supports the use of wild yam cream to ease hot flashes and dry vagina, but "dermal absorption of crude plant hormones is nil," says David Hoffman, author of the *New Wholistic Herbal* and director of the California School for Herbal Studies.[70]

For greatest effect and safety, use wild yam internally, not externally.

Internal use of wild yam during your menopausal years can help:

- *Ease joint pain*
- *Relieve menstrual cramping, ease mittelchmertz (ovulation pain)*
- *Prevent incontinence*

Wild yam's strong anti-inflammatory action stops spasms and reduces swelling in all tissues, offering relief to those dealing with fibromyalgia, arthritis, rheumatism, uterine/ovarian pain, and urinary problems. Its weak estrogenic effect strengthens the sphincter of the bladder, too.

- *Moderate hot flashes and hormonal surges*
- *Decrease erratic bleeding, stabilize menses*
- *Influence fertility*
- *Prevent bone loss*

Wild yam helps "any endocrine imbalance," says American herbalist Amanda McQuade Crawford. Wild yam can be used to prevent pregnancy (3 cups of tea daily) or to increase fertility (dropperful of tincture 1-3 times a day, for the last two weeks of menstrual cycle). It can ease some menopausal symptoms (use as needed, in any form). Postmenopausally, a small amount of tea or tincture several times a week keeps bones, heart, and breasts healthy.

• *Improve digestion, strengthen liver and gallbladder*
• *Treat nausea, increase frequency and ease of bowel movements*
Wild yam eases painful pelvic or digestive system problems such as gall stones, weak liver, diverticulitis, gas, constipation, pelvic adhesions, pelvic inflammatory disease, or endometriosis. It helps the liver, reducing flashes.

• *Lower blood pressure and cholesterol*
• *Improve circulation*
• *Calm nerves*
Wild yam's phytosterols compete with cholesterol for absorption in the intestines, improving your lipid profile. It is a superior nerve tonic.

• *Prevent senility*
• *Nourish longevity, rejuvenate sexuality (especially for men)*
Wild yam is very high in cobalt, zinc, and manganese, perhaps other trace minerals as well. Science can't explain it, but herbalists world-wide insist that wild yam is a superb tonic to brain (and gonads).

Wild yam grows in the tropics. Most roots are from Mexico. Fenugreek seed contains the same steroidal saponins and may be used instead.

Dosage: Tincture of fresh or dried roots, 30 drops/1 ml, 1-3 times daily.
Infusion or tea of dried root, 1-3 cups/250-750 ml daily.

CAUTION: Frequent use may promote enlargement of the uterus.

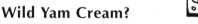

Wild Yam Cream?

Wild yam cream is of no particular value for menopausal women and useless for postmenopausal women. It does not increase progesterone production, nor affect bone mass.[71]

After three months of daily use, women had no more pro-gesterone in their saliva than they did at the start of the study.

Wild yam does not contain progesterone but steroidal saponins which convert into many hormones. If wild yam cream could increase progesterone production, it would also increase production of cortisone and other hormones. It doesn't.

The starting compound for progesterone is cholesterol, not sterodial saponins, so rubbing your belly with butter will pro-duce a stronger and cheaper effect than wild yam cream could.

CAUTION: Real hormones are often added to wild yam creams.

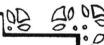

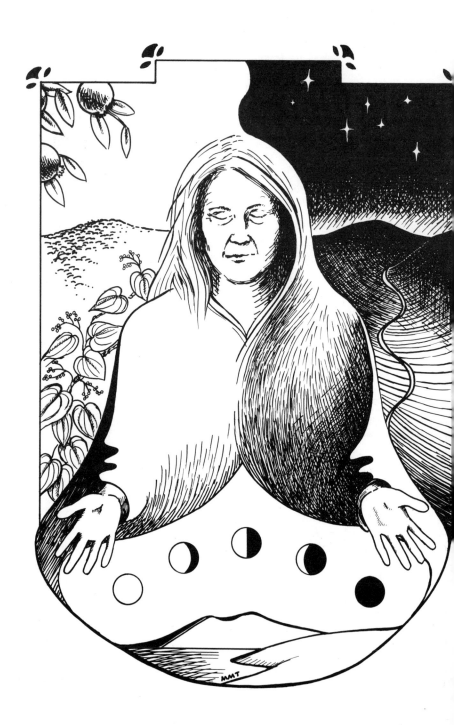

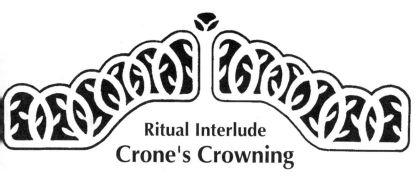

Ritual Interlude
Crone's Crowning

The idea of menopause as a deficiency disease is faltering. More and more women are finding beauty in their menopause and claiming themselves as Crone, woman of wholeness. Let us not replace that story with one even more injurious to women: that the healthy, well-adjusted woman breezes through menopause with scarcely a problem.

The menopausal years, the climacteric years, constitute an enormous **Change**. And change is a challenge. A challenge each woman will meet in her own unique way. You may feel at times like a stranger in your own body, confused by your own feelings, uncertain and afraid of the **Change** taking place in your own being. You may feel, perhaps with fear, the "you" that you have known for so many years dying, as your last menses become memories.

I know of no herbs, no rituals, no special ways of eating or exercising that will prevent the **Change** of menopause. And, as with puberty, pregnancy, and birth, you may change in ways that are dramatic and difficult to live with. This is not a failing on your part.

In menopause, **Change** is normal; but normal may be difficult, painful. Normal, natural menopause may really hurt, for it is a symbolic death as well as an actual rebirth.

When the pain of labor reaches the ultimate intensity, the child begins at last to come down the birth canal. Slowly or quickly the small body pushes head-first toward its new life. The head at last reaches the vaginal opening; it is crowning.

When the distress of menopause reaches its peak, you begin the push toward your new life. As you reach the outer edge of menopause, you crown yourself Crone.

Your Crone's Crowning ritual marks a change as dramatic as the babe's movement from watery womb dependence to air-breathing independence. You will never again be the same woman you were before you stopped bleeding. As you accept this death, you birth yourself as Crone.

The ritual of Crone's Crowning is the stillpoint before the actual emergence. Umbilicus throbbing, psychically connected still to the mother you were, you pause before the final push. Your menstrual cycle is finished, forever. Your role as Mother is at an end. Your role as Crone begins with the next breath, the first breath of your new life. To make way for this first breath, the new life, we give death to ourselves as we were.

The following ritual is one way to experience symbolically the death aspect of your menopausal Change. I envision you doing this ritual alone or with a group of like-minded women. (This particular ritual is a women's mystery and, as such, does not include men.) I suggest that you do this ritual no sooner than thirteen moons after your very last menses.

*   *   *   *   *

On the night of the new (dark) moon make your way to a place where you feel very safe, very secure. Bring with you pictures, poems, objects, and mementos of your life as a bleeding woman, as Mother (even if you have no children).

Create an altar (sacred space) to woman as mother, she-who-bleeds-and-does-not-die, she-who-creates-from-her-own-blood, she-who-gives-birth-to-all-that-is. Make this altar as beautiful as you can, using lots of flowers and colors. Light three candles, one white (the color of death), one red (the color of life), and one black (the color of fertile possibility). Hum or sing a lullaby while you do this. If you like, place a small statue of the Blessed Virgin Mary or some other symbolic mother on your altar.

Face the altar and breathe toward it. As you inhale, fill yourself with the images, feelings, ideas, thoughts of yourself as Mother. If you have not given birth and feel sad, that is appropriate, as is delight in your choice. If you gave your child away, through adoption or abortion, let the feelings of pain or relief come to the foreground. If you have children, focus on how you feel about your role as their mother.

Call upon the energies of the Mothers of the east, those who sing in new life. Ask them to be present with you. Call upon the energies of the Mothers of the south, those who stoke the fires of new life. Ask them to be present with you. Call upon the energies of the Mothers of the west, those who cry and laugh with life. Ask them to be present with you. Call upon the energies of the Mothers of the north, those who form new life. Ask them to be present with you.

Hold your right hand out in front of you. Look at it carefully as you say: "This is the hand of life. This is the hand of beginnings." Imagine that you hold yourself, as mother, in the palm of your right hand.

Hold your left hand out in front of you. Look at it carefully as you say: "This is the hand of death. This is the hand of endings." Imagine that you hold yourself, as crone, in your left hand.

Looking intently at both of your hands, say, in your own words: "The time for the right hand has come to an end for me. I can no longer give life from my own belly, my own breasts. In the great balance of all that is, I enter now the time for the left hand. I am readying myself to be a giver of death. Although death is a gift that is feared, it is utterly necessary to the continuation of life. As woman it is my privilege to give life and call myself mother. As woman it is my duty to give death and name myself Crone."

Slowly, slowly, bring your hands together, left palm up and above the right hand. "I give death to myself as Mother. I claim my power as Crone." Signify the Mother's death by placing your right hand in a waiting container of mud or clay or brown fingerpaint.

With your left hand, snuff out the red candle. Put the black and white candles to one side, then remove everything else from the altar and place it, with love/relief, grief/joy into a fire or a bucket of water or a trash can. Cry out for the death of your Mother self.

Ask the Crones of the east to come and replace the Mothers of the east. Welcome those who sing the songs of death. Ask the Crones of the south to come and replace the Mothers of the south. Welcome those who stir the cauldron of change and lay the feast for the dead. Ask the Crones of the west to come and replace the Mothers of the west. Welcome those who open the door to death, whose tears shine the way to letting go. Ask the Crones of the north to come and replace the Mothers of the north. Welcome those who silently guard the realm of the dead.

On the bare altar place the two lit candles, black and white, and one hair from your head, a silver one. "I claim myself as Crone. I claim my right to name the end of things." Place upon your head a wreath or crown of your own devising. "I crown myself as Crone. I am she-who-holds-her-wise-blood-inside; I am she-who-walks-with-death."

Thank the Crones, the Mothers, and the energies of the four directions. With your left hand snuff out the black and white candles; in the darkness, hum a lullaby.

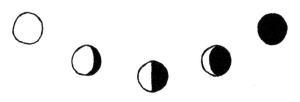

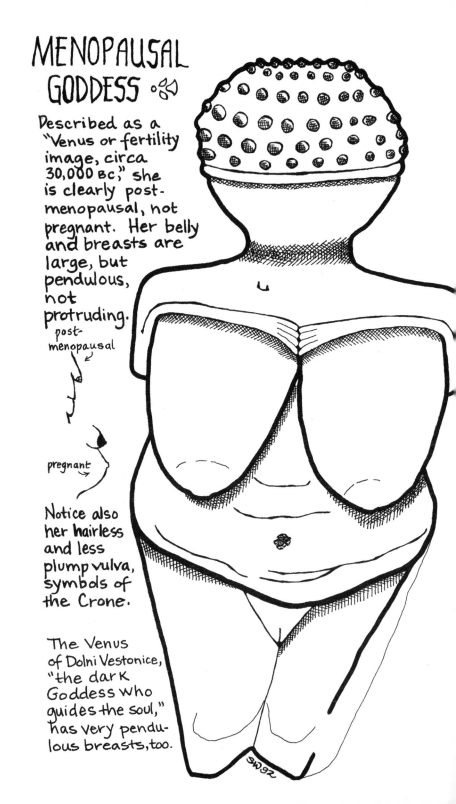

MENOPAUSAL GOODESS

Described as a "Venus or fertility image, circa 30,000 BC," she is clearly post-menopausal, not pregnant. Her belly and breasts are large, but pendulous, not protruding.

post-menopausal

pregnant

Notice also her hairless and less plump vulva, symbols of the Crone.

The Venus of Dolni Vestonice, "the dark Goddess who guides the soul," has very pendulous breasts, too.

SW92

Post-Menopause
She-Who-Holds-
Her-Wise-Blood-Inside

"Soon your voice will merge with my own, dear one," chuckles Grand-mother Growth. "We have journeyed long together through this Change, your menopause. And now it is completed. You are crowned Crone. What I have shared with you is imprinted in your cells. Do not be surprised when you look in the mirror and see yourself resembling me.

"You are no longer a maiden; but always Maiden, filled with blissful, carefree, poetic energies. You are no longer a mother; but ever Mother, abundant with creative, supportive, life-giving energies. You are now, and all the rest of your days will be, Crone, woman of wholeness, woman of wisdom, she who knows death as well as life, impeccable action as well as spontaneous vitality. And, in time, you will be seen as Grand-mother to your community, and Grandmother Growth to new generations of baby Crones.

"It is almost time for me to say farewell, granddaughter. But not before I share a few stories with you: stories of flexible bones, and open hearts, and sensual, sexual old age. And not before I urge you to nourish yourself.

"There is much for you to do, young Crone. As one of millions of women coming to their Change now, you have a very special place in what some call the 'earth changes.' Yes, granddaughter, by 2013, you and your sister Crones will constitute such a great pool of collective wisdom that you will be able to guide Gaia and her human inhabitants into an amazing new era of global wholeness and personal health."

You no longer bleed on a monthly basis. Your outer, visible tie to the rhythms of the moon is gone. Now you follow the inner ebb and flow of your own ocean, knowing full well how intimately connected you are to the swells and contractions of the entire universe. You are a postmenopausal woman and again a virgin (she who is owned by no one; not a sexual innocent), freed from any worry about conception, pregnancy, or mothering.

Most of the distresses of your **Change** have faded. Hot flashes are milder, and far less frequent. Creative juices are willing to flow at ordinary hours, allowing a full night's sleep. Your energy levels and emotional levels seem more solid than they've ever been.

Keep taking great care of yourself. Post-menopause can bring vaginal and bladder changes leading to incontinence, infections, and painful intercourse (herbs and exercises can prevent/relieve these problems); heart disease (Wise Woman ways can greatly reduce your risk); osteoporosis (simple foods and herbs can keep bones strong and flexible); and joints that often ache (herbs offer safe pain relief).

With the help of home remedies, herbal allies, and Grandmother Growth's wise words, your postmenopausal years can be vital and beautiful. Remember, the *ugly* old woman/witch is the invention of male-dominated cultures, and a projection of our own fear of death. In peaceful matrifocal cultures, the beauty of crones is legendary: old women are satin-skinned, softly wrinkled, silver-haired, and awe-inspiring in their truth and dignity.

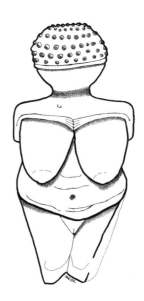

Vaginal/Bladder Changes

"Motherwoman, you flowed, you flowed," sings Grandmother Growth. In rich fertility you flowed. You flowed with blood. You flowed with fertility. As Mother, you flowed with milk, with life.

"Crone woman's blood does not flow. Crone woman's womb bears no children, her breasts fill no more with milk. Are her flowing days over? Not so, not so. Your flow has not ended, young Crone. Your flow has gone underground. Your flow is now internal.

"Listen carefully, great-granddaughter. When your wise blood stays inside, it may make your belly heavy, hot, and dry. To keep your uterus, vagina, and bladder soft and moist, you need to keep your wise blood circulating and your root energies moving. Let the belly relax and sag a bit so the blood and energy can move freely.

"Take time to be with yourself sensuously, pleasurably, lovingly. Stir the cauldron of your belly. And tend the fires at your root. Take time to listen to the memories stirred up when the wise blood flows and spirals inside your belly. Listen with your inner ear to your inner stirrings. Let the spiral move the energy out of your root chakra and up, to sparkle at the crown.

"Listen, listen, listen. Flow like a Crone, and listen."

The pelvic (root) energies of the postmenopausal woman, having no outlet in menstruation or birth, easily become congested. This congestion traps hot energies in the vagina, bladder, uterus, and anus, reducing vaginal lubrication, thinning and irritating the vagina and vulva (vaginal lips), instigating constipation and hemorrhoids, encouraging incontinence, and giving rise, in the worst case, to vaginal atrophy and chronic vaginal yeast and bladder infections.

Thinning and drying of pelvic tissues can occur rapidly (within 6-10 months of the last menses) when menopause is induced, the adrenals/kidneys are weak, or there is insufficient body weight.

Women who achieve menopause naturally, carry enough body fat, and nourish their adrenals/kidneys, will experience few problems with vaginal/bladder weakness in the postmenopausal years.

Dry Vagina

"You have been wet and fertile at the will and whim of your body for most of your years, great-granddaughter," murmurs Grandmother Growth. "But you have changed. You grow moist with readiness for play now only when you truly desire it, not at reproduction's dictates. Have no fear that your springs have run dry. If you consciously call up your flood of pleasure, it will answer. This is one of my greatest gifts to you, young Crone. No longer will you be accessible to those who do not inspire love and trust in you. The great portals of life, your womb, your vagina, now serve only you, now open only at your bidding."

Step 1. Collect information . . .

We are given two contradictory pictures of postmenopausal sex. On one hand, we're to look forward to freedom from conception worries, resulting in more spontaneous, relaxed, joyful sex filled with multiple orgasms. On the other hand, we're to expect dried-up, atrophied vaginas and dyspareunia (painful intercourse).

Thinning and drying of the vaginal tissues in the postmenopausal years is often first noticed during sexual activity when the expected lubrication is slight or absent. Is this normal?

Yes; almost all postmenopausal women will experience a lessening of sexual lubrication. No, you don't have to give up your sexual self. Crones know there are many ways to ecstasy besides intercourse, and many ways to be slippery when we want to be.

(Remedies to ease extreme thinning and drying are on page 187.)

Step 2. Engage the energy . . .

• **Homeopathic remedies** include:

☞ *Bryonia*: root chakra overheated and dry, dry vagina, dry stools/constipation.

☞ *Lycopodium*: lack of root stability, vagina very dry, self-confidence withered, skin dry.

☞ *Belladonna*: vagina painfully dry and too sensitive to tolerate touch.

• This yoga exercise sounds simple, but requires concentration. Squeeze the anal/pelvic floor muscles firmly while inhaling; hold. Breathe out, hold the root lock and add a chin lock. Hold for two seconds. Visualize the nectar of the universe flowing down your spine and between your legs. Relax as you exhale.

★ **Slowly, slowly.** Give yourself plenty of time to warm up before inserting anything into your vagina.

Step 3. Nourish and tonify . . .

★ **Eat more fat**, especially foods rich in essential fatty acids, such as **sardines**, **plantain seeds**, **organic butter**, and fresh **purslane**. Most women notice a difference in a few weeks.

★ **Comfrey root sitz bath** (two quarts/liters of the infusion) is an old favorite for keeping vaginal tissues flexible, strong, and soft. Sitz for 5-10 minutes several times a week.

• Drink more water, not more tea or coffee or juice or soda . . . **water**. Or boil a small handful of rice in two cups/500 ml of water to make a thin broth regarded as an ideal internal moistener for women with dry vaginal tissues or dry mouths. Drink freely.

★ As part of your love play, chew on a small piece of **dong quai root**.

• Pause for the soothing cooling touch of **chickweed** tincture, 25-40 drops in water, several times a day for 2-4 weeks, and see if your hot, dry vaginal tissues don't smile moistly.

• Increase lubrication and the thickness of your vaginal walls by starting your day with: 25 drops of **motherwort** tincture *or* 1 tablespoon/15 ml freshly ground **flax seeds**. Look for results within a month.

★ **Acidophilus capsules inserted vaginally** help prevent yeast infections and create copious amounts of lubrication. Insert one (or two) about 4-6 hours before lovemaking.

★ **Comfrey** ointment is the ally of choice when skin needs flexible strength. Rub in the morning and night and use as a lubricant for love play. The vulva will be noticeably plumper and moister within three weeks.

• If you have access to **slippery elm**, try this soothing vaginal gel. Slowly heat 2 tablespoons/30 ml slippery elm powder in a cup/250 ml of water, stirring until thick. Cool (you can even chill it) before spreading over and inside the vulva and vagina. This gel lubricates, heals, and nourishes.

★ **Exercise, exercise.** Every part of your body will age more gracefully if you work it out regularly. That goes for your vagina and vulva, too. Weekly orgasm is the recommended exercise, but daily **pelvic floor exercises** tonify the vaginal tissues. See box, page 188.

Step 4. Stimulate/Sedate . . .

• Avoid the problem! Try sex without intercourse.

★ **Plantain ointment** helps restore youthful moistness and elasticity to postmenopausal vaginal tissues.

• You are more likely to be troubled by vaginal dryness and the loss of lubrication if your adrenals have been exhausted by overuse of coffee, alcohol, and white sugar; severe stress; or steroid/cortisone drugs.

• Herbalist Rina Nissim suggests applying the essential oil of *Salvia sclarea* to vaginal tissues that have lost their elasticity. Dilute with olive oil; pure essential oils can be fierce on sensitive mucous surfaces.

Step 5a. Use supplements . . .

• Daily doses of 100-200 IU of vitamin E for 4-6 weeks can help you increase vaginal lubrication. You may need to continue with your daily dose for months to maintain your juiciness. Experiment to find the lowest effective dose for you. (See cautions, page 91.)

★ **Astroglide** is favored by those who like to have slippery fun.

Step 5b. Use drugs . . .

• Polycarbophil, the active ingredient in Replens, pulls water into vaginal cells, to restore and maintain healthy lubrication. It also increases alkalinity in the vagina, reducing vaginal infections.

• Estrogen creams really do revitalize vaginal tissue. But they may increase risk of endometrial cancer more than oral estrogen. Occasional, rather than regular, use minimizes risk.

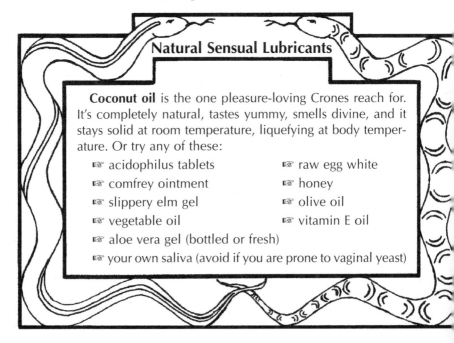

Natural Sensual Lubricants

Coconut oil is the one pleasure-loving Crones reach for. It's completely natural, tastes yummy, smells divine, and it stays solid at room temperature, liquefying at body temperature. Or try any of these:

- ☞ acidophilus tablets
- ☞ comfrey ointment
- ☞ slippery elm gel
- ☞ vegetable oil
- ☞ aloe vera gel (bottled or fresh)
- ☞ raw egg white
- ☞ honey
- ☞ olive oil
- ☞ vitamin E oil
- ☞ your own saliva (avoid if you are prone to vaginal yeast)

Itching, Burning Vulva/Vaginal Atrophy

"Do you feel like you're sitting on a vol . . . cane . . . ohhhhhhh!?"
Grandmother Growth's voice rises shrilly. "Who said Crones weren't hot?!
  "Root chakra energies — anger, sex, power — are hot subjects. And this
Change called menopause fires the root chakra. Can you sit still in
the midst of this rapidly vibrating energy? Can you dance with its searing
touch? Oh granddaughter, what are you itching to do now that you are
crowned Crone? What lights your passion? Shine, young Crone. Burn.
And keep that energy moving so your inner heat doesn't dry you out."

Step 1. Collect information . . .

Postmenopausal vaginal or vulval burning and itching is disre-
spectfully labeled "senile vaginitis," "vulvar dystrophy," or "atrophic
vulvitis." (Also leukoplakia, lichen sclerosis, kraurosis, and sclerotic
dermatosis.) This painful itching and burning (referred to as "pruritus"
in premenopausal women) is caused by irritating, alkaline vaginal
secretions acting on tender vaginal tissues.[72] It is especially bother-
some when the vaginal tissues are thin, dry, and cracked.

The following remedies stop the itching and burning and heal the
crone's sensitive vagina/vulva (which may appear white, shiny, and
clearly abraded or scratched), restoring pinkness, plumpness, and pli-
ability, so long as there are no yeast overgrowths or bacterial infections
to complicate the picture. (See pages 190-192 for yeast remedies.)

Step 2. Engage the energy . . .

• Relax. Lie down. Watch your breath. See yourself breathing out through
your vagina. Visualize yourself breathing cool blue energy in and out.

• **Homeopathic remedies** include:
  ☞ *Belladonna*: Painful, hot vagina, tender, reddened.
  ☞ *Cantharis*: vagina burning and raw.
  ☞ *Natrum mur.*: the entire vagina, inside and out, is intensely painful.

Step 3. Nourish and tonify . . .

★ **Motherwort** tincture (10-20 drops several times a day) quickly restores
thickness and moisture to vaginal walls. So does regular use of **vitex**.

★ I've never met a crone's itch that could hold its own against **plantain** oil or ointment. Relief is immediate; the effect generally lasts for
hours. Continued applications strengthen the skin, hasten healing, discourage infection, and stop inflammation. (See Appendix 2.)

Pelvic Floor Exercises (Kegels)

Begin with fewer repetitions and gradually increase.
Expect results within 4-6 weeks.

◊ While not usually considered an exercise, **sexual excitement** and orgasm is the best way to keep the vagina and vulva well nourished and well lubricated. Sexually active women actually have plumper thicker cells in their bladders and vaginas than celibate women.[73] Don't worry about having a partner; self-love works fine.

◊ **To increase vaginal lubrication**: Breathe out and push down as though you were trying to push something out of your vagina. Hold for 3 seconds. Inhale and relax. Do 25-50 repetitions.

◊ **To tone vaginal muscles** and increase lubrication: Tighten the inner muscles of the vagina tightly around a finger or small smooth marble or crystal egg and hold for 10-13 seconds; pulse (contract and relax) your vaginal muscles rapidly (10-30 times) as you breathe out. Repeat 10-25 times.

◊ To tone **vagina and bladder**: Sit in a basin or bathtub with water up to your hips. See if you can suck water in your vagina and expel it. Suck in as you breathe in; push out as you breathe out. Do 20-50 times.

◊ To **identify and strengthen the muscles that control voiding**: Next time you pee, stop the flow. Hold as long as you can (work up to at least ten seconds) before letting go and peeing again. As soon as you can, stop and hold again.

◊ To **improve bladder control**: Pulse your urine flow by pushing the flow out very strongly, then slackening it off until it barely dribbles out, then push out strongly again, and again slack off. As a variation, push out strongly and increase the flow powerfully, then shut it off completely. Repeat as many times as possible.

★ Applying **aloe vera gel** or any herbal cream or oil directly to the vagina and vulva with attention, care, love, and stroking will help.

• Drink a quart/liter of **nettle** infusion several times a week; or sit in it.

• **Calendula** cream applied morning and night helps strengthen vaginal tissues, heal minor abrasions, relieve pain, and discourage infection.

Step 4. Stimulate/Sedate . . .

★ Take the time to soothe your vulva and yourself with an **oat bath** (see page 260). Regular use encourages healthier tissues.

★ Hygroscopic (water-drawing) honey will moisturize and heal your tender vulva. Apply directly where needed or pour some **honey** on a menstrual pad and wear it.

★ A **comfrey root** or **chamomile blossom** compress will soothe itchy, dry vaginal tissues and promote healthy skin growth. Infuse the comfrey root and soak a towel in the liquid. Or make a cup of chamomile tea and use the teabag (warm, room temperature, or chilled). Apply either compress to your tenderness while in a reclining position.

• Massage in small circles around the inner and outer sides of your ankle bone to stimulate the flow of energy to the pelvic organs.

• Soap, douches, bubblebaths, nylon underwear, and pantyhose encourage itching/burning of the vagina/vulva.

Step 5a. Use supplements . . .

★ **Cod liver oil** (1-2 tablespoons a day) can reverse vaginal thinning and drying, relieve itching and burning, and improve bone health, too.

• Progesterone creams contain active hormones. A friend noted: "Many women who would never think of eating anything that might contain hormones blithely smear this stuff on their ya-yas!"

• Vitamin B_2 supplements may be helpful in relieving crone's itch.

Step 5b. Use drugs . . .

• Use of **hormone creams** (progesterone, estrogen or testosterone) may be the only way to remedy very thin, irritated vaginal tissues in undernourished women. To minimize risk, use one-eighth of an applicator as needed.[74]

• Use vaginal anti-itch creams containing cortisone as a last resort; excess cortisone weakens the bones.

Vaginal Yeast Overgrowth

"Old sour puss, they used to call the spinster." Grandmother Growth closes her eyes and a sly grin spreads over her face. "Well, I guess a crone has right to a sour puss, sure enough. That way she doesn't wind up scratching her privates in public."

Step 1. Collect information . . .

Yeast (*Candida albicans* or *monilia*) is a natural part of a healthy vaginal environment. It helps prevent the growth of infective bacteria.

If the yeast grows too much, it is noticeable as a nice-smelling, white, cottage-cheese-like accumulation on your vaginal walls or in your underwear. This can make your vagina and vulva very irritated, sensitive, sore, and itchy, and can even cause episodes of incontinence.

Lactobacilli (such as acidophilus) also live in healthy vaginas. They prevent yeast overgrowths. (And turn milk into yogurt.) Lactobacilli thrive in acidic vaginas. When vaginal acidity drops, yeasts thrive.

You can check the pH of your vagina with litmus paper. A healthy acidic reading is 4 to 4.5. Yeast overgrowth begins at 5.5 and irritation occurs when the pH reaches 6 or higher (more alkaline).

As estradiol and progesterone stop stimulating the reproductive tissues, vaginal secretions naturally become less acidic and yeast overgrowths are more common. When the **Change** is rapid (as in induced menopause), the upsurge in vaginal yeast causes incredibly intense itching. When the **Change** is slower, the lactobacilli have time to adapt to the less acidic environment and yeast overgrowth is minimized.

Postmenopausal women who take hormones are often bothered by vaginal yeast, as are diabetic crones, and those who take antibiotics.

These tried-and-trusted remedies, from the grandmothers and wise women of today and yesterday, offer fast, effective relief. **Important**: If you experience chronic or repeated vaginal yeast overgrowths, all of your love play partners need to use the remedies, too, not just you.

Step 2. Engage the energy . . .

★ What is the benefit of a vaginal yeast overgrowth? If it gives you an excuse to **say "No"** (to sex), here are some other ways to say it:

☞ Stand in front of a mirror and say "No" at least 25 times.

☞ Yell "No" and stamp your foot ten times. Breathe.

☞ Stand in front of your lover. Keep your eyes open. Say "No!"

☞ Hold your arms at shoulder level, palms out, push against a tree or a wall or the palms of another person, and say "No!"

Step 3. Nourish and tonify . . .

★ Insert one or two capsules of **acidophilus powder** into your vagina every other day for two weeks. Acidophilus is a variety of lactobacillus. If you keep adding lactobacilli to the vagina, the yeast stops growing. Be sure to push the capsule all the way up to the cervix (feels like the tip of your nose).

• If the yeast is persistent, insert the acidophilus capsule *behind* the cervix, in the little pocket between it and the vaginal wall nearest the rectum. (Putting one foot up on a chair, while standing, helps open the vagina and ease insertion.) And **treat all your play partners**, too. Have the male partners soak their members in apple cider vinegar or diluted yogurt for five minutes daily for a month to kill yeast living in and on the glans.

• Other ways to nourish lactobacilli (to the detriment of the yeast):
   ☞ Eat a cup of **plain yogurt** daily. (Organic is best.)
   ☞ Insert 1-2 tablespoons/15-30 ml of plain yogurt in the vagina every day or so. (Be imaginative; you *can* get it in there.)
   ☞ Use a yogurt sitz bath. (Dilute 16 ounces/125 ml yogurt in 2 quarts/500 ml warm water.) Sitz in it 1-4 times a week.

★ Make sure your yogurt contains live cultures (it will say on the label). If it does, your symptoms will usually be relieved within 48 hours.

• Sweets of any kind (sugar, fruit juices, even artificial sweeteners) can change the vaginal pH enough to encourage yeast overgrowth, especially in the postmenopausal years.

★ "So long as I drink my 2 cups of **nettle** infusion daily, my crotch feels fine, no itching, no burning, no yeast."

Step 4. Stimulate/Sedate . . .

• If neither acidophilus nor yogurt curbs your yeast overgrowth, try these ways to reacidify your vagina (in order of increasing strength):
   ☞ **Apple cider vinegar**: Dilute half a cup/120 ml in two quarts/liters of water. Sitz in it once or twice a day for ten days. Results will be evident in 3 days. Okay to alternate with acidophilus every other day for a week.
   ☞ **Lemon juice** or **white vinegar (acetic acid)**: Use 1 tablespoon/15 ml in a quart/liter of water. Sitz daily for 10-14 days.
   ☞ **Lactic acid** (sold as Lactinex powder): as directed.
   ☞ **Boric acid**: a heavy-duty measure. Have the druggist put 600 mg boric acid in 00 gelatin caps (or fill them yourself). Insert one high up in the vagina, by the cervix, every day or so for two weeks.

★ If yeast remedies work, but only temporarily, there are probably bacteria thriving in your vagina creating the alkaline conditions that yeast love. No matter how acidic you make your vagina, the bacteria undo all your efforts. **To eliminate mild bacterial infections**, insert a clove of garlic high up in the vagina, on or behind the cervix, before going to bed every night for 5-10 days. CAUTION: Tender tissues may be burned by garlic, so peel the clove gently. *Your breath and sweat will smell of garlic if you use this remedy.*

• Vaginal penetration in love play when there's a yeast overgrowth causes friction which irritates the vaginal walls and makes the overgrowth more difficult to remedy.

• Yeast loves the hot, moist environment of pantyhose, nylon underwear, swimsuits, tight pants.

• Douches, soap, and bubblebaths make the vaginal environment more alkaline, that is, more friendly to yeast. Women who douche weekly have 4-5 times more vaginal yeast overgrowths.

• Crones may want to avoid using goldenseal or myrrh douches (often recommended to remedy chronic vaginal yeast overgrowth). Both of these herbs are quite drying and may irritate sensitive tissues.

Step 5a. Use supplements . . .

• High doses of **B vitamins** may help remedy chronic overgrowths. Avoid daily consumption of nutritional yeast (often recommended as a source of B vitamins) as it can leach calcium from the bones.

Step 5b. Use drugs . . .

• Despite its innocent name, **gentian violet** is a dangerous, concentrated fungicide (yeast killer). It is very messy, but very effective. Use cotton swabs to paint a one percent aqueous solution on the cervix, vaginal walls, and vulva before going to bed. Wear a sanitary pad to contain the staining. Repeat 4-6 times during the next two weeks. CAUTION: If this causes burning, immediately insert some plain yogurt into your vagina or sit in a tub of vinegared water.

• Nystatin (Nilstat or Mycostatin) is another fungicide. But yeast infections frequently recur after being cured by it.

• Strong drugs — miconazole (Monistat), clotrimazole (Gyne-Lotrimin), or metronidizole (Flagyl) — are prescribed for women with severe, chronic overgrowths. CAUTION: Flagyl causes cancer in animals. Flagyl may cause yeast overgrowth and contribute to depression.

Incontinence

"A sour puss, a crazy lady, and a real pisser, yep, that's me," Grandmother Growth declares with mischief in her sparkling eyes. "And if you don't want to wet your pants, young Crone, come close. Let me teach you how to stir your fluids so they don't leak out at inopportune moments."

Step 1. Collect information . . .

Many women will experience incontinence briefly during menopause. Most women (65-75 percent) will experience one or more occurrences of urinary incontinence in the decades following menopause.[75] And about 11 million American women deal with incontinence on a regular basis.

Stress incontinence refers to urine leakage when the bladder is stressed. Stresses include laughing, sneezing, coughing, picking something up, walking up stairs, running, and other normal activities that put stress on the bladder.

Urge incontinence refers to urine leakage as soon as the urge to void is felt. (This is the kind I had sometimes during menopause. And it was triggered by the sight of the toilet as well as the thought of it. So long as I kept my eyes closed, and my thoughts on other things, I could make it!) Both together is *mixed incontinence.*

The known causes of stress and urge incontinence include: weakened or damaged pelvic floor from pelvic surgery (caesarean section, hysterectomy, laparoscopies, tubal ligation); precipitous birth, repeated pregnancies; thinning bladder wall after menopause; medications (see Step 5); alcoholism; urinary tract infections; overactive bladder; fibroids; and diabetes.

Women over the age of 60 who have had a prior hysterectomy are half again as likely to have chronic incontinence as women who keep their uterus. And 40 percent of the women in industrialized nations have had such surgery.

Isolated incidents of incontinence are usually due to bacteria in the bladder or lack of tone in the pelvic muscles and bladder.

Step 2. Engage the energy . . .

• **Homeopathic** remedies include:
  ☞ *Pulsatilla*: bladder and pelvic floor feel unreliable or weak.
  ☞ *Zincum met.*: there is frequent slight loss of urine.

★ **Biofeedback** helps women with incontinence control the muscles of their bladder and urethra. A success rate of 55-80 percent is common with twice-daily use. Buy your own machine or use one at a clinic. The ultimate biofeedback machine, of course, is your body and its senses.

★ **Empty** the bladder *completely* every time you void by pressing down behind your pubic bone with fingertips or the flat of your palm. This can be a critical move in changing your relationship with your bladder.

Step 3. Nourish and tonify . . .

★ Boil dried **teasel** (*Dipsacus sylvestris*) roots, a tablespoon/15 ml to a cup/250 ml of water for ten to fifteen minutes, and drink daily to strengthen and restore tone to overstretched sphincter muscles. This is a favored and specific cure for incontinence.

★ It's all in the timing. One of the most effective remedies for occasional and even chronic incontinence is **scheduled toileting**. Go to the toilet on a regular schedule, say every 60-90 minutes. After 3-4 consecutive dry days, increase the interval by 15-30 minutes, and continue increasing until you can handle intervals of four hours or more.

• Some women report a daily eye-opener of **cranberry juice** (not "cocktail," *real* juice) helps relieve urge incontinence.

★ The very best cure for any kind of urinary incontinence, even when caused by surgical damage or postmenopausal thinning of the bladder walls, is regular **pelvic floor exercises** (Kegels). Women who do 8-12 Kegels three times a day improve more than those on all other treatment. Directions for doing Kegels are on page 188. Like any tonic, they give the best effect when done regularly and repeatedly for months or years. Once you're accomplished, you can Kegel your way through that overwhelming urge and sedately stroll to the toilet. Whew!

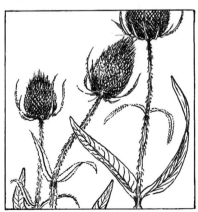

Teasel - *Dipsacus sylvestris*

Step 4. Stimulate/Sedate . . .

★ Push hard on the very top of the head to relieve urge incontinence on the spot.

• **Antispasmodic herbs** such as black cohosh, ginger, catnip, and cornsilk may help when incontinence comes from a hyperactive bladder (more frequent with urge incontinence than stress incontinence). Use 10-20 drops of **black cohosh** tincture once or twice daily for several weeks or as needed. A tea of any of the others may be taken freely. **Ginger** will warm and help relieve constipation (which may contribute to urge incontinence). **Catnip** is so relaxing that it can be sleep-inducing. **Cornsilk** is an excellent herb for strengthening the bladder and removing minor infections; however, it is also a diuretic, which might cancel its benefits for some women.

• Limit coffee to one cup or less a day to limit incontinence. Avoid alcohol and white sugar; they aggravate both stress incontinence and urge incontinence. And beware of bladder irritants: cayenne, hot peppers, artificial sweetners, citrus, tomatoes, iced drinks, very cold foods, pineapple, and carbonated drinks.

★ Cross your legs before you sneeze or cough.

• Regular use of tobacco increases your risk of developing stress incontinence by 350 percent.

• The **water cure** aims to pump energy into the pelvic floor and strengthen the bladder. Set out two shallow basins: one with very hot water and one with icy cold water. Start by relaxing for three minutes in the hot one. Then lower yourself up and down, in and out of the icy water for one minute. Repeat 3-4 times; do it several times a week. (My mother would call this the kind of remedy where the cure is worse than the problem!)

★ Wear clothes that come down or go up easily so you don't have to fiddle when you want to piddle. Forget girdles, jumpsuits, and tight pants. And reconsider high heels; they appear to make incontinence worse.

★ Women with stress incontinence who leak only during certain activities may find dryness with a pessary or tampon to support and lift the neck of the bladder temporarily.

• Women with stress incontinence who tried the NeoControl Pelvic Floor Therapy System not only improved (77 percent) but stayed improved for at least four months (48 percent). You sit, fully clothed, on a special chair while magnetic fields in the seat stimulate pelvic-floor muscles to contract. (I wouldn't make this up!) Treatment is by prescription only: two 30-minute sessions a week for eight weeks.

• Similar, but simpler, is the probe that you place in your vaginal canal twice a day for 15 minutes. It electrically stimulates Kegels. Wow!

• The Physiostim machine expands the concept. It stimulates pelvic floor contractions electrically. Then you try to duplicate the motion yourself while a biofeedback machine tells you how close you're getting.

Step 5b. Use drugs . . .

★ Behavioral treatments (Kegels, biofeedback, scheduled toileting) are significantly more effective (81percent) in reducing urge incontinence than drugs (68 percent) such as Detrol (tolterodine tartrate) and Ditropan (oxybutin chloride). You also avoid side effects such as dry mouth, severe memory impairment, and blurred vision.

★ Common prescription and non-prescription drugs that can provoke incontinence: antihistamines; diuretics; antidepressants; hypertension drugs including beta-blockers, Minipress (prazosin), reserpine, ACE inhibitors; sleeping pills, tranquilizers, sedatives; anticholinergics, and urinary tract anti-infectives.

• Hormone creams can reverse incontinence; hormone replacement does not seem to prevent it however.

Step 6. Break and enter . . .

★ Surgery is a risky cure for incontinence. Newer techniques, such as TVT (tension-free vaginal tape) resolve stress incontinence for 87 percent of women, and they remain dry for years. Older techniques only helped about 50 percent of women; and half of those were left so continent, they could not empty their bladders at all after the surgery.

• Injectable bulking agents (collagen, fat, or carbon-coated beads) can reduce leakage for some women with stress incontinence. If this works, you have to keep doing it, as the material resorbs.

★ Protect your hips! Invest in a chamber pot. Women with urge incontinence are 34 percent more likely to break a bone than women with little or no incontinence. When? Rushing to the bathroom at night.

"Having experienced episodes of urge incontinence all my life, I have watched carefully to see what triggers them. And for me it is clearly linked with sub-clinical urinary tract infections. So long as I'm totally infection-free, I don't go until I'm ready to go."

Bladder Infections

"If you let that fiery wise blood just sit there in your belly, great grand-daughter," admonishes Grandmother Growth, "you'll get the urge to quench that heat. You'll get a tickle, a twinge, an urgent call. But you won't have the moisture you need. It's boiled away. It's gone up in steam.

"So I'll say it once more: circulate your wise blood, granddaughter. Spiral it around and up to your crown. Take action on your anger. Pleasure yourself. And you'll be one of those old crones, like me, whose eyes sparkle with mirth and flash with intention."

Step 1. Collect information . . .

Bladder infections are also known as cystitis, urethritis, and UTIs (urinary tract infections). When bacteria grow in the bladder, the result-ing infection usually causes symptoms such as: a burning sensation during voiding, overwhelming urgency, frequent but minuscule urina-tions, incontinence, bloody urine, and pelvic pain. *Up to 25 percent of bladder infections in postmenopausal women are asymptomatic.*[76]

Bacteria enter the bladder in three primary ways: when feces are spread to the bladder opening (such as wiping from back to front after toileting), when the tube leading to the bladder is irritated or bruised (as from use of a diaphragm, pelvic surgery, or prolonged/vigorous vaginal penetration), or when there is an in-dwelling catheter.[77]

The thinning and shrinking of reproductive and bladder tissues that may occur in the postmenopausal years contributes to bladder infec-tions in older women, as does lessening of vaginal acidity.

Sometimes tiny ulcerations appear in the wall of the bladder; this is called interstitial cystitis (IC). Some of the remedies in this section are contraindicated for women with interstitial cystitis. (IC remedies on pages 200-202.)

Step 2. Engage the energy . . .

• **Flow, flow, flow.** Head off that bladder infection by drinking a glass of water hourly as soon as you feel the first urgency or burning. It is tempting to stint on drinking if you find yourself unexpectedly inconti-nent, but don't. Bladder infections only make incontinence worse.

• Urine is ideally neutral to slightly acidic (pH 5.8-pH 7). Very acidic urine (below pH 5.5) encourages infections. An established infection gives rise to alkaline urine (pH 7.5 or higher) which causes stinging and burning. Test your urine with pH paper at any time *except* first thing in the morning. Cranberry juice lowers pH; vitamin C raises it.

• *Cantharis* is a homeopathic remedy for scalding urine.

Step 3. Nourish and tonify . . .

• **Cranberries** (*Vaccinium macrocarpon*) contain substances that kill bacteria *and* make your bladder wall so slippery that bacteria can't live there. Unsweetened cranberry juice (or concentrate) is the most effective. (Sugars in cranberry cocktails and juice blends feed the infection.) Drink freely, at least a glass a day, up to a quart/liter a day for acute infections unless your urine's pH is already low.

★ Pelvic floor exercises help prevent and relieve bladder infections too! See page 188 and try this one: After urinating, close your eyes, relax, breathe out, and see if you can squeeze out an extra dribble.

• An overgrowth of vaginal yeast may be irritating your bladder or urethra. Eat one cup of plain yogurt 4-5 times a week.

Step 4. Stimulate/Sedate . . .

★ **Uva Ursi** (*Arctostaphylos uva ursi*) is an old favorite for strengthening the bladder and ending chronic infections. I infuse the dried leaves, but know women who have successfully used cold water infusions, tinctures, even vinegars. A dose is 1 cup/125 ml of infusion; 10-30 drops of tincture; 1 tablespoonful/15 ml of vinegar; 3-6 times a day initially, then 1-3 times a day for 7-10 days. In very chronic cases, eliminate all forms of sugar (even fresh fruit, fruit juice, and honey) as well.

★ **Yarrow** is a urinary disinfectant with a powerful antibacterial action and an astringent effect. A small cup of the infusion, once or twice a day for 7-10 days, tones up weak, lax bladder tissues. Combines well with uva ursi. Results may be felt within hours.

★ In my experience, *Echinacea purpurea* and *E. augustifolia* are as effective as antibiotics in clearing bladder infections (and, unlike

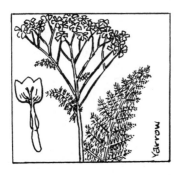

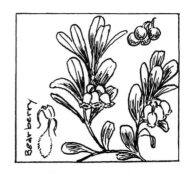

antibiotics, do not contribute to vaginal yeast). A dose is 1 drop tincture per 2 pounds/1 kilo body weight. In acute cases, I take a dose every 2 hours. As the infection clears, lengthen the amount of time between doses. Continue with 2 doses a day for another 2-10 weeks.

• Women who wash their vulva with soap and water are four times *more* likely to get vaginal and bladder infections. Douches, bubblebaths, tampons, nylon underwear, and pantyhose may also irritate the urethra and contribute to bladder infections.

• Known **bladder irritants** include: alcohol, black tea, coffee, sodas, citrus juices, chocolate, cayenne, and hot peppers. (An herbal tincture in an alcohol base won't irritate the bladder if you take it diluted in a glass of water or a cup of herb tea.)

•**Urinating after love play** flushes out bacteria and cuts down on UTIs. Urinating before love play increases your risk of a bladder infection.

Step 5a. Use supplements . . .

• Ascorbic acid wrings the kidneys, flushes the bladder, and raises urinary pH. Try 500 mg hourly for 6-8 hours. (*IC sufferers — avoid!*)

• Avoid calcium supplements. They increase bacterial adherence to the bladder wall, increasing bladder infections.

Step 5b. Use drugs . . .

• Antibiotics are standard treatment for bladder infections. But taking antibiotics frequently causes vaginal yeast overgrowth (which can lead to bladder infection). Nitrofurantoin (Macrodantin) often causes microscopic scarring and ulceration of the bladder wall, precipitating IC.

Step 6. Break and enter . . .

• Avoid dilation of the urethra. It is expensive, painful, and causes tiny scars on the urethra which may lead to interstitial cystitis. I have seen it referred to as "the rape of the female urethra."

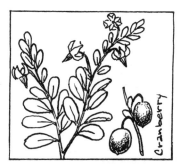
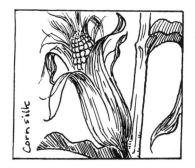

Interstitial Cystitis

Step 0. Do nothing . . .

• Getting a diagnosis of interstitial cystitis (IC) is not easy. It is under-diagnosed and the diagnostic procedure itself carries risk. (See Step 6.) If you have had recurrent bladder infections for more than ten years, especially if you do not respond to antibiotic therapy, you may have IC.

★ Relaxation techniques are quite helpful in relieving both chronic and acute pain from IC. Breathe out. Close your eyes. Let your body send pain-blocking hormones to your bladder.

Step 1. Collect information . . .

"Interstitial" means "in the interspaces of a tissue." Interstitial cystitis is a chronic inflammation of the space between the lining of the urinary bladder and its muscle, leading to ulceration and scarring.

Since women with bladder infections have bacteria in their urine, antibacterial drugs and herbs (such as yarrow or uva ursi) usually restore health quickly. Women with IC, however, have no bacteria in their urine, and antibacterial agents fail to relieve the distress.

Women with IC may have symptoms similar to those signaling a bladder infection. But in IC the symptoms become chronic and intensify into spasms, throbbing, and electric shock-like sensations that prevent sleep and interfere greatly with life. IC can scar and stiffen the bladder, decrease capacity, trigger incontinence and leaking, cause pinpoint bleeding, and even ulcerate the bladder lining.

There are about 550,000 people with IC in North America, 90 percent of whom are women between the ages of 40-60. The cause of IC is currently a mystery. One theory says it may occur in women exposed to heavy metals at very young ages.

Step 2. Engage the energy . . .

• **Cranial-sacral adjustments** gently adjust the flow of energy, relieving IC pain for some women.

• **Thoughts of suicide** were reported by 55 percent of women diagnosed with IC. While it is understandable to want to end such pain, don't do it. My teachers tell me that dying (naturally or by suicide, no matter) is like stopping the movie: wherever I am, whatever I feel, is where I will be, and what I will feel, until my next rebirth. Instead, try Stephen Levine's meditations on opening to pain in *Who Dies?* And read page 116 in this book, "Thoughts of Suicide."

Step 3. Nourish and tonify . . .

★ **Mallows** of any kind make a delightfully soothing infusion for irritated bladders. Marsh mallow (*Althea officinalis*) is the classic, but I've also used *Malva sylvestris*, *rotundifolia*, and *neglecta*. Soak a small handful of the fresh root or 2 tablespoons/12 grams of the dried in 8 ounces/250 ml water overnight; strain and drink next morning.

• Most women with IC find correlation between symptoms and foods. This is highly individual, but the most **problematic foods** seem to be: avocados, bananas, cranberries, peaches, strawberries, tomatoes, tofu, fava beans, lima beans, nuts, vinegar, yogurt, sharp cheeses, white flour products, and brewer's yeast.[78]

• Vegetables that tend not to aggravate symptoms include carrots, celery, green beans, and zucchini.

★ Regular use of **Kegel exercises** (see page 188) strengthens the muscles surrounding the bladder, increases circulation of lymph and blood, tonifies the bladder wall, and reduces symptoms.

★ **Comfrey leaf infusion** (2-4 cups a day for several weeks) eases burning sensations in the bladder and vagina. If you don't like the taste, add some mint — or use it as a sitz bath.

★ **Barley broth** brings fast, soothing results. Cook one cup/250 ml barley in 8 cups/2 liters water until soft. Drink 1 cup/250 ml at least every other day for a month or more.

Step 4. Stimulate/Sedate . . .

• **Anti-inflammatory herbs** provide powerful pain relief. But be cautious; remember, any new substance can increase distress. Be sure to use tinctures or glycerates, not capsules.

☞ **Osha root** (*Ligusticum porteri*) tincture, 3-5 drops at a time, repeated up to four times a day, stops swelling in the mucous tissues; try it when your belly feels heavy and full.

☞ **Poke root** (*Phytolacca americana*) tincture, 1-2 drops at a time and only once a day, has a special affinity for women and the pelvis; try it when your pain is cyclical.

☞ Tincture of the fresh flowering tops of **St. Joan's wort** (*Hypericum perforatum*), 20-30 drops as many as six times a day, relieves nerve pain; try it when the pain is electric.

☞ **Black cohosh root** (*Cimicifuga racemosa*) tincture, 10-15 drops, up to three times a day, is a menopause herb that is also an antispasmodic. Just the thing to relieve pain that is sharp and stabbing.

• Stimulants such as coffee, black tea, green tea, alcohol, tobacco, chocolate, and sex (even with oneself) may exacerbate symptoms, alas. Food preservatives, food dyes, carbonated drinks, aspartame, and saccharine do too.

★ **Acupuncture** treatments may relieve IC. According to one expert, Dr. Matthew Lee, half of those who will experience relief will do so in three sessions, and 95 percent of those who will benefit will do so in six sessions. Similarly, a few visits (but only a few) to a chiropractor may be helpful. CAUTION: In my experience, many chiropractors and acupuncturists believe you must wait for months before seeing improvement. Women with interstitial cystitis should expect results within weeks.

Step 5a. Use supplements . . .

• Dyes and binders in most supplements aggravate symptoms of IC.

• Women with IC who took **L-arginine** supplements (500 mg three times a day) had half as many symptoms as those who took a placebo.

Step 5b. Use drugs . . .

• Ibuprofen is useful for occasional symptomatic relief of mild discomfort. Avoid aspirin; it is associated with bleeding of the mucosal membranes, a potentially dangerous side effect for those with IC.

• Prescription antidepressants taken in small doses (10-40 mg a day at bedtime) can block pain, calm spasms, and decrease inflammation.

• Estrogen replacement, especially vaginal estrogen creams, can reduce symptoms for some menopausal women according to Dr. Elizabeth Lee Vliet. She cautions that progesterone tends to inhibit formation of the protective lining of the bladder and is therefore contraindicated, or to be used in the lowest possible dose, by women with IC.

Step 6. Break and enter . . .

• Definitive diagnosis of IC in the Scientific tradition requires general anesthesia so the bladder may be entered with fluids, gases, and instruments and examined.

• Intravesical treatments deliver steroids, anti-inflammatory agents such as dimethyl sulfoxide (DMSO), and the mild anti-clotting drug sodium pentosanpolysulphate by catheter directly into the bladder, often on a weekly basis. Only half of the women treated will experience any lessening of pain, and that may take 6 months to a year.

• Unfortunately, women who have their bladder removed in hopes of removing the source of their pain frequently suffer from "phantom bladder" pain. Women who undergo hysterectomy find it aggravates the symptoms of IC. Nearly half (44 percent) of women with IC have had a prior hysterectomy.

Postmenopausal Bleeding

"Crones hold their wise blood inside," declares Grandmother Growth. "Crones stir their wise blood inside. Your menses have stopped. Crones hold their wise blood inside."

Step 1. Collect information . . .

Vaginal bleeding in a postmenopausal woman is generally cause for alarm, but not for panic. There are a few benign causes: A sudden increase in optimum nutrition, such as the addition of nourishing herbal infusions to your diet, may tickle one or two last eggs into developing, causing a "normal" menstrual cycle. So can falling in love, they say. Blood spots during or after love play generally come from slight tears in more delicate older vaginal tissues or small cervical polyps (generally benign), commonly found among crones.

If you rule out these possibilities, seek help from someone experienced in women's health care.

Dry Mouth

"Yes, you must learn to spit it out, great-granddaughter. Say it out loud, sing it, express it for all to hear," says Grandmother Growth, licking her lips. "What? Mouth dry with stage fright? Chew this over with me, young Crone. Loosen your lips (speak your heart), expand your tongue (learn another language) and find the strength in your jaw (stand up for your rights). Is your mouth moist now?"

Step 1. Collect information . . .

Dry mouth is not caused by aging. Salivary gland function remains strong in healthy people, no matter what their age. However, dry mouth may be a temporary problem during the menopausal years.

Decreased saliva production is a minor annoyance but a major health hazard. Without adequate saliva, teeth and gum tissues quickly become abraded, infected, and demineralized. As oral health declines, so does heart health and the ability to take in adequate nourishment. Use these remedies to help prevent such problems in your Crone years.

Step 2. Engage the energy . . .

• Fear is the emotion connected with dry mouth. (See pgs. 121-124.) Remember that fear is the messenger of hidden desires.

Step 3. Nourish and tonify . . .

★ Drink rice or barley water. Boil a handful of grain in 4 cups/1000 ml water for an hour. These soothing grain beverages nourish deeply, supporting the body's ability to keep the mouth moist.

•Sip nourishing and soothing herbal brews such as **sassafras** leaf tea, **violet** leaf infusion, **marsh mallow** root tea, or **comfrey** leaf infusion throughout the day.

• Begin your day with a bowl of mouth-watering oatmeal and slippery elm. Replace up to 1 tablespoon/15 ml of 1/2 cup/125 ml dry oatmeal with slippery elm bark powder before cooking in 2 cups/500 ml water.

Step 4. Stimulate/Sedate . . .

★ The easiest way to stimulate and encourage saliva production is to suck or chew on something. Try slippery elm lozenges, malt-sweetened hard candies (available in health food stores), a piece of dong quai, or licorice root (not licorice candy).

• Smoking slows saliva output; so does consumption of alcohol.

• Massage under the jaw, along the center of the bone, to relieve spasms in the salivary glands.

Step 5a. Use supplements . . .

• Dry mouth is related to deficiencies of iron, calcium, potassium, B_6.

Step 5b. Use drugs . . .

★ Medications are the major cause of dry mouth. Nearly 400 commonly prescribed drugs — including antihistamines, decongestants, antidepressants, and high blood pressure medications — list dry mouth as a side effect. With the exception of licorice root, which may be contraindicated for those taking blood pressure medicines, the remedies in Steps 2, 3, and 4 are effective and safe to take with medications.

Postmenopausal Vaginal/Bladder Changes
References & Resources

Bergner, Paul. "Herbal/alternative management of urinary tract infections." *Medical Herbalism,* Fall 1991

Chalker, Rebecca & K. Whitmore. *Overcoming Bladder Disorders: Compassionate, Authoritative Medical* and *Self-Help Solutions for Incontinence, Cystitis, Interstitial Cystitis, Prostate Problems, Bladder Cancer.* HarperCollins, 1991

DeMarco, Carolyn, MD. *Take Charge of Your Body.* Well Woman Press, 1994

Gardener, Joy. *The New Healing Yourself.* Crossing Press, 1989

HIP: Help For Incontinent People from PO Box 544, Union, SC 29379
  • Audio tape and booklet on pelvic floor exercises; also, *Resource Guide for Continence Aids & Services* for $3

Home Remedies for Vaginitis. Santa Cruz Women's Health Center, 250 Locust St., Santa Cruz, CA 95060 ($.50 plus SASE)

Interstitial Cystitis Association, PO Box 4178, Great Neck, NY 11207

Interstitial Cystitis Association of America, 51 Monroe St., Suite 1402, Rockville, MD 20850, 800-HELPICA

Interstitial Cystitis Network, 4773 Sonoma Hwy, #125, Santa Rosa, CA 95409, 707-548-9442

Interstitial Cystitis Society, PO Box 28625, Burnaby, BC, Canada, V5C 6J4

National Association for Continence, 800-BLADDER

pH paper (ColorpHast) by mail from EM Science, 480 S. Democrat Rd., Gibbstown, NJ 08065 800-222-0342

Porcino, Jane. "Urinary Incontinence" in *Growing Older, Getting Better.* Addison-Wesley, 1983

Simon Foundation for Continence, Box 835-F, Wilmette, Illinois 60091, 800-23SIMON • www.simonfoundation.org

Vliet, Elizabeth Lee, MD. *Screaming to be Heard, Hormonal Connections Women Suspect and Doctors Ignore.* M. Evans & Co., 1995

"Urinary Incontinence in Adults." NIH Consensus Program Information, PO Box 2577, Kensington, MD 20891 • Free

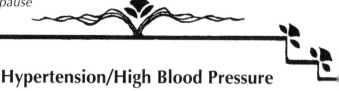

Hypertension/High Blood Pressure

★ Deep relaxation and yoga breathing, such as alternate-nostril breath calms the sympathetic nervous system, thus relaxing the small arteries and permanently lowering blood pressure.

★ Use the tincture of **hawthorn**, **motherwort**, or **dandelion** to reduce hypertension, tonify your heart (and blood vessels), and eliminate excess fluid. Regular use for 2-3 months may be necessary before results are measurable. (These tonifying herbs literally rebuild your blood vessels and heart muscle, and that takes some time.)

★ **Potassium** is the critical mineral for maintenance of healthy blood pressure. The great majority of hypertensives (80-85 percent) who eat six portions of potassium-rich foods daily reduce their need for medication by half or more. See Appendix 1 for sources of potassium.

★ Eat 1/2 clove of raw **garlic** a day and watch your blood pressure drop. My favorite raw garlic dishes:
  ☞ Scrambled eggs topped with minced raw garlic.
  ☞ Tomato sauce with chopped raw garlic added just before eating.
  ☞ Yogurt cheese with minced raw garlic on whole wheat crackers.
  ☞ Minced raw garlic on a baked potato.
  ☞ Herb vinegar and minced raw garlic on cooked greens like dandelion, spinach, kale, collards, mustard, amaranth, or lamb's quarters.

★ **Ginseng** is well documented as a highly effective blood pressure regulator. So is seaweed.

• Hypertensive medications lower blood pressure by draining fluids from circulation (diuretics) or by blocking the nerve signals that constrict the arteries (beta blockers). But diuretics may actually increase the risk of heart attack by leaching potassium salts needed by the heart; and the heart may respond to blocked nerve signals by trying harder, and harder, until it fails.

   If you currently take blood pressure medications, and wish to experiment with easing off them, do it gradually, monitor your blood pressure several times a day, and use one or more of the above remedies for several weeks first.

• Regular consumption of meat, coffee, table salt, and more than one alcoholic drink a day increases blood pressure. To lower it: Eat meat once a week, drink nourishing herbal infusions daily, use seasalt and seaweed.

Heart Healthy

"Open your heart to me, my own," whispers Grandmother Growth so softly you aren't certain you hear her. "Open the wisdom way of compassion here in your heart and draw me inside. Let Grandmother Growth be inside you, helping you encompass the whole, in the beat of your own heart, my heart, Crone's heart."

Step 0. Do Nothing

• Thinking of taking hormones to keep your heart healthy? Think again. Retrospective studies do show a connection between ERT/HRT use and less mortality from heart disease, but no double-blind study (a more dependable measure) does. In fact, two recent studies — the Heart and Estrogen/Progestin Replacement Study (HERS, 1998) and the Women's Health Initiative (2000) — found the oppostite to be true.

Estrogen does lower LDL and increase HDL cholesterol, but the connection between cholesterol and women's heart disease is weak. (Most heart attack patients don't have high cholesterol levels.)

Estrogen raises blood pressure (one of the top three reasons for heart attacks in women), increases triglycerides, promotes clotting (a leading factor in heart attacks and strokes), and raises levels of C-reactive protein (a marker for inflammation associated with heart disease). Taking progestin/progesterone increases the risk even more.

For a healthy heart, don't take hormones.

Step 1. Collect information . . .

". . . during the first two years of postmenopausal hormone replacement therapy there is a slightly greater risk of heart attack, stroke and blood clots."   — Women's Health Initiative, April, 2000

Heart disease is America's top killer of men and women. We are told postmenopausal women are as likely as a man to die from heart disease. But, according to Susan Love, MD, women in their sixties and seventies have 45 percent less heart disease than men their age. Menopause does not increase heart disease — age and lifestyle do.

The women in the often-cited Nurses Health Study who were least likely to die of heart disease not only took hormones, they ate well, exercised regularly, and did not smoke — behaviors that are critical to heart health. The simple truth is **more than 90 percent of all heart disease is preventable with lifestyle choices**.

The three top risk factors for heart disease in women are belly fat, smoking, and untreated hypertension. High cholesterol is one of the top three risk factors for men, but not for women. (After menopause, women make heart healthy hormones from cholesterol.)

The Nurses Health Study — which followed 86,000 women for 14 years — shows what happens to those wise old Crones who follow heart healthy behaviors:

☞ Those who ate more fish than meat, plus plenty of **whole grains**, beans, leafy greens, fruits, and vegetables reduced their risk of heart disease by one-third compared to those who ate a "normal" diet. (One serving a day of whole-grain foods reduced heart attacks by 34 percent in another study of 34,000 postmenopausal women.)

☞ Those who ate at least 5 ounces of **nuts** a week were only half as likely to have a heart attack as those who ate none.

☞ Those who **walked** a total of three hours per week or who exercise vigorously for at least 90 minutes a week had one third fewer heart attacks than those who got no exercise. Those who walked more cut their risk in half. (Another study found walking for even one hour a week halved the risk of coronary artery disease, even for high-risk women.)

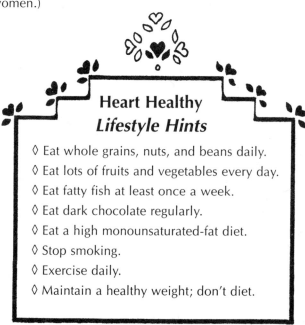

Heart Healthy Lifestyle Hints

◊ Eat whole grains, nuts, and beans daily.

◊ Eat lots of fruits and vegetables every day.

◊ Eat fatty fish at least once a week.

◊ Eat dark chocolate regularly.

◊ Eat a high monounsaturated-fat diet.

◊ Stop smoking.

◊ Exercise daily.

◊ Maintain a healthy weight; don't diet.

Step 2. Engage the energy . . .

• **Rose** flower essence and rose quartz essence engage heart energy.

• Do you attack your heart? Do you close it to protect it? Try Stephen Levine's meditation "Opening the Heart" in *Who Dies?*

• Give yourself plenty of nice strokes so you won't have a bad stroke.

• People in Hawaii, New Mexico, and Arizona have the healthiest hearts in the United States. Imagine you live there.

★ **Smile!** Depression increases your risk of both heart attack and stroke. In fact, severe depression is more strongly linked to stroke risk than high blood pressure, high cholesterol, smoking cigarettes, being overweight, and nine other known risk factors. When you smile, your brain makes hormones that make you, and your heart, feel good. So, smile.

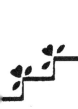 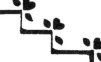

Healthy Heart Hints
Stop Smoking

Tobacco is highly addictive and you can beat it. Get an extra edge on quitting by nourishing yourself with a handful of freshly toasted sunflower seeds and a cup of nettle or oatstraw infusion daily for 4-6 weeks before you stop smoking. Sunflower seeds reduce cravings for nicotine by filling the nicotine receptor sites. Nettle and oatstraw strengthen nerves and cushion the impact of withdrawal.

Nourish yourself the Wise Woman way when you want tobacco:

◊ Take an oatstraw bath. (See Appendix 2, page 253.)
◊ Get a massage.
◊ Eat a wild salad (even if it's only one dandelion leaf).
◊ Bring home a flower.
◊ Let someone cook dinner for you.
◊ Go to a yoga class or a martial arts class.
◊ Buy something for yourself instead of cigarettes.
◊ Miss your smoke break? Take a break for pleasure!
◊ A weight gain of 15 pounds/7 kilos is normal for quitters.
◊ Nicotine withdrawal causes constipation (remedies page 44).
◊ Read, get, buy *The No-Nag, No-Guilt, Do-It-Your-Own-Way Guide to Quitting Smoking* by Tom Ferguson, MD, Ballantine, 1987.

Step 3. Nourish and tonify . . .

★ **Touch and be touched.** People who are touched lovingly every day have significantly fewer heart problems than those who aren't.

• Environmental Nutrition Newsletter (52 Riverside Dr, NY, NY 10024) lists the "Top Ten for Preventing Heart Disease": nuts, fish, whole grains, garlic, soy, psyllium, B vitamins, vitamin C, vitamin E, and plant sterols.

★ **Nuts** to heart attacks. Volunteers on diets with 35-40 percent of calories from nuts (and olive oil) lower LDL cholesterol by 13-17 percent. Greek women eat this way, and have one of the lowest rates of heart disease in the world. Monounsaturated fats in nuts are released more slowly into the blood and cleared more completely than those in oils.

• **Essential fatty acids** (EFAs) are essential for a healthy heart. Get them from fish (salmon, sardines, trout, herring are highest), seeds, whole grains, beans, and nuts. EFAs are especially abundant in wild seeds such as **plantain** (related to psyllium), **lamb's quarter**, and **amaranth**. And in **cod liver oil**. Women whose diets are rich in alpha-linolenic acid (an EFA) have the lowest risk of fatal heart attacks.[79]

★ If you eat meat, also eat foods rich in folates and other **B vitamins**, such as leafy greens, whole grains, and beans. Animal proteins require a lot of B vitamins (especially B_6) for complete utilization. Without them, homocysteine (an amino acid found abundantly in meat) is concentrated in the blood. Postmenopausal women with the highest levels of homocysteine have twice the coronary risk of those with the lowest levels (and more dementia, too).

★ Many studies have shown that daily use of vitamin E supplements (200 IU) cuts heart attack risk in half. A study of 34,486 post-menopausal women found "those with the highest **vitamin E intake from food** (not supplements) had the lowest heart disease risk.

• **Garlic**, Knoblauch, Ail (*Allium sativum*) is a great friend to old hearts. Several cloves a day of fresh, raw garlic (see page 206) can lower blood pressure, reduce phospholipids and cholesterol, strengthen heart action, increase immune response, reduce platelet clumping and clotting (thus reducing strokes), and stabilize blood sugar levels.

Don't like raw garlic? Use powdered! A four-year study found women who ingested 900 mg (1/4 teaspoonful) of garlic powder daily had 18 percent less arterial plaque than those taking a placebo.

"What emerges is a clear association of heart disease with . . . consumption of devitalized, processed, fabricated food items, including sugar and fructose, soft drinks, fortified white flour, milk and egg powders, caffeine, synthetic vitamins, vegetable oils, and hydrogenated fats." — Sally Fallon

★ **Seaweeds** are superior for the heart. Their clinically proven cardiotonic effects include: stabilization of blood pressure; regulation of triglycerides, phospholipids, and cholesterols; prolongation of the life of the heart muscle; and maintenance of a steady heartbeat.

★ **Motherwort**, that dear friend of menopausal women, is a favorite heart tonic. A dose of 10-20 drops of the tincture of the flowering tops, taken up to three times a day, helps lower blood pressure, strengthen heart action, ease palpitations and irregular heartbeats, and makes room in the heart for compassion.

• Women who regularly eat foods rich in **carotenes** cut their risk of stroke by 40 percent. Women who eat **broccoli** at least once a week have roughly half the risk of heart disease as women who eat none.

★ **Hawthorn** berry tincture is the standard herbal heart tonic, and for good reason. It is broadly effective, virtually without overdose, and easy to make from fresh or dried berries. An elegant shrub or small tree, hawthorn is frequently cultivated in the suburbs. Injectable forms were used by MDs up until the 1950s to treat vascular heart disease, high blood pressure, inflammation of the heart muscle, and arteriosclerosis. The action of hawthorn is slow but complete. It strengthens the heart, establishes a regular heartbeat, relieves water build-up around the heart, and resolves stress throughout the cardiovascular system. Dose is 25-40 drops of the berry tincture, up to 4 times a day. Expect results no sooner than 6-8 weeks. CAUTION: Hawthorn potentiates the action of digitalis, warns herbalist Chris Hobbs.

★ Keep your heart healthy by eating **chocolate**. Sound too good to be true? Despite its reputation, chocolate is loaded with heart healthy phytochemicals. Cocoa's *tretramers* curb oxidation of the blood vessel walls, short-circuiting the build-up of atherosclerotic plaque; they also help keep the vessels relaxed, keeping blood pressure down. Chocolate's *flavonoids* are more powerful than vitamin C in limiting oxidation of LDL; they protect all lipids in the blood from free-radical damage. Procyanidins are flavonoids that work like mild aspirins, keeping the blood thin and free-flowing.

Polyphenols are heart-healthy substances found abundantly in red wine, green tea, and chocolate. Daily use may prevent stroke by delaying blood clotting time. (.75 ounces/20 grams of dark chocolate = one-half cup tea = one glass red wine.)

Chocolate also prevents blood platelet fragmentation (which occurs when platelets get sticky), and boosts HDL (good) cholesterol. No wonder it often comes in heart-shaped boxes!

• **Lemon balm** is so strengthening to the heart, it is said those who drink it daily will live forever. Brew fresh or dried leaves in a cup of water for 5-10 minutes. Or steep fresh leaves in a glass of white wine for 1-2 hours and drink with dinner. Or enjoy 1-2 tablespoons/15-30 ml of the vinegar.

• You don't have to sweat, but you do have to **move**! to keep your heart healthy. Even ten minutes a day helps. You can do it. Do it! No excuses.

• **Dandelion root** tincture is a friend to the heart as well as the liver. Regular use lowers blood pressure and keeps your heart and cardiovascular system healthy and happy. A dose is 10-25 drops with meals.

★ Eliminating refined flour and sugar, and **limiting total carbohydrates** has halved the cholesterol of several friends with totals above 400.

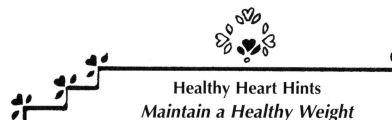

Healthy Heart Hints
Maintain a Healthy Weight

Postmenopausal women nourish healthy hearts by making desired weight changes very slowly. Chinese herbalists consider it dangerous to the heart to *lose* weight after the age of forty. "Eat right; do not worry about weight," sums up their attitude and mine.

◊ **Up**: Once you have attained your full size as a Crone (usually one size bigger than premenopause), maintain that weight. You don't need a scale. Take a pinch of belly fat. Less than two inches? You're fine.

◊ **Down**: Easiest way to lose weight? Move more! And eat more: whole grains, vegetables, fruits. To melt off excess, you have to make "no" effort. That is, you have to say "no" to white sugar and white flour in any form.

◊ **All over**: Restricted diets promote heart attacks. Frequent dieting, fasting, bingeing and purging unbalance electrolyte levels, weaken the heart muscle, and damage blood vessels.

◊ **Just right**: Drink water and herbal infusions as your daily beverages. Enjoy green, black, and herbal teas whenever you wish. Use fruit and vegetable juices sparingly. Limit coffee to no more than a cup a day. Avoid all soda pops, carbonated waters, diet drinks, fruit drinks, and sweetened beverages.

Step 4. Stimulate/Sedate . . .

★ **Blood thinners**, like aspirin, reduce the incidence of strokes and diminish mortality from heart disease by reducing platelet aggregation and inflammation. Blood-thinning herbs — **alfalfa** (*Medicago sativa*), **birch** (*Betula*), **sweet clover** (*Melilotus*), **bedstraws** (*Galium*), **poplar** (*Populus*), **red clover** (*Trifolium pratense*), **willow** (*Salix*), and **wintergreen** (*Gaultheria procumbens*) — do the same. A dose of two teaspoons/10 ml of a vinegar made from the leaves, buds, and/or flowers of any of these provides the benefits of aspirin, plus bone healthy minerals and acids to improve digestion.

★ Instead of aspirin or blood-thinning herbs, have a drink. A review of 25 studies done over the past two decades found a direct link between moderate **alcohol** consumption (for women, no more than one drink a day) and reduction of death from ischemic stroke and heart attack. All kinds of alcohol reduce platelet aggregation and increase HDLs. As an added benefit, postmenopausal women who have 2-3 drinks a week have better bone density than teetotalers.

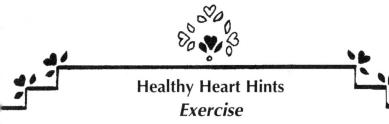

Healthy Heart Hints
Exercise

Your heart and circulatory system thrive on vigorous movement. Frequent small doses of physical activity are more heart healthy than infrequent heavy workouts. Thirty minutes of exercise a day will do, and you can do it in little pieces. **Nettle** infusion increases stamina and energy. A cup for breakfast and another at lunch will make you want to exercise, you'll be so full of get-up-and-go.

◊ Take a five-minute stretch break for every hour of work.
◊ Use the stairs (down counts, too).
◊ Park farther away; walk the extra distance.
◊ Keep a jump rope, light weights, or a frisky dog handy.
◊ Stand up when you talk on the phone; stretch, move.
◊ Turn on dance music while you wash dishes and sweep up.
◊ Go on a hike or camp out at least once this year.
◊ Become friends with someone who loves to exercise.

★ A bacterial infection (*Chlamydia pneumoniae*) may trigger arterio-sclerosis. For heart health, take a dropperful of an **anti-infective herb** — such as echinacea, hyssop, St. Joan's wort, usnea, or yarrow — for 10-20 days, twice a year.

Step 5a. Use supplements . . .

• Women aged 55-69 who took 500 mg of **calcium** daily were 44 percent less likely to die from heart attack and 35 percent less likely to develop heart disease than those who did not.[80]

• Get your **magnesium** from food. In one study, those taking 360 mg magnesium supplements were *more likely* to suffer a second heart attack, need a bypass, or die a sudden death than those taking the placebo.

★ Rice fermented with **red yeast** is prescribed by Chinese herbalists for those with high cholesterol and triglycerides. Interestingly enough, this remedy (sold as **Cholestin**) is chemically identical to the drug lovastatin (Mevacor), which blocks cholesterol production. In conjunction with exercise and good diet, two 600 mg capsules of Cholestin daily can lower blood cholesterol by as much as 40 points in eight weeks. CAUTION: Avoid if you have a liver problem or drink heavily.

★ **Niacin** supplements (*not niacinamide*) reduce mortality from heart problems. The recommended dose is 500 mg with meals (three times a day). CAUTIONS: Niacin causes a hot-flash-like flush lasting about 30 minutes after ingestion. The more regularly you take it, the less often this happens. Discontinue if you become nauseated or have gastrointestinal distress. Do not use if you have gout, diabetes, liver disease, gastric ulcers, or coronary heart disease. Avoid time-release capsules.

Step 5b. Use drugs . . .

• Postmenopausal women who took 1-6 aspirins a week reduced cardiovascular disease by 32 percent. But daily use can contribute to cerebral hemorrhage and gastrointestinal disorders, including bleeding ulcers.

★ Women who take lovastatin or pravastatin increase their risk of breast cancer. (In one study, 12 of the women taking pravastatin developed breast cancer while only 1 of those taking the placebo did.)

Step 6. Break and enter . . .

★ Have your blood tested for factors that signal danger. High levels of **homocysteine** are strongly associated with hardening and blocking of blood vessels. A three-year study of 28,000 postmenopausal women found those with the highest **C-reactive protein** levels four times more likely to have heart disease then those with the lowest levels.[81] Postmenopausal women who take hormones have very high CRP levels.[82] High levels of **lipoprotein (A)** triple your risk of heart attack and stroke.

★ A postmenopausal woman is one-and-a-half times more likely to die of a heart attack than a man. What makes heart attacks so deadly for women?

☞ Women's symptoms are not as severe as men's. No crushing chest pain for us. We feel short of breath or have difficulty breathing, have an ache in our jaw or neck, get cramps similar to gas pains, or feel suddenly exhausted. (Both men and women have nausea, vomiting, intense anxiety, or headache as the heart attack occurs.)

☞ Woman are reluctant to call an ambulance. It takes most women an hour longer to get to the hospital than men.

☞ Women are not treated with the same sense of urgency when they do get to the hospital. "Gender based inequities exist in the utilization of hospital resources . . . and may ultimately reflect important differences in adjusted hospital mortality."[83]

★ Think you're having a heart attack? Call for help *immediately*. (Worried about raising a false alarm? Better embarrassed than dead.) Chew and swallow an adult aspirin. Go to the *nearest* hospital, even if it does not have a special cardiac care unit. A heart attack does the most damage in the first two hours.

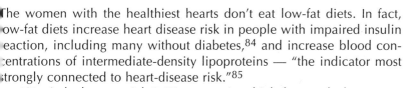

Healthy Heart Hints
Eat the Right Fats

The women with the healthiest hearts don't eat low-fat diets. In fact, low-fat diets increase heart disease risk in people with impaired insulin reaction, including many without diabetes,[84] and increase blood concentrations of intermediate-density lipoproteins — "the indicator most strongly connected to heart-disease risk."[85]

Worried about weight? Dieters eating high-fat meals lose more weight. For heart health, eat more — monounsaturated — fat, please.

◊ Eat fatty fish at least once a week.
◊ Eat organic meat, and eat less of it.
◊ Use only olive oil; other oils increase inflammation.
◊ Enjoy your eggs: they're full of heart-healthy lecithin.
◊ Eat bittersweet chocolate, organic if possible.
◊ Eat freshly roasted almonds and sunflower seeds.

Memory Loss/Dementia/Alzheimer's

"Touch my face, granddaughter," murmurs Grandmother Growth. "Feel the lines that time has worn. Each line tells a story. Feel the lines in my palms. Every line is a memory.

"Close your eyes and travel with me to your ovaries, real or energetic. They are your memory baskets. When you feel forgetful, close your eyes and journey to the place of memories. Touch your face, your palms, return to this place, and retrieve the memory you want.

"And, dearest," Grandmother's voice sighs with the wind, "remember for yourself. You are busy now with Change, and truly do not need to remember for others. Remember for yourself. Remember yourself."

Step 0. Do nothing . . .

• Improve your memory fast with meditation. Start with five minutes a day. You can do it! Breathe out.

Step 1. Collect information . . .

• Does ERT/HRT reduce the incidence of Alzheimer's disease? A double blind study of 120 women found 80 percent of those taking ERT had less memory, less ability to perform daily tasks, and less cognitive functioning after fifteen months of hormones.[86]

• Neurobiologist Fred Gage overturned conventional wisdom by proving that fresh cells grow in our hippocampus — a brain region critical to learning and memory — our entire lives.

Step 2. Engage the energy . . .

• Double-blind studies on drugs against memory loss, dementia, and Alzheimer's consistently find a very strong placebo response. Use this to your advantage. Label a pill bottle "Memory Pills," fill it with almonds (or any placebo of your choice), and take one a day to improve memory.

Step 3. Nourish and tonify . . .

★ **Ginkgo biloba** tincture has been well studied as an ally for people dealing with Alzheimer's and dementia. In one study, among those who took the leaf extract, 27 percent maintained cognitive functioning and memory, while 86 percent of the placebo group lost functioning. CAUTION: Ginkgo increases aspirin's blood-thinning effects.

• Seafoods contain dimethylaminoethanol (DMAE), believed to help nourish the brain.

★ Herb researcher Dr. James Duke says the **mint family** can help prevent memory problems and reduce dementia. His favorites are oregano, rosemary, savory, and thyme (all rich in rosmarinic acid); peppermint and spearmint (which also contain the anticholinesterase compound 1,8-cinerole); and self-heal (*Prunella vulgaris*). Eat them; drink them!

★ **Mental exercise** (word puzzles, reading, writing) and **physical exercise** tonify the brain and memory. Memorize poetry; participate in community theater. The more you use your memory, the stronger it is.

• Low levels of **B vitamins**, especially B_{12} and folate, are strongly associated with dementia and Alzheimer's disease. Fish, meat, milk, and eggs are the best sources of B_{12}; nourishing herbal infusions supply generous amounts of folate.

Step 4. Stimulate/Sedate . . .

• **Lower your blood pressure** and improve your memory. Women with even moderately high blood pressure (164/89) have slower reaction times and more memory problems than those with normal blood pressures. A dose of 1 dropperful/1 ml of motherwort tincture daily, an increase in exercise, and a cup of nourishing nettle infusion four or five times a week will lower blood pressure and improve memory.

Step 5a. Use supplements . . .

★ **Vitamin E** has a powerful reputation as a brain booster. One trial found daily doses of up to 2000 IU (a staggeringly large dose) did not improve memory, but did delay institutional care. My father started using vitamin E supplements (first 200 IU, then 400 IU, finally 800 IU a day), and ginkgo (2-4 dropperfuls/2-4 ml a day) at the fist signs of his dementia, delaying his need for drugs by 10-15 years according to his doctor. (For cautions, see page 91.)

• Supplements of choline have not been found to be effective in slowing the progression of cognitive and memory problems.

Step 5b. Use drugs . . .

• Selegiline is a known anti-oxidant with powerful effects on the brain. Like all drugs, it can have nasty side effects.

• Anti-inflammatory drugs, such as prednisone and colchicine, are somewhat successful in moderating memory loss and dementia.

Osteoporosis Risk Factors

Every "yes" increases your risk. If you have four or more "yes"es, read this chapter carefully.

◊ I am white-skinned with a fair complexion.
◊ I am thin/petite.
◊ I smoke cigarettes every day.
◊ I have 10 or more alcoholic drinks (including beers, wine) a week.
◊ I drink at least three cups of coffee daily.
◊ I eat animal protein at least twice a day.
◊ I eat salty, processed food (chips, meats) regularly.
◊ I drink carbonated soda (even "healthy" kinds) daily.
◊ My ovaries were removed (or ceased functioning) before I turned 40.
◊ I breast-fed two or more children before the age of 25.
◊ I have given birth to more than six children.
◊ I have never been pregnant.
◊ I frequently diet or fast; was/am anorexic/bulimic.
◊ I was malnourished as a child or as a teenager.
◊ I am a vegan/vegetarian who eats a lot of tofu and soy beverage.
◊ I work sitting down/am restricted to a wheelchair or bed/ don't exercise.
◊ I have exercised to the point where I lost my period.
◊ I have not eaten dairy for ten or more years.
◊ I did/do receive long-term adrenal steroid/cortisone therapy.
◊ I take diuretics on a regular basis.
◊ I take anticonvulsants such as Dilantin or phenobarbitol.
◊ I have kidney disease/am on dialysis.
◊ I have chronic diarrhea/often take antacids/am a gastrectomy patient.
◊ I am hyperthyroid/hyperparathyroid/take thyroid medication.
◊ I am diabetic.

Note: *High-risk women benefit from exercise, yogurt, and nourishing herbal infusions, even if, especially if, they elect to use drug therapy.*

Osteoporosis

"Metamorphosis means complete Change, great-granddaughter," says Grandmother Growth, in time to her drum beat. (Or is that your heart?) "And menopause is metamorphosis. To change completely, you must dissolve the old outline, then fill in the new one. As a baby Crone, you saw your rigidity soften, your willpower dissolve, your very bones growing open. Now you are ready to re-form yourself, to recast yourself, to create a new standing for yourself in your community."

Step 1. Collect information . . .

There is a certain chill slide of fear in thinking about the dreadful sound of bone breaking, the horror of being a stooped old lady, the slip that breaks a hip, landing you in a wheelchair, or even the grave. (As many as 30 percent of those over sixty who break a hip die as a result.)

And that fear starts with the word *osteoporosis* (loss of bone mass). Osteoporosis means thin bones. Does that mean more prone to breakage? No. We are led to believe it is so, but osteoporosis does not equal broken bones. Studies of women aged sixty and older consistently find that low bone mass does *not* correlate with higher fracture rates.[87] The American College of Physicians says: "The majority of women with hip fracture have a density of the hip that is within the normal range."

That's really frightening. If preventing osteoporosis isn't the key to preventing fractures, what is?

"Dear daughter," chuckles Grandmother Growth, "the answer is simple, though it may surprise you: consume plenty of protein and fat, eat mineral-rich grains and beans, grow and eat your own vegetables (and the weeds), become friends with nettle, oatstraw, and seaweed, take time to enjoy yourself, and, whenever you can, chop wood, carry water."

Nourishing the whole woman, not just the bones, is the goal of the Wise Woman Tradition. Calcium supplements, drugs, and hormone replacement may prevent or halt osteoporosis, but they don't create healthy women. Regular exercise, whole foods, and nourishing herbs not only prevent and halt osteoporosis, but also create healthy women free of heart disease, breast cancer, and depression.

Improving bone mass does not improve a woman's health. There is a negative correlation between bone mass and breast cancer: post-menopausal women whose bone mass is the highest have four times more breast cancer than those whose bone mass is the lowest.

Even healthy women lose some mass during the menopausal years. Demand for minerals is so high that the bones rarely get enough, and the changing hormones may disrupt utilization. But once your menopausal **Change** is complete, bone mass is easily rebuilt.

Step 2. Engage the energy . . .

• **Safety first.** Preventable falls are the biggest cause of broken bones, especially after the age of seventy, when 90 percent of all hip fractures occur.[88] Install safety bars in the bathroom. Test vision and hearing regularly. Wear sensible shoes. Make carrying a cane fashionable. Beware the effects of alcohol and prescription drugs. Wear protective underwear with **hip shields**: among frail patients 80 and older, falls were 84 percent less likely to cause a hip fracture if a protector was being worn.

★ Counter early warning signs of osteoporosis (see box, **next page**) with this **visualization**. Envision yourself as a skeleton. Your bones as very white. They are a thick milky white, dense cooked-egg white, blank piece of paper white, thick, flexible white.

• Is osteoporosis hereditary? No. Genetic factors do play a part in determining bone mass, but genetics do not predict fractures.

• The homeopathic cell salt *Silica* strengthens bones.

Step 3. Nourish and tonify . . .

★ Motivated menopausal and postmenopausal women, even those diagnosed with osteoporosis, can increase bone mass by as much as six percent in six months with this four-step plan:

☞ Eliminate all soy products except tamari and miso. (Unfermented soy prevents you from utilizing calcium.)

☞ Drink a quart of nourishing herbal infusion (nettle, oatstraw, red clover, or comfrey leaf) at least four times a week.

☞ Use at least 2 tablespoons of *Old Sour Puss Mineral Mix* on your food daily. (The minerals in greens are specialists in building bone, especially when coaxed into solution in vinegars and infusions.)

☞ Eat a quart or more of yogurt a week. (See next page.)

For optimum bone health, also:

☞ Eliminate all foods containing white sugar or white flour.

☞ Drink no more than two cups of coffee or two soft drinks a week.

Surprised I suggest dairy? Many sources maintain that meat and milk *cause* osteoporosis. Not so.

Meat and milk, butter and cheese are mainstay foods of the healthiest people of all races. When these products come from animals on pasture, and are part of a diet rich in fruits, vegetables, legumes, and whole grains, calcium flows freely to the bones, and fractures are rare. High protein diets correlate strongly with a decreased risk of hip fracture in women.[89,90] High-protein, mineral-rich nourishing herbal infusions give us double protection for bone health.

But herbs and greens don't contain enough fat for true bone health. All fat soluble vitamins — A, D, E, K — are critical to bone health, and deficiencies in any of them lead not only to osteoporosis but to brittle, breakable bones. It is important to get minerals from green sources, but when we add animal fats to them, the nutrients are far better utilized.[91] (Did your granny put a piece of fatback in her collards as they cooked?)

To my mind there is no more perfect food than organic full-fat whole-milk yogurt. It's rich in bone-building minerals (a cup supplies one-third of your daily postmenopausal need for calcium). It contains fats to aid absorption of those minerals. And, because it is fermented, yogurt contains little or no lactose, and improves digestive functioning. It is an immune system booster, as well.

Some animal protein (dairy or meat) is critical for optimum bone health. Postmenopausal women who eat equal amounts of protein from animal and vegetable sources have the least bone loss and the lowest fracture rates.[92]

Optimum bone health requires nutrients from animals and plants.

Early Signs of Osteoporosis

◊ Persistent backache, especially in the lower back.
◊ Severe or sudden periodontal disease, gum infections, loose teeth.
◊ Sudden insomnia and restlessness.
◊ Frequent leg and foot cramps.
◊ Gradual loss of height. Check yearly by measuring from fingertip to fingertip (arms outstretched) then down your back from head to heels. The measurements should be equal.

• **Exercise** (a vigorous 50 minute walk four times a week) and a **calcium-rich diet** (1650 mg daily) reversed osteoporosis in a year-long study of 36 postmenopausal women. Bone mass increased in those who exercised, irrespective of calcium levels (non-exercisers lost 7 percent).[93]

★ **Weight training** builds strong flexible bones (but gardening is even better). Begin with 1 pound/.5 kilo weights. Sit in a sturdy hard-backed chair (wheelchair is fine). Lift one weighted foot or hand straight out in front of you. Hold for 1-3 seconds; lower *slowly* and rest for 1-3 seconds. Repeat. Work up to a set of 10 lifts for each arm and leg.

★ **Yoga, tai chi,** and stretching exercises promote balance and flexible, break-proof bones. But get a clock. Stretch for 60 seconds. It increases flexibility and range of motion twice as fast as stretching for 30 seconds.

•Women who get 1500 mg of **calcium** daily from food reduce their fracture rate by as much as 75 percent. But those who exercise, even if they get little calcium are no more likely to break a bone than those who exercise little and consume lots of calcium.[94]

★ **Horsetail** is a favorite herb for restoring bone density and healing fractures. One woman in her 60s successfully healed three broken vertebrae (from a skiing accident) with a horsetail/comfrey leaf infusion and was back on the slopes, cautiously, in less than three months.

• Older stomachs may not produce enough hydrochloric acid to free calcium and other minerals from foods. **Dandelion** root tincture, 10-25 drops taken before meals, will remedy this.

★ Include in your daily diet at least three of these bone builders:
☞ 1 cup/250 ml of yogurt or whey
☞ A big mug/300 ml of calcium-rich herbal infusion (see page 261)
☞ 2 cups/500 ml fresh or 1 cup/250 ml cooked dark greens
☞ 1 tablespoon/15 ml herbal vinegar (see page 261)
☞ 2 tablespoons/30 ml blackstrap molasses
☞ 1 teaspoon/5 ml seaweed such as kelp or wakame

★ Natural **vitamin D** is critical for flexible, strong bones. Women with osteoporosis lack it. Up your levels with a daily dose of **sunlight** (10-15 minutes between 8 a.m. and 4 p.m.) or **cod liver oil**. Sunblock blocks production of vitamin D almost completely.

★ Keep your thyroid healthy (see pages 52-56). It produces **calcitonin**, an important hormone that maintains bone density.

"My grandmother started doing these weighted lifts last year when she turned 100. This year, at 101, she fell backwards over a planter and landed hard on her hips, suffering no more than a bruise and some loss of dignity."

Anyone for an Old-Fashioned Stroll?

Exercise is a postmenopausal woman's most powerful ally. It makes bones thicker, more flexible, resistant to breaks. And walking is one of the easiest and best ways to do it.

Active postmenopausal women have the fewest fractures; sedentary ones have the most, irrespective of diet.

Moderate exercisers reduce hip fracture risk by 42 percent and vertebral fracture risk by 33 percent. Two hours of exercise per week can be done in 4 thirty-minute sessions, 8 fifteen-minute sessions, 12 ten-minute session, or 24 five-minute sessions.

Even one hour a week of low intensity activities (walking, gardening, dancing) significantly reduces fracture risk.

Any exercise, even non-weight-bearing exercise, is a lot better than nothing. *Go for it,* no matter how much you do.

Weight-Bearing Exercise

◊ walking
◊ jogging
◊ bicycling
◊ hiking
◊ tai chi
◊ jumping rope
◊ arm and leg lifts with weights

◊ X-country skiing
◊ gardening
◊ weight training
◊ snow shoeing
◊ climbing stairs
◊ playing tennis

◊ bowling
◊ golfing (no cart)
◊ yoga postures
◊ rowing
◊ dancing

◊ Start or join a women's **walking** club. Make friends, increase heart and lung capacity, strengthen bones, enjoy the scenery.
◊ Start or join a **dance** group. Dance with your girl friends; don't be shy.

Non-Weight-Bearing Exercise

◊ swimming (though it's good for your back)
◊ riding a horse (walking and grooming it is weight bearing)
◊ love-making (unless you stand up to do it)

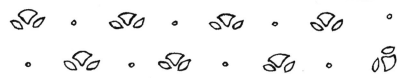

★ **Micronutrients** such as selenium, chromium, copper, boron, silicon, zinc, cobalt, and sulfur are vital for flexible strength in bones. Rich sources include seaweeds, nettles, dandelion, and horsetail.

Step 4. Stimulate/Sedate . . .

• Women who drink 2-3 cups of coffee daily, whether regular or decaffeinated, increase their risk of osteoporosis-related fractures by 69 percent; those who drink more increase their risk by 82 percent.[95]

"Osteoporosis-related fractures are easy to prevent: just decrease coffee and alcohol, increase exercise and calcium."   — New York City gynecologist

• **Weak electrical charges** (therapeutic EMFs) stimulate bone growth, increasing mass and healing fractures. Machines make them, so do:
☞ weight-bearing exercise   ☞ massage
☞ hands-on energy treatments   ☞ crystals
☞ sexual tension and release   ☞ tai chi and chi gung
☞ pressing with fingertips into the middle undersides of both feet

★ Women with high systolic **blood pressure** (148 or above) lose bone mass twice as fast as those with systolic pressures under 124.

Step 5a. Use supplements . . .

• Thinking of using **progesterone cream**? Think again. Dr. Lee's studies show benefit from ProGest cream.[96] All other studies have found negligible effects in healthy menopausal and postmenopausal bones.[97]

★ **Microcrystalline hydroxapatite** deposits minerals into the bones, reversing osteoporosis and healing compression fractures of the spine.

★ **Vitamin D** from sunlight is harder to make as we age. Vitamin D supplements can help old bones. The dose is high: 400-600 IU if younger than 70; 600-800 IU if older. (Vitamin D toxicity for elders begins at 2000 IU.)

• **Calcium supplements** are not nearly as effective as a calcium-rich diet.[98] Women who took 1500 mg of calcium daily for four years had denser neck, back, and thigh bones, but significantly *more* arm, leg, wrist, rib, and hip *fractures* than a control group.[99]

• For every milligram (3,333 IU) of **vitamin A** as retinol consumed in supplements, cod liver oil, and fortified foods the risk of hip fracture rises "a staggering 68 percent." Carotenes do not have this effect.

"Osteoporosis can be induced by a diet deficient in any of about ten micronutrients."   — From a study on dietary causes of osteoporosis

• **Fluoride** increases bone density. In one study, women who drank fluoridated water had fewer hip and spine fractures. In another, post-menopausal women whose drinking water contains 4 parts fluoride per million incurred more than twice as many fractures as those whose drinking water had little or none (regardless of calcium ingestion).[100]

• If boron-rich organic produce and grains are not part of your diet, you may wish to supplement with 3 mg of **boron** daily.

Step 5b. Use drugs . . .

★ Use of long-acting tranquilizers or antidepressants increases falls among the elderly by 200 percent or more, and these falls are more likely to result in fractures.

• Low doses of doxycycline or minocycline (types of tetracycline) show promise in slowing age-related bone loss.

• **Hormone replacement** can reduce the risk of osteoporotic fractures by as much as fifty percent, if combined with exercise and adequate calcium intake. But exercise and adequate calcium intake alone reduce postmenopausal fracture rates by fifty percent and do not increase cancer risk.

New "designer hormones" seek to avoid estrogen's cancer-promoting effects on the breasts and uterus. Collectively known as SERMs (selective estrogen receptor modulators), they include tamoxifen, raloxifene (Evista), droloxifene, idoxifene, and levormeloxifene. While SERMs seem effective in helping postmenopausal women maintain bone mass their use increases the risk of blood clots and death from stroke. **The risks of taking hormones almost always outweigh the benefits.**

• Other drugs that are used to slow or halt osteoporosis include:

☞ A synthetic version of **calcitonin** is used to decrease vertebral fractures and increase bone density in women more than five years past menopause. (It has little effect earlier.) It can also cause flushing, nausea, and diarrhea; and you can become resistant to it.

☞ Bisphosphonates, such as Didronel (etidronate), Actonel (risedronate) and **Fosamax** (alendronate) stop bone cells from breaking down by coating them in a crystalline covering. This decreases new fractures and stops height loss. The downside is severe irritation of the esophagus unless taken following strict rules. The Fracture Intervention Trial found 5mg (half the usual dose) as effective as 10 mg. When you stop taking bisphosphonates (seven years is the upper limit for use), bone "density will not decline as fast as it does when you quit HRT."

☞ **Ipriflavone** is a synthetic derivative of isoflavones. Although it is currently used in more than two dozen countries as a treatment for osteoporosis, recent double-blind studies conclude that in post-menopausal women, ipriflavone neither prevents bone loss, nor reduces fracture risk. And it lowers the level of lymphocytes (white blood cells), making women more vulnerable to infection.

• Even a slight **overdose of thyroid hormone weakens bones**. If you take thyroid hormone, aim for the lowest effective dose.

• **Parathyroid hormone** is a natural protein that signals the body to make new bone cells. Among 1600 women with osteoporosis, those who took 20-40 mg daily for 2 years reduced fractures by two-thirds.

Step 6. Break and enter . . .

• Do you need a bone scan? Since 75 percent of all white women and 84-90 percent of women of color will not develop osteoporosis,[101] and since exercise and good diet are both prevention and cure, I say: "Skip the test and start walking."

• In the future, we may monitor bone health by testing saliva (or blood or urine) for bone loss markers such as interleukin-6 or osteocalcin.

"Research evidence does not support bone density testing of well women at or near menopause as a means to predict future fractures."
— British Columbia Office of Health Technology Assessment, 1998

Mending Broken Bones

"Knowing a woman's age is almost as good in predicting her risk of fracture as is measuring her bone mass."   — AMA, 1989

Step 1. Collect information . . .

Obviously, it is preferable to keep your bones strong rather than heal them, but many women simply don't until they break a bone. Even if you have osteoporosis, these remedies will help you heal more quickly and with fewer complications. They are wonderful allies for women undergoing total hip replacement as well.

If you suspect a broken bone, and don't want, or don't have access to, X-rays, try this. Place a vibrating tuning fork at one end of the bone in question. Then at the other end. If the bone is intact, the vibration will be pleasant; if broken, the vibration will be painful or uncomfortable.

In many instances, bones mend better in a splint rather than a cast. Ask your helper/doctor for a splint you can remove easily, so poultices and massages can be used to promote healing.

Step 2. Engage the energy . . .

• Shine a **blue light** on the broken bone, or visualize blue light surrounding it. This can significantly reduce the pain.

• Hatha yoga postures help the mending bones and muscles stay strong and vital. Find an experienced teacher and ask for help.

★ Bones lay down new cells best when there is a weak electrical charge passing through them. (See page 224.) Even imagining that you are exercising the broken limb increases the electrical flow!

• Is this a *breakthrough* for you at a basic/bone-deep level?

Step 3. Nourish and tonify . . .

★ **Horsetail** herb sparks bone cell growth. Add a tablespoon/3 grams to an ounce/30 grams of any one of the following bone-menders, infuse in 1 quart/liter of boiling water for 4 hours. Drink 2-4 cups a day.

◊ nettle leaves   ◊ raspberry leaves
◊ comfrey leaves   ◊ oatstraw grass
◊ red clover blossoms   ◊ mullein leaf

• Insure infection-free healing and prevent nerve damage by using 25-30 drops of **St. Joan's wort** (*Hypericum*) tincture once or twice a day.

Step 4. Stimulate/Sedate . . .

★ **Skullcap** tincture eases pain from broken bones. Try 3-5 drops every 30 minutes at first, then use as needed. Large doses are sleep-inducing, but not habit-forming. **Boneset** (*Eupatorium perfoliatum*) relieves bone pain too, but doesn't taste as good. A dose is a dropperful/1 ml.

★ Stimulate repair of muscles, tendons, ligaments, and bones with **comfrey**. Pour boiling water over the fresh or dried leaves. Steep for at least an hour. Place a cloth on the injury, then the warm comfrey leaves, a layer of plastic wrap, and finally a thick layer of towels. Remove when cool. Drink a cup or more of comfrey leaf infusion daily.

(Steps 5a, 5b, and 6 omitted on purpose.)

My Aching Joints

"Keep moving, keep moving, bend and flow, bend and flow, sweet sister," the ever-so-faint whisper of Grandmother Growth's voice plays around your ears. "Keep your wise blood circulating in your belly, moving through your spine, and flowing into action. Stay loose, stretch, reach, retain your flexibility. Move, flow, bend, and grow, sweet sister, grow."

Step 1. Collect information . . .

Whether it is age or changing hormones, more than half of all postmenopausal women experience occasional to severe joint pain. (Twice as many women as men suffer from aching joints.)

Aching knees, elbows, and shoulders are the most frequent aching joints at menopause. Aching hips, lower back, wrist joints often indicate deeper distresses such as worsening osteoporosis, kidney weakness or immune system dysfunction.

Don't ignore aching, swollen joints. Osteoarthritis (stiff, achy, lumpy, swollen, hot, noisy) can degenerate the joints. Rheumatoid arthritis (swollen, tender joints, sometimes accompanied by fever or fatigue) is an auto-immune disorder that can progressively deform joints until function is lost. But early treatment, especially when the joint begins to ache, can effect a cure and forestall further occurrences of arthritis.

Step 2. Engage the energy . . .

★ Sit or lie in a comfortable position and **visualize** your aching joints getting hotter and hotter. When they are as hot as you can bear, imagine them getting colder and colder. Go back and forth at least four times, ending at a temperature that feels just right.

• To help aching hips, shoulders, knees, elbows, find a **hatha yoga** teacher and attend class regularly. Joint mobility increases rapidly with the focused attention and gentle stretching of yoga postures.

• The majority of postmenopausal women who exposed their painful joints to light shining through a blue filter for 15 minutes a day experienced significant pain relief from their rheumatoid arthritis.

• Homeopathic *Hypericum* is the general remedy for sore joints.

Step 3. Nourish and tonify . . .

• **White birch**, Weissbirke, Boleau blanc (*Betula alba* and most other species) is an ally for the postmenopausal woman troubled by arthritis, uric acid build-up in the joints (gout), calcium spurs in the heels and feet, heart/kidney edema, arteriosclerosis, high cholesterol, hypertension, obesity, and chronic cystitis. A dose of the tincture of fresh leaves and buds is 1-2 dropperfuls 1-3 times a day; or you can use tea of the dried leaves freely.

• **Black currant** bud macerate soothes the pain of arthritis, rheumatism, allergies, headaches, and persistent hot flashes. A dose is 30-50 drops as needed.

★ Exercise is now advised for everyone with joint pain. Be gentle with yourself. **Swim in warm water** to safely exercise sore joints.

★ **Moxibustion** tonifies sore joints. The smoky warmth of the burning *Artemisia* eases pain and keeps joints open and flexible.

★ Massage **arnica** or **St. Joan's wort** oil into the painful joint for amazing relief. Or apply a fresh **chickweed poultice**.

• Vegetable oils promote inflammation through the action of their omega-6 EFAs. For supple joints, use only olive oil.

Step 4. Stimulate/Sedate . . .

★ Terrible as it may sound, getting stung by **nettle** on an aching joint can bring instant relief and help prevent further distress.

• Cold vegetables on hot joints are a great blessing. Try a poultice of tofu, grated raw potato, or squash.

• **Acupuncture** treatments have effectively relieved chronic joint pain for centuries. If you're afraid of needles, look for a doctor who uses transcutaneous electrical nerve stimulation (TENS).

★ **Ginger baths**, soaks, and compresses bring soothing, warm relief to sore and aching joints.

★ Sweat lodges, saunas, steam baths, mud baths, and mineral soaks penetrate the joints with intense heat and initiate healing energy and movement in the area.

• Some women report dramatic improvement in joint mobility and less pain when they eliminate one or all of these foods from their regular diet: sugar, nightshades (potatoes, tomatoes, eggplant, peppers), citrus, processed meats, vegetable oils (excluding olive), MSG, alcohol.

• **Poke** (*Phytolacca americana*) and **devil's club** (*Oplopanax*) are unusual plants of the east and west coasts of North America, respectively. The roots of both have long-lived reputations for easing joint pains, especially from rheumatoid arthritis. Dose of either root tinctured (*do not use dried poke root*) is 1-4 drops daily. Poke berries may be taken as well: 1-2 dried whole berries each morning. (The toxic seeds pass harmlessly through the digestive tract if you swallow the berries without chewing.) CAUTION: Poke root and poke berry seeds are considered highly toxic. I have used the low doses recommended here for more than fifteen years with highly favorable results.

★ A poultice of **cayenne** interferes with the body's perception of pain and triggers the release of endorphins (natural pain-relievers), offering instant relief from joint pain.

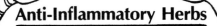

Anti-Inflammatory Herbs

Herbs that relieve joint pain, like drugs that relieve joint pain, may be rich in salicylates (aspirin is acetylsalicylic acid) and/or rich in steroids (cortisone is a steroid). Herbs, unlike drugs, also provide bone-building minerals, immune-strengthening micronutrients, and endocrine-nourishing glycosides. Why settle for less?

Salicylates are found in abundance in the bark, buds, and leaves of many herbs. Vinegar is the best medium for extraction; 1 teaspoonful/5 ml equals one aspirin. My favorites:

◊ willows (*Salix*)   ◊ poplars (*Populus*)
◊ birches (*Betula*)   ◊ black haw (*Virbunum*)
◊ true wintergreen (*Gaultheria procumbens*)

Steroids are found in the roots of many plants. Vodka tincture of the fresh roots of one or more of these steroid-rich herbs (10-25 drops as a dose) helps ease sore joints.

◊ wild yam (*Dioscorea*)   ◊ black cohosh (*Cimicifuga*)
◊ sarsaparilla (*Smilax*)   ◊ poke (*Phytolacca*)
◊ ginseng (*Panax*)   ◊ devil's club (*Oplopanax*)

Step 5a. Use supplements . . .

★ **Glucosamine sulfate**, alone or combined with **chondroitin**, gives miraculous relief to some arthritis sufferers. A naturally occurring substance made from sugar, it plays a significant role in the creation and maintenance of connective tissues, especially cartilage.

• **MSM** (methylsulfonylmethane) provides extra organic sulfur, a key building block of glucosamine sulfate and other joint components. Its pain relief is equal to that of over-the-counter nonsteroidal anti-inflammatories. It can prevent pain if taken before exertion.

★ **Fish oil supplements** can lessen joint tenderness, swelling, and stiffness within a few days.

Step 5b. Use drugs . . .

• Instead of non-steroidal anti-inflammatory drugs (NSAIDs), such as aspirin and ibuprofen, try salicylate-rich herbs (page 230); they don't cause internal bleeding, but they do reduce inflammation and pain. And instead of steroids, try steroid-rich herbs (same page); they don't promote osteoporosis and suppress the immune system, but they do relieve swelling and pain.

Step 6. Break and enter . . .

• Injection of cortisone into the affected joint may sometimes offer prompt relief. The trade-off is the deep harm done to the immune system. And sometimes it doesn't work at all.

• Ditto for gold injections.

Foot and Leg Cramps, Numbness

Step 1. Collect information . . .

Frequent leg and foot cramps or numbness of the extremities may be an annoying minor problem during or after menopause, or a symptom of some deeper distress. (Box, page 232.) The two most common causes of night cramps in postmenopausal women are use of tobacco and inactivity of the legs. Also see pages 233-34: Restless Legs Syndrome.

Step 2. Engage the energy . . .

• Try a warm **foot bath** with a few drops of essential oil of **peppermint** or **rosemary** right before bed.

Step 3. Nourish and tonify . . .

★ Ingest more **calcium**-rich foods. (See page 24.)

★ **Black haw** tincture or tincture of **St. Joan's wort** blossoms helps prevent and relieve muscle cramps. Try 20-25 drops just before bed.

Step 4. Stimulate/Sedate . . .

• A **hot bath** right before bed soothes muscles, increases blood flow, and can help you get through the night smoothly. Add **valerian** to the bath to promote deep sleep.

• Quinine is an old standby that still helps wonderfully well. Yes, it is in tonic water.

"As a pubescent girl, I had terrible foot cramps that would bring me bolt upright out of my sleep. I kept a cola bottle under my bed, and got relief in seconds by pressing and rolling the bottle on the floor with my foot."

Step 5a. Use supplements . . .

• A **calcium/magnesium** supplement (500 mg) taken at bedtime often relieves foot and leg cramps during the night.

• If that doesn't do it, add a 100 mg niacin supplement.

• Vitamin E supplements also help relieve cramping of the legs at night. See page 91 for doses and cautions.

• Numbness and cramping of the legs can be symptoms of an overdose or depletion of vitamin B_6.

Step 5b. Use drugs . . .

• Drugs can cause writhing and aching sensations deep in the legs.

Numb/Cramped Feet and Legs

Numb legs and cramped calves and feet could be caused by:

◊ Heart problems; use cardiotonic herbs, see pages 207-215.

◊ Osteoporosis; see pages 219-227.

◊ Smoking tobacco; hints for stopping on page 209.

◊ Inactivity; five-minute exercises on page 213.

◊ Hypothyroidism (low thyroid activity); use seaweed to increase available iodine. Read pages 52-56.

Restless Legs Syndrome

Step 0. Do nothing . . .

• Observe the feelings in your legs. Remain the observer. No need to move. Nothing to do. Mind serene. Emotions at peace.

Step 1. Collect information . . .

Legs that twitch and tremble. Legs that shake and ache. Creepy, crawly, tingly, burning, tugging, itching, prickling sensations that make you want to move your legs. It could be restless legs syndrome (RLS), especially if it strikes when you try to go to sleep and wakes you in the night. (Yes, it can include your arms.)

Also called leg jitters, *Ekbon syndrome*, *anxietas tibialis*, or *hereditary acromelalgia*, RLS may make a brief appearance during menopause, but is more likely to become a problem afterwards. It is fairly common, affecting about 15 percent of Americans, most of whom are over 50 years of age. It affects 20 percent of all pregnant women. RLS is both a movement and a sleep disorder, and tends to run in families.

Restless Legs Syndrome Foundation (877-463-6757) has more info.

As does Virginia Wilson's book describing her dance with RLS: *Sleep Thief: Restless Legs Syndrome*, Galaxy Books, 1996.

Step 2. Engage the energy . . .

• The movement of chi (life force energy) through the body is variously described as flowing, flaring, vibrating, and pulling. These are also descriptions of the sensations of RLS. Chi flow in the body increases notably (and sometimes uncomfortably) during and after menopause; it is possible that what you are experiencing is "merely" that. Try channeling the energy out of your legs and into creative or healing endeavors. This yoga pose can help: Sit on the floor with your legs in front of you and feet against a wall. Push your feet against the wall for a count of ten. Release. Repeat three more times.

Step 3. Nourish and tonify . . .

★ Muscles that lack minerals — especially **calcium** and **magnesium** — go into spasms and quiver. If this sounds like your legs, reach for a big glass of nourishing **oatstraw** infusion or a cup of **yogurt**.

★ Tired legs are more likely to stay quiet at night. So **exercise** it is. If you're stuck behind a desk, run in place sitting in your chair for several minutes every hour and take a walk during your lunch break.

★ Low blood levels of **iron**, with or without anemia, are strongly linked to onset and worsening of RLS. See page 9 and Appendix 1 for best sources. Or drink nourishing **nettle** infusion. It builds iron and strengthens the kidneys, too. (More than half of all patients with end-stage kidney failure have RLS.)

• RLS is also associated with **folic acid** anemia and a deficiency of **B vitamins**. Red clover infusion is rich in both, as are oatstraw, nettle, and comfrey leaf infusions. Rather than mix them, I alternate, drinking one each day.

• Losing sleep because of RLS? Consult pages 128-132 for sleep-inducing hints. A dropperful/1 ml of **St. Joan's wort** (*Hypericum*) tincture, taken 5-10 minutes before lying down, can help prevent spasms all night.

Step 4. Sedate/Stimulate . . .

★ A **warm bath** before bed can keep your limbs quiet all night.

★ **Massage** definitely helps, but doesn't cure, those with RLS.

• When RLS wakes you in the night: **Stretch**hhhhhhh those muscles by pointing your toes away from you and imagining someone is pulling on your leg. Think relaxing thoughts.

★ **Eliminate coffee and alcohol** for at least one month. Sometimes this effects a complete "cure."

• Alternate hot and cold packs on your legs for 30 minutes before sleep.

★ A cup or two of **kava kava** with dinner will relax your legs by bedtime and give you giggles in your dreams.

Step 5. Use drugs . . .

• Some evidence points to drugs as the trigger for the onset or worsening of RLS. Which ones? Calcium channel blockers, anti-nausea drugs, tricyclic antidepressants, serotonin reuptake inhibitors (SSRIs), lithium, some cold and allergy medications, and the anticonvulsant drug phenytoin.

• **Dopaminergic agents** (such as levodopa) are used occasionally or intermittently to relieve RLS, but can worsen symptoms over the long run. **Dopamine agonists** are effective for those with severe RLS. Long-term effects remain unknown. **Opiates** are addictive, but incredibly effective in calming restless legs. **Anticonvulsants** and benzodiazepines may be tried when all else fails. No single drug or dosage works best. Keep looking until you find what helps you.

References & Resources
Chapter 3: Post-Menopause

Periodicals

Crone Chronicles, back issues. PO Box 81, Kelly, WY 83011
HealthFacts, Center for Medical Consumers, 237 Thompson St., NY, NY 10012
Johns Hopkins Medical Letter on Health After 50, 550 North Broadway, Suite 1100, Baltimore, MD 21205
Sage Woman, PO Box 641, Point Arena, CA 95468

Books

Adams, Caroline Joy. *A Woman of Wisdom*. Celestial Arts, 1999
Bissinger, Margie. *Osteoporosis: An Exercise Guide*. Cornell, 1998 (Booklet #IMP 145, $10 from 800-762-7720)
Bolen, Jean. *Goddesses in Older Women*. HarperCollins, 2001
Budapest, Z. *Grandmother of Time*. Harper & Row, 1989
Calyx, ed. *Women and Aging: An Anthology*. Calyx, 1990
Doress, Paula. *Ourselves, Growing Older*. Simon & Schuster, 1990
Fisher, M.F.K. *Sister Age*. Vintage Books, Random House, 1983
Gardiner, Ruth. *Celebrating the Crone*. Llewellyn Pub., 1999
Hardin, Paula Payne. *What Are You Doing with the Rest of Your Life?* New World Library, 1992
Herself. *Peace Pilgrim*. Ocean Tree, 1982
Long, Christina & L. Quinn. *No Stone Unturned: The Life and Times of Maggie Kuhn*. Ballantine, 1991
Macdonald, Barbara. *Look Me in the Eye: Old Women, Aging and Ageism*. Spinsters/Aunt Lute, 1983
Martz, Sandra (ed.) *When I am an Old Woman I Shall Wear Purple*. Papier Mache, 1990
Morrison, Dorothy. *In Praise of the Crone*. Llewellyn Publications, 1999
Nelson, Miriam. *Strong Women, Strong Bones*. Putnam's Sons, 2000
Noble, Vicki. *Shakti Woman*. Harper, 1991
Porcino, Jane. *Growing Older, Getting Better*. Addison Wesley, 1983
Seaman, Barbara. *Women and the Crisis in Sex Hormones*. Bantam, 1978
Snowdon, David, Ph.D. *Aging with Grace*. Bantam, 2001
Starlanyl, Devin J. *The Fibromyalgia Advocate*. New Hampshire Publications, 1998
St. Armand, Paul & C.C. Merek. *What Your Doctor May Not Tell You About Fibromyalgia*. Warner Books, 1999
Walker, Barbara. *The Crone*. Harper, 1986

Organizations

Insure a happy cronehood for yourself and others; consider joining:

• Gray Panthers, 733 15th St. NW, Suite 437, Washington DC 20005
• Women's Initiative of AARP, 601E St. NW, Washington, DC 20049

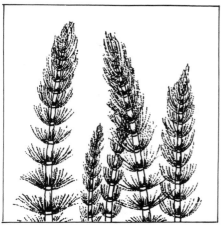

Horsetail — *Equisetum arvense*

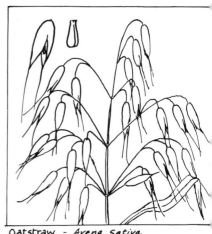

Oatstraw - *Avena Sativa*

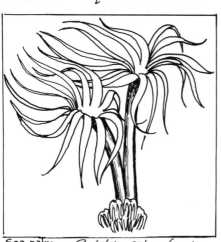

Sea palm — *Postelsia palmæformis*

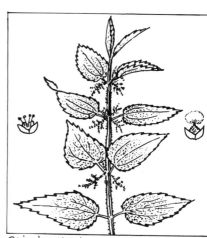

Stinging Nettle - *Urtica dioica*

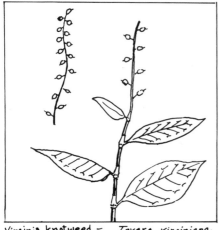

Virginia knotweed - *Tovara virginiana*

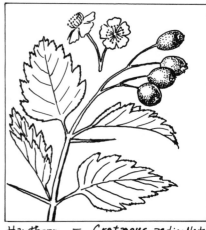

Hawthorn — *Cratægus pedicellata*

Herbal Allies for Postmenopausal Women

My favorite herbs for postmenopausal women are horsetail, oatstraw, red clover, stinging nettle, seaweeds, and the plants rich in flavonoids. These gentle green allies are more like foods than drugs; they offer bone-creating, heart-protecting, disease-preventing, sex-enhancing optimum nourishment to the woman in the second half of her life.

Horsetail
Equisetum arvense
Ackerschachtelhalm, Prêle des champs

Horsetail is particularly rich in glycosides which nourish hormones, heart, and bones, making it a special ally for postmenopausal women.
Use spring-picked horsetail, as a tea or infusion, to:

- *Reverse osteoporosis*
- *Stimulate fracture-mending and bone repair*

Mineral-rich horsetail feeds the bones, increasing mass and flexibility. No matter how old or thin, bones respond to consistent use of horsetail.

- *Stabilize and reverse chronic periodontal disease*

Gum problems can lead to heart problems. Brush, floss, and try a daily cup of horsetail tea. It acts as a catalyst to healthy gums and teeth.

- *Relieve cystitis*

Horsetail has been used since the sixteenth century to tonify the bladder and ease irritation anywhere in the urinary tract. Plants harvested when too old may aggravate rather than soothe.

- *Reduce bloat*
- *Check menstrual hemorrhage*
- *Prevent clogged arteries, strengthen veins*
- *Ease persistent hot flashes*

Horsetail's astringent components, trace minerals (including chromium), saponins, and flavonoids are responsible for these effects. Add horsetail to your nettle infusion to magnify the benefits of both.

- *Increase energy, reduce fatigue*

Horsetail supplies peppy potassium, merry magnesium, and strong-as-nails iron for building Crone power.

• *Nourish strong, healthy hair and fingernails*

Horsetail is frequently found in expensive shampoos and rinses. Instead, use leftover horsetail tea (alone or with nettle) as your final rinse. Leave it in. And drink a cup now and then for lovely nails.

Horsetail is locally abundant in the wild, so rarely cultivated. The small horsetail that looks like a soft baby pine tree is preferred over the rigid, leafless kind. To avoid silica problems, pick horsetail early, during the first 4-6 weeks of its growth.

A tea of dried herb works great, as does the vinegar. When buying horsetail, look for good green color and a rich sparkle of vitality.

Dosage: Tea of dried herb, 1 cup/250 ml, 1-2 times a day.
Vinegar of fresh herb, 1 tablespoon/15 ml daily.

CAUTIONS: If you experience nervous sensitivity or urinary irritability after use, discontinue.

Oatstraw Fan Club

Angela continued her pattern of premenstrual upset into her menopause, and was dubious that drinking the pleasant-tasting, mellow brew of oatstraw could have any effect on her "killing rage." Angela combined her oatstraw with a weekly yoga class and discovered she really wanted to paint. Two years later, she had her first piece in a show. "Rage is so much more interesting slashed across canvas," she told me, raising her cup of oatstraw with a wink.

"After three weeks of drinking oatstraw infusion I realized that I felt more emotionally resilient, more capable in stressful situations, more on-center than I thought was possible."

Vaginal dryness bothered Anne, but she was even more concerned that she seemed to have "misplaced my libido." Anne bought a big bag of sweet-smelling green oatstraw, drank her infusion morning and night, and did a sitz bath once a week. "Makes me too mellow to complain," she noted after the first week. Six weeks later, she called to say she felt sexier than she ever had, with plenty of lubrication. "Maybe it was the oatstraw," she mused, "and maybe I just needed to slow down and catch up with myself."

Oatstraw
Avena sativa
Gruen Hafer, Avoine cultivée

This is the grass of the very same oats you eat for breakfast. Best known as a cholesterol-lowering food, oats is also a special ally to women who wish they wouldn't "fly off the handle" so easily, to women who want to be sexy old ladies, and to women who treasure their bones. All the benefits of eating oatmeal are to be had from drinking oatstraw infusion (but not from tea, tincture, or capsules).

Let lovely Avena help you to:

- *Build strong, pliable, flexible bones*
- *Maintain firm, reliable teeth*

Rich in calcium — and the synergistic minerals and vitamins needed for best use of calcium — oats have a well-deserved reputation for building tough, hardy folks with tough, hardy bones.

- *Stabilize blood sugar levels*
- *Relieve depression and ease emotional uproar*

A cup of oatstraw infusion in the morning provides steroidal saponins to nourish your pancreas, liver, and adrenals and help prevent erratic blood sugar levels from playing havoc with your emotions.

- *Reduce cholesterol and risk of heart disease, improve circulation*

Oats and oatstraw can make your blood vessels more elastic, more vital. How will you notice? Your hemorrhoids and varicose veins will shrink, your heart rate will slow, and disturbances in your heart rate (such as palpitations and tachycardia) will diminish or disappear.

- *Nourish strong nerves*
- *Help you engage high energy currents*

Oatstraw and oats, both superior sources of the vitamin B complex, are exceptionally capable allies for women under stress.

- *Reduce frequency and duration of headaches*
- *Maintain restful sleep patterns*
- *Ease bladder spasms, incontinence, uterine pain, vaginal dryness*

Oatstraw infusion in your teacup and your bathtub (ahhh!) relieves physical and emotional pains and energy disturbances, and strengthens vaginal, bladder, and urethral tissues. (Oatstraw Bath, page 260.)

- *Be an outrageously sexy old lady.*

Dosage: Infusion of dried herb, 1-4 cups/250-1000 ml, daily.

CAUTIONS: None.

Seaweeds

The weeds of the ocean have so much to give. Let them help you:

- *Prevent and relieve osteoporosis*
- *Maintain strong, flexible bones*

Seaweeds contain lavish amounts of every mineral needed to create and maintain solid bone mass. Kelp is an exceptionally rich source.

- *Lower blood pressure and cholesterol, increase cardiac efficiency*
- *Eliminate varicose veins and hemorrhoids*

Japanese research confirms the cardiotonic and hypotensive effects of seaweeds.

- *Maintain healthy thyroid function*
- *Relieve incontinence, vaginal dryness, and persistent hot flashes*
- *Nourish the glandular and urinary systems*

Seaweeds are superb sources of the nutrients most needed by the endocrine, circulatory, and immune systems. Regular use helps maintain adequate production of all hormones, especially thyroid hormones. Lavish use may reverse hypothyroidism.

- *Increase immune functioning*
- *Increase stamina*
- *Minimize the effects of stress, chemicals, and radiation*
- *Lengthen life span*

Algin in seaweed escorts damaging compounds harmlessly out of the body. Free radicals are also eliminated. Vitamins E, C, and A are found abundantly in seaweeds. I use seaweed to protect myself from air pollution, chemicals in my food, and the thinning ozone layer. It can be used freely for several days before and after any X-ray, from dental ones to mammograms.

- *Improve digestion*
- *Restore sexual interest and enjoyment*
- *Ease sore joints*
- *Bring a glossy glow to hair and skin*

As befits denizens of the ocean, seaweeds are especially good at nourishing juices: digestive juices, joint juices, emotional juices, erotic juices. Seaweed helps them all flow.

All seaweeds are edible. Gather your own, if you wish. Kelp, wakame, kombu, dulse, hijiki, and arame are sold at health food stores.

**Dosage: As a vegetable, 1/2 ounce/15 grams dry weight, weekly.
As a condiment, unlimited daily use.**

CAUTIONS: Kelp's iodine may aggravate hyperthyroid conditions.

Stinging Nettle
Urtica dioica, Urtica urens
Brennessel, Ortie

Some postmenopausal women tell me stinging nettle is so nourishing and energizing they find themselves unexpectedly having a normal menstrual flow after regular use of it.

The more usual effects of nettle are to:

- *Nourish, strengthen, rebuild kidneys and adrenals*
- *Ease and eliminate cystitis, bloat, and incontinence*
- *Rehydrate dry vaginal tissues*

Nettle has a miraculous ability to heal and restore adrenal/kidney functioning. Stories continue to make their way to me of women who have avoided dialysis, gotten off dialysis, and so repaired their kidneys that replacement surgery was canceled, thanks to sister stinging nettle. Nourish your postmenopausal adrenals with nettle infusion and they'll produce enough estrogen to keep you looking and feeling juicy.

- *Nourish and energize the endocrine glands*
- *Nourish and rejuvenate the cardiovascular system*
- *Normalize weight*
- *Ease and prevent sore joints*
- *Relieve constipation and reduce hemorrhoids*
- *Nourish supple skin and healthy hair*

Nettle's super supplies of vitamins, minerals, proteins, and micro-nutrients nourish every bit of you, encouraging optimal functioning in all aspects of your being. Nettle influences hormones through its wealth of lipids (triglycerides, fatty acids, tocopherols, sterols, galactosyl-diglycerides) and restores health to the cardiovascular system burdened with cardiac edema and venous insufficiency.[102]

- *Create strong, flexible bones*

Nettle infusions, vinegars, and soups are fantastic sources of calcium, magnesium, potassium, silicon, boron, and zinc: the strong bone sisters. Nettles are also a source of vitamin D, a crucial nutrient for flexible, healthy bones.

- *Stabilize blood sugar*

Rich in chromium, manganese, and other nutrients restorative to glandular functioning, nettles, I suspect, help prevent adult-onset diabetes.

- *Reduce fatigue and exhaustion; improve stamina*

Nettles nourish your energy at the deepest possible levels with intense supplies of iron, chlorophyll, and copper.

• *Reduce and eliminate headaches*
• *Nourish and support the immune system, prevent cancer*
• *Nourish and heal the digestive system*
• *Nourish and strengthen the nervous system*

Nettles are an optimum source of the vitamins critically important for health: vitamin B complex (especially thiamine, riboflavin, and niacin), carotenes (vitamin A), and vitamin C (ascorbates and bioflavonoids).

Enjoy cooked nettle greens all spring, but be sure to harvest and dry enough for winter-time infusions, too. I pick nettles only before they flower. Fresh leaves steeped in olive oil impart a rich taste and innumerable healing qualities to the oil. Nettles make a great vinegar, too.

Dosage: Infusion of dried herb, 1-4 cups/250-1000 ml, a day.

CAUTIONS: Do not use flowering nettle for food or medicine.

Bioflavonoids

Plants containing flavonoids (from the Latin, *flavus*, yellow) were originally valued as dye plants. Today we appreciate them because we know they are *anti-inflammatory, antihepatotoxic, antimicrobial, anti-tumor, antiviral, antioxidant, antiallergic, anti-ulcer, analgesic,* and *strengthening to the entire circulatory system,* from capillaries to heart.

Flavonoids have an estrogenic effect, scientifically established as 1/50,000th the activity of estradiol. Bioflavonoids in foods are essential to our ability to absorb ascorbic acid. No wonder plants exceptionally rich in flavonoids are such important allies for post-menopausal women.

Regular use of bioflavonoid-rich herbs helps:

☞ restore vaginal lubrication   ☞ decrease or end hot flashes
☞ improve pelvic tone   ☞ improve liver activity
☞ strengthen the bladder   ☞ lower risk of stroke & heart attack
☞ reduce water build-up in tissues   ☞ reduce muscle cramping
☞ ease sore joints   ☞ improve resistance to infection

★ The richest source of bioflavonoids is the **inner skin of citrus** fruits. "Peel Power" is a lovely way to start the day. (See Appendix 2.)

★ **Buckwheat greens**, Buckweizen, Sarrasin (*Fagopyrum esculentum*) are an exceptional source of bioflavonoids. Grow them at home, like alfalfa sprouts, or buy them dried and made into tablets. (Kasha, the grain of buckwheat, does not contain bioflavonoids.) The wild equivalent is the leaves of yellow dock (*Rumex crispus*) or any knotweed (*Polygonum* species in the *Polygonaceae* family).

★ **Elder**, Holunder, Sureau (*Sambucus nigra* and other species) is rich in bioflavonoids. I use the berries in jelly and wine, and the flowers for tinctures and wines.

★ **Hawthorn**, Weissdorn, Aubépine (*Crataegus oxycantha* and other species) offers berries, flowers, and leaves full of bioflavonoids. I use the berries to makes jellies, wines, and a heart-strengthening tincture. The flowers and leaves, dried, make a wonderful tea.

★ **Horsetail**, Ackerschachtelhalm, Prêle des champs (*Equisetum arvense*) is best picked in the spring. I use it fresh in soups (not salads) and dried as a tea. (See page 237.)

• **Knotweeds**, Vogelknöterich, Renouée des oiseaux, Ho Shou Wu (*Polygonum* species) are well known for their abundance of bioflavonoids. In addition to buckwheat and yellow dock leaves, try the greens of any other knotweed local to your area.

• **Roses**, Hagrose, Rosier (*Rosa canina* and other species) are sisters to hawthorn and similarly abundant in bioflavonoids. I use fresh rose hips in jellies and wines and dry them for winter teas and soups. We eat the blossoms in salads and use glycerin to draw out the healing qualities of flowers and leaf buds.

★ **Shepherd's purse**, Hirtentäschel, Capselle (*Capsella bursa-pastoris*) leaves are wonderful in salads. When it flowers, I use the whole fresh plant to make vinegar and vodka tinctures, capturing bioflavonoids for later use. (A dose is 25-50 drops three times daily.)

• **Sea buckthorn**, Sanddorn, Argousier (*Hippophae rhamnoides*) leaves are rich in many nutrients needed by postmenopausal women: bioflavonoids, carotenes (vitamin A), vitamin C, vitamin E, and the B vitamin complex, especially B_6. If you live where it grows, try the tender baby leaves in salads.

• **Toadflax**, Frauenflachs, Linaire commune (*Linaria vulgaris*) flowers add flavonoids to salads. They can also be tinctured. (A dose is 15-20 drops.)

• **White dead nettle**, Weisse Taubnessel, Lamier blanc (*Lamium album*) doesn't sting, so try it in salads. Or dry bunches when it's flowering and get your bioflavonoids from the infusion; or make a vinegar.

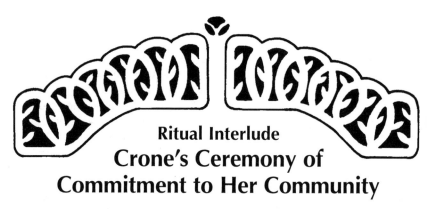

Ritual Interlude
Crone's Ceremony of Commitment to Her Community

As the menopausal years draw to a close and you find yourself more stable in your new self, feeling more like your "old self" as you become your older self, it is time to manifest the last stage of initiation: rebirth.

You've spent time in some form of isolation as you journeyed the unpredictable years of menopause. You have given death to your images of yourself as Maiden, as Mother. You have crowned yourself, or been crowned as, Crone. Your metamorphosis is complete. Now comes the time to return to your community. To assume your new roles.

You return as Crone. You hold your wise blood inside. You have learned how to spiral the updrafts of hot flashes. You have learned detachment in the midst of emotional hurricanes. You have submitted yourself to chaos and have witnessed the most ancient of all mysteries. How can you share this with your community?

In the days of the matriarchy, and in some matrifocal cultures yet, a woman who has completed her menopausal metamorphosis initiates young men into the ways of love play most pleasing to women. She is honored as the teller of truth and the keeper of peace. She is the tradition keeper and the people's link to the spirit world.

Today, there are no givens. We are each free to choose our own role as Crone. A ritual of commitment helps others know what your new roles will be. Here is one example to guide you.

*   *   *   *   *

For this ritual, gather an audience of friends, family, and significant others, the more the better. You could compare it, at least in mood, to a wedding or a christening. Wait until at least thirteen moons after your Crone's Crowning ceremony before doing this ritual.

Let there be music and sweet scents as you gather. At the appointed time, call everyone together to join hands. You alone remain outside the circle.

When the circle is complete, begin a hum, vibrating from the feet. Let it move and spiral until the group energy feels whole. With the hum of the group supporting you, ask nourishment, breath, and inspiration, the powers of the east, to be present. Ask heat, protection, and excitement, the powers of the south, to be present. Ask emotion, fluidity, and compassion, the powers of the west, to be present. Ask stillness, patience, and wisdom, the powers of the north, to be present. Ask the above and the below to be present. Ask the inner core of each person to be present.

Ask the circle to open and include you, symbolizing your return to community life. In your own words affirm: "I stand before you as self-initiated Crone, woman of wholeness. Though I have lived for many years, I expect to live for many more. Today, and for the rest of my life, I ask you to accept and honor me as Crone. And I wish to commit to you, my community and family, my intention as Crone to. . . ." (Speak your intent.)

The oldest woman present gives you a ball of yarn; she holds the end. You move around the circle, unwinding a long continuous thread into everyone's outstretched hands. When you're done, ask everyone to stretch the yarn taut between their hands, close their eyes and think of something they would like to end. After a minute of silence, begin to move to your right around the circle, cutting the yarn between their hands and saying, in your own words: "I am She-Who-Holds-Her-Wise-Blood-Inside. I have crowned myself Crone and accepted the responsibility of giving death. I cut the thread. I set it free." When you finish, invite each person to keep the yarn or to place it in a special basket, to be left outdoors as a give-away.

To close, hum as before, asking the entire circle to join you. Thank the energies and attributes of the seven directions (inside, below, above, north, west, south, and east). Then, let there be feasting and dancing, music and pleasure, flowers and feathers, spring water and herbal wine, lit candles and lovely clothing. You have completed your menopausal years. You are truly Crone, woman of wholeness.

*   *   *   *   *

This ceremony marks the beginning, of your new identity as Crone. Most older women I spoke with felt they didn't fully settle into their new self image until the age of 60, or after their second Saturn return.

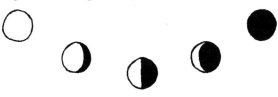

Herbal References

Bethel, May. *The Healing Power of Herbs.* Wilshire Books, 1978
Boon, Heather & M. Smith. *Botanical Pharmacy.* Quarry Health, 1999
Crawford, Amanda. *Herbal Menopause Book.* Crossing Press, 1996
Erichsen-Brown, Charlotte. *Use of Plants.* Breezy Creek, 1979
Felter & Lloyd. *King's American Dispensatory* (1898). Eclectic, 1983
Fleming, Thomas (ed). *PDR for Herbal Medicines,* 2nd ed. Medical
    Economics, 1999
Grieves, Maude. *A Modern Herbal.* Dover, 1971 (Orig. 1931)
Hoffmann, David. *The New Holistic Herbal.* Element, 1983
Holmes, Peter. *Energetics of Western Herbs.* Artemis, 1989
Hudson, Tori. *Women's Encyclopedia of Natural Medicine.* Keats, 1999
Hutchens, Alma. *Indian Herbalogy of North America.* Merco, 1969
Krochmal, A. & C. Krochmal. *Guide to Medicinal Plants.* Quadrangle, 1973
Lewis, Memory & W. Lewis. *Medical Botany.* Wiley & Sons, 1977
Levy, Juliette de B. *Common Herbs for Natural Health.* Ash Tree, 1997
Lust, John. *The Herb Book.* Bantam, 1974
Mabey, Richard. *The New Age Herbalist.* Collier/Macmillan, 1988
Mills, Simon. *Dictionary of Modern Herbalism.* Healing Arts, 1988
Nissim, Rina. *Natural Healing in Gynecology.* Pandora, 1984
Parvati, Jeannine. *Hygieia, A Woman's Herbal.* Freestone, 1978
Weed, Susun S. *Healing Wise.* Ash Tree, 1989

Mail Order Herbs

Avena Botanicals • "Lovingly grown and wildcrafted"
    219 Mill St., Rockport, ME 04865 (207-594-0694)
    www.avenaherbs.com
Blessed Herbs • "Serving the highest spirit in all."
    109 Barre Plains Rd., Oakham, MA 01068 (800-489-4372)
    www.blessedherbs.com
Catskill Mountain Herbal • "This work is a labor of love."
    PO Box 1426, Olivebridge, NY 12461 (845-657-2943)
    www.catskillmountainherbals.com
Frontier Herbal Coop • "Dedicated to much more than our own
    success." 2000 Frontier, Norway, IA 52318 (800-669-3275)
    www.frontiercoop.com
Green Terrestrial • "In co-creation with the devas."
    1449 Warm Brook Road, Arlington, VT 05250 (802-375-8087)
    www.greenterrestrial.com
Red Moon Herbs • "Wildcrafted and organic herbal medicines."
    1039 Camp Elliot Rd., Black Mt, NC 28711 (888-929-0777)
    www.redmoonherbs.com

Appendix 1
Vitamins and Minerals
For the Menopausal Years

Lists are arranged thusly: Most important sources, in decreasing order, are first. Other excellent sources follow the semicolon.

Vitamin A: Vitamin A is formed in the liver from ingested carotenes and carotenoids. No plants contain it. Liver, milk, and eggs do. In pill form, vitamin A can cause birth defects, hair loss, and liver stress.

Depleted by: Coffee, alcohol, cortisone, mineral oil, fluorescent lights, liver "cleansing," excessive intake of iron, lack of protein.

Vitamin B complex: For healthy digestion, good liver function, emotional flexibility, less anxiety, sound sleep, milder hot flashes with less sweating, steady heartbeat.

Depleted by: Coffee, alcohol, tobacco, refined sugar, raw oysters, hormone replacement, birth control pills (especially B_6).

Food Sources of B vitamins: Whole grains, well-cooked greens, organ meat (liver, kidneys, heart), sweet potatoes, carrots, molasses, nuts, bananas, avocados, grapes, pears; egg yolks, sardines, herring, salmon, crab, oysters, whey.

Herbal Sources of B vitamins: Red clover blossoms, parsley leaf, oatstraw. See also specific factors, following.

Vitamin B_1, Thiamine: For emotional ease, strong nerves.

Food Sources of B_1, Thiamine: Asparagus, cauliflower, cabbage, kale, barley grass, seaweeds, citrus fruits.

Herbal Sources of B_1, Thiamine: Peppermint, burdock, sage, yellow dock, alfalfa, red clover, fenugreek seeds, raspberry leaves, nettle, catnip, watercress, yarrow leaf/flower, rose buds and hips.

Vitamin B_2, Riboflavin: For more energy, healthy skin, less cancer.

Depleted by: Hot flashes, crying jags, antibiotics, tranquilizers.

Food Sources of B_2, Riboflavin: Beans, greens, onions, seaweeds, yogurt, cheese, milk, mushrooms.

Herbal Sources of B_2, Riboflavin: Peppermint, alfalfa greens, parsley, echinacea, yellow dock, hops; dandelion root, ginseng, dulse, kelp, fenugreek seed, rose hips, nettles.

Vitamin B$_6$, Pyridoxine: For improved immune functioning; especially needed by women using hormone replacement.

Food Sources of B$_6$, Pyridoxine: Baked potato with skin, broccoli, prunes, bananas, dried beans, lentils; meat, poultry, fish.

Vitamin B factor, Folic acid: For strong, flexible bones, easy nerves.

Food Sources of folic acid (folate): Leafy greens, liver, kidney, lentils, whole grains, seeds, nuts, fruits, vegetables.

Herbal Sources of Folic acid: Leaves: Nettles, alfalfa, parsley, sage, catnip, peppermint, plantain leaf, comfrey, chickweed.

Vitamin B factor, Niacin: For relief of anxiety and depression, decrease in headaches, reduction of blood cholesterol levels.

Food Sources of Niacin: Asparagus, cabbage, bee pollen.

Herbal Sources of Niacin: Hops, raspberry leaf, red clover; slippery elm, echinacea, licorice, rose hips, nettle, alfalfa, parsley.

Vitamin B$_{12}$: For healthy metabolism, stronger eyes, better memory, more energy, less cancer, osteoporosis, arthritis, fibromylagia, and depression. Aids absorption of all other minerals, especially calcium.

Depleted by: Unfermented soy, lack of animal foods in the diet.

Food Sources of B$_{12}$: Liver, kidney, yogurt, cheese, milk, eggs, meat, poultry, shellfish.

Herbal Sources of B$_{12}$: None.

Bioflavonoids: For healthy heart and blood vessels, easier hot flashes and night sweats, less menstrual bleeding, unlumpy breasts, less water retention, less anxiety, less irritable nerves.

Food Sources of Bioflavonoids: Citrus pulp and rind.

Herbal Sources of Bioflavonoids: Buckwheat greens, elder berries, hawthorn fruits, rose hips, horsetail, shepherd's purse, chervil.

Carotenes: For a well-lubricated vagina, strong bones, protection against cancer, healthy lungs and skin, strong vision, good digestion.

Food Sources of Carotenes: Well-cooked red, yellow, or green vegetables/fruits: carrots, winter squash, tomatoes, seaweeds, cantaloupe.

Herbal Sources of Carotenes: Peppermint, yellow dock, uva ursi, parsley, alfalfa, raspberry, nettles, dandelion greens; kelp, green onions, violet leaves, cayenne, paprika, lamb's quarters leaves, sage, chickweed, horsetail, black cohosh roots, rose hips.

Vitamin C complex: For less intense hot flashes, less insomnia and night sweats, stronger bones, fewer headaches, better resistance to infection, smoother emotions, less heart disease, rapid wound healing. Critical to good adrenal functioning, especially during menopause.

Depleted by: Antibiotics, aspirin and other pain relievers, coffee, stress, aging, smoking, baking soda, high fever.

Food Sources of Vitamin C: Freshly picked foods, cooked potatoes.

Herbal Sources of Vitamin C: Rose hips, yellow dock root, raspberry leaf, red clover, hops; pine needles, dandelion greens, watercress, echinacea, skullcap, plantain, parsley, cayenne, paprika.

Vitamin D: For very strong, very flexible bones, hormonal ease, cancer prevention, regulation of glucose metabolism, reduction of risk of adult onset diabetes.

Depleted by: Mineral oil used on the skin, frequent hot baths, sunscreen with SPF8 or higher.

Food Sources of Vitamin D: Sunlight, butter, egg yolk, cod liver oil; liver, shrimp, fatty fish (mackerel, sardines, herring, salmon, tuna).

Herbal Sources of Vitamin D: None. Vitamin D is not found in plants.

Vitamin E: For milder hot flashes, fewer night sweats, protection from cancer, fewer signs of aging, fewer wrinkles, moist vagina, strong heart, freedom from arthritis.

Depleted by: Mineral oil, sulfates, hormone replacement.

Food Sources of Vitamin E: Freshly ground whole-grain flours, cold-pressed oils; fresh nuts, peanut butter, leafy greens, cabbage, asparagus.

Herbal Sources of Vitamin E: Alfalfa, rosehips, nettles, dong quai, watercress, dandelion, seaweeds, wild seeds (lamb's quarters, plantain).

Essential fatty acids (EFAs), including GLA, omega-6 and omega-3. For a healthy heart, less severe hot flashes, strong nerves, strong bones, well-functioning endocrine glands, fewer wrinkles.

Food Sources of EFAs: Flax seeds, cod liver oil, wheat germ oil, whole grains; seeds such as borage, evening primrose, black currant, hemp, safflower, and their oils.

Herbal Sources of EFAs: All wild plants, but very few cultivated plants, contain EFAs; fresh purslane is notably high.

Folic Acid: See vitamin B factor, folic acid.

Vitamin K: For less menstrual flooding, stronger bones.

Depleted by: X-rays, radiation, air pollution, enemas, frozen foods, antibiotics, rancid fats, aspirin.

Food Sources of Vitamin K: Healthy intestinal bacteria produce vitamin K; green leafy vegetables, yogurt, egg yolk, blackstrap molasses.

Herbal Sources of Vitamin K: Nettle, alfalfa, kelp, green tea.

Minerals

Boron: For strong, flexible bones.

Food Sources of Boron: Organic fruits, vegetables, nuts.

Herbal Sources of Boron: All organic garden weeds including all edible parts of chickweed, purslane, nettles, dandelion, yellow dock.

Calcium: For sound sleep, dense bones, calm heart, strong muscles, less irritable nerves, lower blood pressure, sound blood vessels, regular heartbeat, freedom from depression and headaches, less bloating, fewer mood fluctuations.

Depleted by: Coffee, sugar, salt, alcohol, cortisone, enemas, unfermented soy products, antacids, too much phosphorus.

Food Sources of Calcium: Yogurt, raw-milk cheese, dark green leaves; nuts, seeds, tahini, seaweeds, vegetables (especially sweet potatoes, cabbage), dried beans, whole grains, whey, salmon, tuna, sardines, shellfish.

Herbal Sources of Calcium: Valerian, kelp, nettle, horsetail, peppermint; sage, uva ursi, yellow dock, chickweed, red clover, oatstraw, parsley, black currant leaf, raspberry leaf, plantain leaf/seed, dandelion leaf, amaranth leaf/seed, lamb's quarter leaf/seed.

Chromium: For less fatigue and lots of energy, fewer mood swings, stable blood sugar levels, higher HDL; less risk of adult onset diabetes.

Depleted by: White sugar.

Food Sources of Chromium: Barley grass, prunes, nuts, mushrooms, liver, beets, whole wheat, bee pollen.

Herbal Sources of Chromium: Oatstraw, nettle, red clover tops, catnip, dulse, wild yam, yarrow, horsetail; roots of black cohosh, licorice, echinacea, valerian, sarsaparilla.

Copper: For supple skin, healthy hair, strong muscles, easy nerves, less water retention, less menstrual flooding, lower blood cholesterol.

Food Sources of Copper: Liver, kidney, seafood, organically grown grains, beans, nuts, leafy greens, seaweeds, bittersweet chocolate, mushrooms.

Herbal Sources of Copper: Skullcap, sage, horsetail; chickweed.

Iodine: For fewer breast lumps, less fatigue, healthier thyroid function, stronger liver.

Depleted by: Unfermented soy products.

Food Sources of Iodine: Seafood, seaweed, sea salt, spinach, beets, mushrooms.

Herbal Sources of Iodine: Kelp, parsley, celery, sarsaparilla root.

Iron: For fewer hot flashes, less menstrual flooding, fewer headaches, better sleep with fewer night sweats, easier nerves, more energy, less dizziness.

Depleted by: Coffee, black tea, alcohol, aspirin, carbonated drinks, lack of protein, enemas, unfermented soy, processed dairy.

Food Sources of Iron: Liver, red meat, canned salmon, sardines, egg yolk, leafy greens, molasses, dried fruit (cherries, raisins, prunes, dates, figs), yellow/orange/red vegetables, bittersweet chocolate; whole wheat, oatmeal, brown rice, mushrooms, potatoes, honey, seaweeds.

Herbal Sources of Iron: Chickweed, kelp, burdock root, catnip, horsetail, *Althea* root, milk thistle seed, uva ursi, dandelion leaf/root; the roots of yellow dock, dong quai, black cohosh, echinacea, licorice, valerian, and sarsaparilla; nettles, plantain leaf, fenugreek seed, peppermint.

Magnesium: For deeper sleep, less anxiety, easier nerves, flexible bones and arteries, lower cholesterol, lower blood pressure, stronger heart, more energy, less fatigue, fewer headaches/migraines.

Depleted by: Hot flashes, night sweats, crying jags, alcohol, chemical diuretics, enemas, antibiotics, "soft" water, excessive fat intake.

Food sources of Magnesium: Leafy greens, seaweeds, nuts, whole grains, yogurt, cheese; potatoes, corn, peas, squash, beans, figs.

Herbal Sources of Magnesium: Oatstraw, licorice, kelp, nettle, dulse, burdock root, chickweed, Althea root, horsetail; sage, raspberry leaf, red clover, valerian, yellow dock, dandelion greens, carrot tops, parsley leaf, evening primrose.

Manganese: for keen hearing, flexible bones, reduction of dizziness, prevention of diabetes.

Depleted by: Chemical fertilizers used agriculturally.

Food Sources of Manganese: Any leaves or seeds from plants grown on healthy soil; seaweeds.

Herbal Sources of Manganese: Raspberry, uva ursi leaf, chickweed, milk thistle seed, yellow dock; ginseng, wild yam, echinacea and dandelion roots, nettle, catnip, kelp, horsetail, hops flowers.

Molybdenum: for fewer hot flashes, prevention of anemia.

Food Sources of Molybdenum: Organically raised dairy products, legumes, grains, leafy greens, seaweeds.

Herbal Sources of Molybdenum: Nettles, dandelion greens, sage, oatstraw, fenugreek seeds, raspberry leaves, red clover blossoms, horsetail, chickweed, kelp.

Nickel: For milder hot flashes, easy nerves.

Food Sources of Nickel: Chocolate, nuts, dried beans, cereals.

Herbal Sources of Nickel: Alfalfa, red clover, oatstraw, fenugreek.

Phosphorus: For strong, flexible bones, more energy.
Depleted by: Antacids.
Food Sources of Phosphorus: Whole grains, seeds, nuts.
Herbal Sources of Phosphorus: Peppermint, yellow dock, milk thistle, fennel, hops, chickweed; nettle, dandelion, parsley, dulse, red clover.

Potassium: For more energy, less fatigue, less water retention, easy weight loss, steady heartbeat, lower blood pressure, better digestion.
Depleted by: Frequent hot flashes, sweating, night sweats, coffee, sugar, salt, alcohol, enemas, vomiting, diarrhea, chemical diuretics, dieting.
Food Sources of Potassium: Celery, cabbage, peas, parsley, broccoli, bananas, carrots, potato skin, whole grains, pears, citrus, seaweed.
Herbal Sources of Potassium: Sage, catnip, peppermint, skullcap, hops, dulse, kelp, red clover; horsetail, nettles, plantain leaf.

Selenium: For clear vision, slower aging, strong immunity, less irritability, more energy, healthy hair/nails/teeth, less cardiovascular disease.
Food sources of Selenium: Liver, raw milk cheeses, seaweeds, whole grains, garlic, kidneys, fish, shellfish, meat, yogurt, beans.
Herbal Sources of Selenium: Catnip, milk thistle seed, valerian root, dulse, black cohosh and ginseng roots; uva ursi leaf, hops flowers, kelp, raspberry leaf, rose buds and hips, hawthorn berries, fenugreek seed, roots of echinacea, sarsaparilla, and yellow dock.

Silicon: For strong, flexible bones, less irritable nerves.
Sources of Silicon: Unrefined grains, root vegetables, spinach, leeks.
Herbal Sources of Silicon/Silica: Horsetail, dulse, echinacea, cornsilk, burdock, oatstraw, licorice, chickweed; uva ursi, sarsaparilla.

Sulfur: For relaxed muscles, soft skin, healthy nerves, strong liver, glossy hair.
Sources of Sulfur: Eggs, dairy products, cabbage family plants, onions, garlic, parsley, watercress.
Herbal Sources of Sulfur: Sage, nettles, plantain, horsetail.

Zinc: For slower aging, better digestion, stronger bones, healthy skin, cancer prevention, increased sex drive.
Depleted by: Alcohol, air pollution, hormone replacement.
Sources of Zinc: Liver, meat, sardines, oysters, eggs, yogurt, leafy greens, beans, pumpkin seeds, nuts, whole grains.
Herbal Sources of Zinc: Skullcap, sage, wild yam, chickweed, echinacea, nettles, dulse, milk thistle; sarsaparilla.

Appendix 2
Recipes and Pharmacy

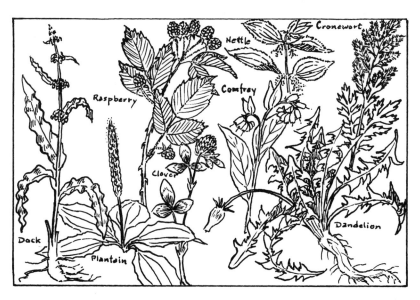

How To Make an Herbal Infusion

A **tea** is a small amount of fresh or dried herb brewed for a short time. An **infusion** is a large amount of dried (not fresh) herb brewed for a long time. An infusion extracts more nutrients than a tincture and more medicinal qualities (and nutrients) than a tea. Most infusions are short-lived; they stay good for only two or three days.

Prepare infusions in pint/half-liter and quart/liter jars with tight lids. A teapot is not as good, but acceptable.

Usual dose of infusion is 1-2 cups/250-500 ml a day, taken hot, chilled, or at room temperature. Infusions may be seasoned with sweeteners, tamari, milk, or any other additions that please your taste. Infusions can also be used as soup stocks, bath waters, hair rinses, facial washes.

Summary of Infusion Data

Plant Part	Amount	Jar/Water	Length of Infusion
Roots/barks	1 oz/30 g.	**pint/500 ml**	8 hours minimum
Leaves	1 oz/30 g.	**quart/liter**	4 hours minimum
Flowers	1 oz/30 g.	**quart/liter**	2 hours maximum
Seeds/berries	1 oz/30 g.	**pint/500 ml**	30 min. maximum

Bonny Bony Brew

Nettle (*Urtica dioica*), 1 ounce/30 grams, dry
Horsetail (*Equisetum arvense*), 1 tablespoon/2 grams, dry
Sage (*Salvia officinalis*), 1 tablespoon/2 grams, dry

Crush sage between palms and drop into a quart/liter container with the other two herbs. Fill jar with water just off the boil, cap tightly, and set in a cozy corner to brew for at least four hours (overnight is fine). Strain; drink as is or heat and add honey. Also nice iced. You can substitute red clover or oatstraw or raspberry for the nettles.

Each cup contributes as much calcium as a cup of milk.

How To Make an Herbal Tincture

Fresh plant material steeped in alcohol makes alkaloid-rich (but nutrient-poor) herbal remedies called tinctures. If you cannot find the fresh herb, you may use dried herbs, but in my experience, only dried roots, seeds, and berries are worth the effort. (Flowers and leaves lose too much in the drying.) Tinctures remain effective for long periods of time and are easily transported. Vinegar does not extract the same properties from plants as alcohol.

To tincture: Identify and pick the plant. Chop the plant material coarsely; do not wash. Fill any size jar with plant material, then pour 100-proof vodka (or grain alcohol) over it, filling the jar to the top. Cap tightly. Label with date and name of plant. Your tincture will be ready to decant (strain) and use in six weeks but can sit there as long as you wish.

Summary of Tincture Proportions

• Tincture **one ounce/30 grams fresh** plant material in approximately **one ounce/30 ml** spirit for 6 weeks.

• Tincture **one ounce/30 grams dried** plant material in **five ounces/ 150 ml** spirit for 6 weeks.

Jiffy Motherwort Tonics

Put fresh flowering motherwort (*Leonurus cardiaca*) through a juicer. Mix 4 tablespoons/60 ml of this fresh motherwort juice with:

vodka, 4 tablespoons/60 ml *or*
honey, 1 cup/250 ml *or*
vinegar, 1/2 cup/125 ml.

Motherwort tincture takes six weeks. If you're in a hurry, try this. But put up some tincture, too. This doesn't work as well.

Keep refrigerated.

How To Make an Herbal Vinegar

Natural vinegars, such as apple cider vinegar, wine vinegar, and rice vinegar are especially effective mediums for extracting the mineral richness of plants. Most vitamins, some alkaloidal components and many essential oils dissolve in vinegar as well. Fill a jar with fresh leaves, roots, and/or flowers. Then fill with vinegar, label, and cap. Use fresh plant materials only.

Beware vinegar's ability to corrode metal; use plastic lids or corks for your herbal vinegars (or put a piece of plastic wrap or waxed paper over the jar before screwing on the lid). Ready to use in six weeks.

Old Sour Puss Mineral Mix

☞ **Yellow Dock** (*Rumex*) leaves/roots
☞ **Dandelion** (*Taraxacum*) leaves/roots
☞ **Plantain** (*Plantago*) leaves
☞ **Nettle** (*Urtica*) leaves
☞ **Raspberry** (*Rubus*) leaves/canes/berries
☞ **Cronewort/Mugwort** (*Artemisia vulgaris*) leaves
☞ **Comfrey** (*Symphytum*) leaves/flower stalks
☞ **Red Clover** (*Trifolium pratense*) blossoms

Completely fill a quart/liter jar with one (or more) of these calcium-rich herbs. Use only fresh plant material. One clean **eggshell** or bone may be added, but will cause the vinegar to foam up wildly and smell strange.

Pour apple cider vinegar over the herbs until the jar is full. Cover with a plastic lid and let sit for six weeks.

Use this calcium-rich vinegar as a refreshing drink before meals by mixing a tablespoon/30 ml in up to a cup of water. For the hardy, and those in need of iron, add a tablespoon/30 ml of molasses. (Adds 150 mg more calcium, too.)

Also great added to soups and bean dishes, and as a salad dressing.

Vinegar has the amazing ability to dissolve calcium (and other materials) and hold it in solution, ready for your ingestion and assimilation. A tablespoon/30 ml of this vinegar will supply about 150-200 mg calcium. Taken before or with your meals, this vinegar increases the digestibility of the minerals in your entire meal.

Menopausal Root Brew

Black Cohosh (*Cimicifuga racemosa*) roots
Black Haw or Cramp Bark (*Viburnum prunifolium, V. opulus*)
Burdock (*Arctium lappa*) roots
Dandelion (*Taraxacum off.*) roots
Devil's Club (*Oplopanax horridum*) root bark
False Unicorn (*Chamaelirium luteum*) roots
Ginseng (*Panax*) roots
Osha (*Ligusticum porteri*) roots
Peony (*Paeonia*) roots
Rehmannia (*R. glutinosa*) roots
Sarsaparilla (*Smilax species*) roots
Spikenard (*Aralia species*) roots
Wild Ginger (*Asarum canadensis*) roots
Wild Yam (*Dioscorea species*) roots
Yellow Dock (*Rumex crispus*) roots

Gather fresh **any three** of these hormone-rich roots/root barks. Substitute local species as desired; there are many varieties of yellow dock, wild yam, and wild ginger to choose from, for example.

Nearly fill any jar with chopped pieces of these fresh roots. You may add one dried **ginseng** or **dong quai** root, if desired. Fill jar to the top with 100-proof vodka. Let sit for six weeks. Then use 10-30 drops, once or twice a day, in a cup of water or garden sage tea. This brew will help you through your menopausal climax years and into a healthy, happy Cronehood.

How To Make an Herbal Glycerine Macerate

Glycerine, a by-product of soap-making, is used to extract hormonal precursors and glycosides from plants. You can buy glycerine at the drugstore. This procedure for macerating plants in glycerine is exactly the same as the procedure for making a tincture. Use fresh plants only. Fill a jar with your plant material; completely cover with glycerine diluted 1:1, 1:2, or 1:3 with water; and macerate, tightly capped, for at least six weeks.

Strong Bone Stew
Serves 3-4

In a large, heavy-bottomed pot, heat 2 tablespoons/30 ml **olive oil**. Sauté in warm oil 1 cup/250 ml organically grown **chopped onions**, 1-3 cloves **chopped garlic**, and 1 cup/250 ml **quartered mushrooms**. When onions are soft, add 1 quart/liter **vegetable stock** (or water), and bring to a boil.

Then add 1 cup/250 ml each of at least four of these organically grown vegetables, cubed, unpeeled: **sweet potato, carrot, turnip, winter squash, potato**, parsnip, **burdock/gobo**. Also add 1/2 cup/125 ml **dried wakame seaweed**, cut small. Simmer for 45 minutes, adding more water or broth if needed.

While the stew simmers, mix together in a large measuring cup or bowl: 2 tablespoons/30 ml **miso**, 2 teaspoons/10 ml **tamari**, 1/3 cup/80 ml **tahini**, 2 tablespoons/30 ml **peanut or almond butter**, 1 tablespoon/15 ml **cronewort vinegar**. (See page 256.)

Just before serving, ladle enough hot broth into the measuring cup or bowl to make a mixture thin enough to pour into the stew. Add this mix and 1 cake **tofu**, cubed, to your stewpot. Continue to cook on very low heat for 5 minutes. Serve hot, with whole grain bread or brown rice.

Thirteen great calcium-rich foods all in one pot. Many thanks to "New Recipes from Moosewood" for sparking the creation of this delight.

Fruit Fix

Simmer together in 8-10 cups/2000-2500 ml water:
1 pound/450 grams pitted dates
1 pound/450 grams dried figs
1 pound/450 grams pitted prunes
1 1/2 pounds/675 grams raisins

When soft, mash together (or put in food processor) and add 2-4 tablespoons rose hip powder. Use this calcium-rich, estrogen-enhancing spread in place of jams and jellies. Try it on a whole wheat cracker when you think you want a cookie.

To relieve constipation, cook in prune juice instead of water.

Four Roots Tonic

Dong Quai (*Angelica sinensis*), 1/2 ounce/15 grams dried root
Burdock (*Arctium lappa*), 1/2 ounce/15 grams dried root
Peony (*Paeonia off.*), 1/2 ounce/15 grams dried root
Dandelion (*Taraxacum off.*), 1/2 ounce/15 grams dried root

Put your roots in a pint/60 ml jar and fill it up to the top with 100-proof vodka or apple cider vinegar. Cap well and label. Wait at least six weeks before using. If you have fresh burdock, dandelion, or peony root (yes, it's the one in your garden), substitute 2 ounces/60 grams fresh for 1/2 ounce/15 grams dried. To take, put a dropperful into a cup of water or fenugreek seed (*Trigonella foenum-graecum*) tea.

CAUTION: Grannies say there's a baby in every cup of fenugreek.

Menopausal First Aid

Eases hot flashes, palpitations, insomnia, night sweats, and anxiety.

Chickweed (*Stellaria media*) leaf and flower tincture
Motherwort (*Leonurus cardiaca*) tincture of flowering tops

Combine equal parts of these tinctures in a one-ounce/30 ml dropper bottle. Use 10-20 drops, as needed, in some water or, better yet, a cup of sage infusion or fenugreek tea.

Easy Homemade Yogurt

1 gallon/4 liters milk, any kind
1 cup/250 ml plain yogurt with active cultures

Heat milk over a low flame in a glass or enamel pot. Stir and feel frequently. When milk feels just a little warm (105°F/37°C), remove from heat. Put yogurt into a glass bowl or quart/liter measuring cup. Add a cup/250 ml of warmed milk. Stir well. Pour this mix into a one-gallon glass jar. (Ask a local restaurant or deli for one.) Add all the rest of the warmed milk, stir well with a wooden spoon, cap, and set to rest in a warm place (100-110°F/37-39°C) for 8-24 hours. The longer it sits, the easier it will be to digest. Keeps refrigerated for four to six weeks.

Springing Soup
Serves 4

To 8 cups/2 liters **water** or vegetable broth, add fresh **nettle greens**, 2 cups/500 ml, and fresh **horsetail**, one handful. Chop 4 **potatoes** and add. Bring to a boil and simmer until potatoes are done. Garnish with wild onions finely minced.

Oat Bath

Make 2 quarts/liters of oatstraw infusion. Add to a hot bath and soak your tensions away. Or put a handful of rolled oats in a kitchen towel, tie it closed loosely, and toss it in a hot bath. When it softens, rub it down all your limbs, from thighs to toes and shoulder to fingertips.

Peel Power

A spoonful of bioflavonoid-rich citrus peels is delicious this way.

Juice **2 organic oranges** and 1 **organic lemon**. Cut the peels (together with inner membranes) into very thin slivers of any length. Heat with 1 cup/250 ml of **honey** until it just boils. Pour immediately into jar, filling it to the brim. Cap. You can use this the very next day, but it does improve with age.

Plantain Ointment

Collect fresh, dark green **plantain** leaves. Chop coarsely and put into a clean, dry jar. Don't quite fill the jar. Pour enough **olive oil** over the leaves to come to the top of the jar. Cap well. Label. Leave on a wooden counter for six weeks. (Some of the oil may leak out.) Squeeze oil from leaves. Add 1 tablespoon/1 gram grated beeswax per ounce/30 ml oil and heat gently. Pour in a jar; cool.

How To Make an Herbal Compress or Poultice

Any fresh herb chewed or crushed and applied to the body is a **poultice**. A **compress** uses dried herbs. To make a compress, first make an herbal infusion. Then strain the liquid off the plant material and put the wet plants in a cloth. Apply, hot or cold, to the painful area. Dip the cloth in the liquid as needed to keep the compress moist.

Appendix 3
Healthy Bones the
Wise Woman Way

Selected mineral data for fourteen frequently used Wise Woman herbs. **Data is for 100 grams dry weight** and does not include all the minerals found in each herb. Approximately 10 percent of the total minerals is extracted into 250ml (one cup) of infusion if 35 grams of dried herb is brewed in one liter of boiling water; approximately 4 percent of the total minerals is extracted into 15ml (one tablespoon) of vinegar if 400 grams fresh herb is infused in 400ml vinegar for six weeks.

Herbs Used Mainly As Nourishing Infusions

• Stinging nettle: calcium (2900 mg), magnesium (860 mg), phosphorus (447 mg), potassium (1750 mg), and zinc (4.7 mg)

• Oatstraw: calcium (1430 mg), phosphorus (425 mg), and potassium (352 mg)

• Red clover blossoms: calcium (1310 mg), magnesium (349 mg), and potassium (2000 mg)

• Comfrey leaves (safety considerations, page 61): calcium (1130 mg), chromium (0.8 mg), manganese (6.7 mg), phosphorus (211 mg), potassium (1590 mg), selenium (0.57 mg), and zinc (0.28 mg)

Herbs Used Mainly As Medicinal Vinegars

• Peppermint: calcium (1620 mg), manganese (6.1 mg), magnesium (661 mg), phosphorus (772 mg), potassium (2260 mg), and selenium (1.1 mg)

• Garden thyme: calcium (1350 mg), chromium (2.0 mg), iron (147 mg), magnesium (436 mg), manganese (6.4 mg), selenium (1.6 mg), silicon (20.2 mg), and zinc (1.5 mg)

• Yellow dock root: calcium (1000 mg), magnesium (320 mg), phosphorus (757), potassium (1220 mg), selenium (2.5), and silicon (1.3 mg)

• Garden sage: calcium (1080 mg), chromium (0.3 mg), magnesium (285 mg), manganese (3.0), potassium (2470 mg), silicon (3.1 mg), and zinc (5.9 mg)

• Burdock root: calcium (733 mg), chromium (2.0 mg), iron (147 mg), magnesium (537 mg), manganese (537), phosphorus (437 mg), potassium (1680 mg), selenium (1.4 mg), silicon (22.5 mg), and zinc (2.2 mg)

• Dandelion root: calcium (614 mg), chromium (0.9 mg), iron (96 mg), magnesium (157 mg), manganese (6.8), phosphorus (362), potassium (1200 mg), selenium (0.86 mg), silicon (4.7 mg), and zinc (1.3 mg)

Herbs Used Mainly As Vegetables

• Kelp: calcium (3040 mg), magnesium (867 mg), manganese (7.6 mg), phosphorus (249 mg), potassium (2110 mg), selenium (1.7 mg), silica (7.6 mg), and zinc (0.6 mg)

• Amaranth greens: calcium (1210 mg), phosphorus (324 mg), and potassium (1864 mg)

• Chickweed: calcium (1210 mg), magnesium (523 mg), manganese (15.3 mg), phosphorus (448 mg), and zinc (5.2 mg)

• Dulse: calcium (632 mg), chromium (2.7 mg), magnesium (593), potassium (2270 mg), selenium (3.3), silicon (36.8), and zinc (3.9)

Sources

Bergner; Paul. *Healing Power of Minerals.* Prima, 1997
Gail, Peter. Wild food activist
Pedersen, Mark. *Nutritional Herbology.* Pederson Publishing, 1987
USDA. Handbook Number 8, 1975

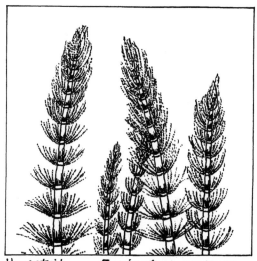

Horsetail — *Equisetum arvense*

Glossary

Adaptogenic: An agent that helps us adapt, especially to stress. Adaptogens tend to be tonifying and nourishing rather than stimulating.

Adenomatous hyperplasia: Benign tumor-like growth of a glandular origin in the lining of the uterus.

Bioflavonoids: Brightly colored substances frequently found in fruits and vegetables in association with ascorbic acid (vitamin C). Also known as vitamin P. Bioflavonoids are required for absorption of vitamin C. Citrin, hesperidin, rutin, flavones, and flavonals are bioflavonoids.

Chakra: Sanskrit word meaning "wheel." The chakras of the human body are energy wheels or energy centers.

Corpus luteum: A mound of yellow, hormone-producing tissue that occurs in the wall of the ovary when (and where) an egg has just been released. It encourages production of progesterone.

Endometrial hyperplasia: Overgrowth of the lining of the uterus. See hyperplasia.

Endometriosis: Endometrial tissue growing somewhere other than inside the uterus where it belongs. It may cause menstrual pain, mid-cycle spotting, flooding, and infertility, but it is unlikely to be life-threatening or cancerous. Endometriosis is progesterone-dependent, and usually disappears after menopause.

Endometrium: The lining of the uterus. It grows each cycle and is shed in menstruation.

ERT: Estrogen replacement therapy.

Estrogen: A group of more than two dozen closely related steroidal hormones produced primarily by the ovaries, adrenals, fat cells, testicles, placenta and fetus. *Estropipate, estrone, estradiol,* and *estriol* are forms of estrogen. Estrogen levels in most 60-year-old women are indistinguishable from estrogen levels in most 40-year-old women. Menopause is not a result of estrogen deficiency. High levels of estrogen are thought to be responsible for many reproductive cancers. *Estrogenic*, adj.

Fibroid: A benign growth in the uterus or breast.

Flavonoids: See Bioflavonoids.

FSH: Follicle stimulating hormone. Produced primarily by the pituitary, FSH triggers ovulation. Levels of FSH rise dramatically in the menopausal years and remain high postmenopausally.

GLA: Gamma linoleic acid; an essential fatty acid, that is, a fat that must be consumed to maintain good health. Flaxseed oil contains linoleic and linolenic acids; most vegetable oils contain only linolenic.

Glycoside: A carbohydrate that breaks down into a sugar and a nonsugar. Plant glycosides affect hormone-producing tissues powerfully.

HRT: Hormone replacement therapy; that is, the replacement of both progesterone and estrogen by pills or injections.

Hyperplasia: Literally an increase in the number of cells in an area or organ. Menopausal women who take supplemental estrogen (ERT) frequently experience *adenomatous hyperplasia* and *endometrial hyperplasia*. Hyperplasia itself is not cancer.

Hysterectomy: Removal of the uterus, leaving ovaries intact.

LH: Luteinizing hormone; produced primarily by the pituitary. In combination with FSH, LH stimulates the ovaries to secrete estrogen, which in turn triggers ovulation. LH is also responsible for changing the ovum follicle into the corpus luteum. LH levels rise dramatically during the menopausal years, and stay elevated through postmenopause. Over-production of melatonin by the pineal gland can stop release of LH.

Luteal phase: The thirteen-day interval between ovulation and menstruation. There is no luteal phase if pregnancy occurs.

Moxibustion: Burning (com*bustion*) of *moxa* (the dried "wool" of *Artemisia vulgaris*). Moxibustion warms, eases pain, relaxes sore muscles, and aids the movement of chi or energy throughout the body.

Palpitations: A pounding, racing heart. See also tachycardia.

Pedunculated: Having, growing on, or being attached by a narrow stalk (peduncule).

Polyp: A small growth emerging from a mucous membrane surface such as the cervix, vagina, or rectum.

Precursor: Comes before, or is easily transformed into. Glycosides and bioflavonoids are hormonal precursors.

Progesterone: A group of pro-gestational steroidal hormones primarily produced by the corpus luteum, adrenals, and placenta. Ovulation increases progesterone production.

Progestin: Synthetic progesterone may be called *progestin, progestogen*, or *progestagen*. Natural progesterone is called progestin, too.

Prostaglandins: Hormone-like fatty acids that act in many ways: they influence hormone production, tonify smooth muscles (heart, uterus, intestines), and nourish the autonomic and central nervous systems.

Phytosterols: Hormones (sterols or steroids) found in plants.

Saponins: Soap-like substances found in plants. Saponins emulsify (combine oil and water) like soap, thus improving the body's absorption of hormones (fat-soluble substances). They also increase the permeability of cellular membranes, hastening and encouraging the absorption of all nutrients and the death of unwanted bacteria.

Solar plexus: Literally sun (solar) center (plexus). Located in the front center of the lower edge of the ribcage, this chakra is associated with digestion, the liver and kidneys, feelings of self-worth and personal power, and bright yellow flowers like dandelion and sunflower.

Tachycardia: Literally "speedy heart." These episodes of very rapid heartbeats, often accompanied by breathlessness, and a lightheaded sensation may occur in healthy people during strenuous exercise. Tachycardia while in a resting state may be due to overuse of coffee, or to fever, heart disease, or menopausal hot flashes.

Yang: Oriental term referring to warm, bright, expanded, active energy; originally, the sunny side of the river.

Yin: Oriental term referring to cool, dark, concentrated, meditative energy; originally, the shaded side of the river.

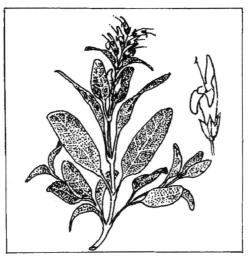

Sage — *Salvia officinalis*

Endnotes

(1) O'Brien, K., B.Caballero. *Nutrition Reviews.* 55(7):284
(2) *JAMA.* Schairer, C., et al. "Menopausal Estrogen and estrogen-progestin replacement therapy and breast cancer risk." January, 2000
(3) Feskanich, D., et al. "Milk, dietary calcium, and bone fractures in women: A 12-year prospective study." *Am J Pub Health.* 87:992-997, 1997
(4) Campbell, T.C., et al. "Dietary calcium and bone density among middle-aged and elderly women in China." *Am J Clinical Nutrition.* 58:219-227, 1993
(5) Campbell, T.C., et al. "Bone density and lifestyle characteristics in premenopausal and postmenopausal Chinese women." *Osteo-porosis International.* 4:288-297, 1994
(6) *British Medical Journal.* 299, 1989
(7) Cumming, R.G., et al. "Calcium intake and fracture risk: Results from the study of osteoporotic fractures." *Am J Epidemiology.* 145:926-934, 1997
(8) *JAMA.* April 28,1999
(9) *Am. J. Epidemiology.* May 15, 1997
(10) *Amer. J. Clin. Nutr.* 69:74, 1999
(11) *Sci. News.* 157:277, 2000
(12) Wing, R.R., et al. "Weight gain at menopause." *Arch Int Med.* 151:97-102, 1991
(13) McCabe, Randi, et al. "The Myth of Dieting: Confronting Weight Gain in the Menopausal Years." *A Friend Indeed.* Volume XVI/2, May, 1999
(14) Ernsberger, P. "Exploding the myth: Weight loss makes you healthier." *Healthy Wt J.* 13:4-6, 1999
(15) Berg, F. *Health Risks of Weight Loss,* 3rd edition. Healthy Living Institute, Hettinger, ND. 1995
(16) *Women's Health Network News.* May/June, 2001
(17) Russell, I.J., et al. "Platelet 3H-imipramine Uptake Receptor Density and Serum Serotonin Levels in Patients with Fibromyalgia/Fibrositis Syndrome." *Journal of Rheumatology.* 19:104-109, 1992
(18) Bennett, R.M. "Low Levels of Somatomedin C in Patients with the Fibromyalgia Syndrome: A Possible Link Between Sleep and Muscle Pain." *Arthritis & Rheumatism.* 35(10):1113-1116, 1992
(19) Russell, I.J., et al. "Elevated Cerebrospinal Fluid Levels of Substance P in Patients with Fibromyalgia Syndrome." *Arthritis & Rheumatism.* 37(11):1593-1601, 1994
(20) Private correspondence from Ellen Weaver (quote is from her). Shamanic massage therapist, treats women with, and has herself, fibromyalgia.
(21) Bacci, Ingrid. "Closing the Door on Pain." *Natural Health Magazine.* April, 2001
(22) "The Comfrey Controversy." *Journal of the Northeast Herbalists Association.* Winter, 1994
(23) Awang, D.V.C. "Comfrey." *Canadian Pharm Journal.* 101-4, 1987
(24) Rao, et al. "Diosgenin—A growth stimulator of mammary gland of ovariectomised mouse." *Indian J Exp Biol.* 30:367-370, 1992
(25) Aldercreutz, H., et al. "Effect of dietary components, including lignans and phytoestrogens, on enterohepatic circulation and liver metabolism of estrogens, and on sex hormone binding globulin." *J Steroid Biochem.* 27:1135-1144, 1987
(26) Aldercreutz, H., et al. "Determination of urinary lignans and phytoestrogen metabolites, potential antiestrogens and anticarcinogens, in urine of women on various habitual diets." *J Steroid Biochem.* 25:791-797, 1986
(27) Folman, et al. "Effect of norethisterone acetate, demethylstilboestrol, genistein, and coumestrol on uptake of estradiol by uterus, vagina, and skeletal muscle of immature mice." *J Endocrinol.* 44:213-218, 1969
(28) Mäkelä, S. et al. "Role of plant estrogens in normal and estrogen-related altered growth of the mouse prostate." *Euro Food Tox III.* Schwerzenbach, Switzerland: Institute of Toxicology. 135-139, 1991

(29) Aldercreutz, H., et al. "Dietary phytoestrogens and cancer: in vitro and in vivo studies." *J Steroid Biochem Mol Biol.* 41:331-337, 1992

(30) Joannou, G.E., et al. A urinary profile study of dietary phytoestrogens. The identification and mode of metabolism of new isoflavonoids. *Journal of Steroid Biochemistry and Molecular Biology.* 54:167-184,1995

(31) Aldercreutz, H., et al. "Excretion of the lignans enterolactone and enterodial in omnivorous and vegetarian women and in women with breast cancer." *Lancet 2.* 1295-1299, 1982

(32) Aldercreutz, Herman. "Phytoestrogens: Epidemiology and a Possible Role in Cancer Protection." *Enviro Hlth Perspc.* 103 (7):103-112, 1995

(33) Trickey, Ruth. *Women, Hormones & the Menstrual Cycle: Herbal and Medical Solutions.* Allen & Unwin. 313, 1998

(34) Weihrauch, J.L., et al. "Sterol content of foods of plant origin." *J AM Diet Ass.* 73:39-47

(35) Whitten, P.L., et al. "Effects of normal, human concentration, phytoestrogen diet on rat uterine growth." *Steroids.* 57:98-106, 1992

(36) Subbiah, M.T.R. "Dietary plant sterols: current status in human and animal metabolism." *Am J Clin Nutr.* 26:219-225, 1973

(37) Rao, A.V., et al. "The role of dietary phytosterols in colon carcinogenesis." *Nutr Cancer.* 18:43-52, 1992

(38) Verdeal. R., et al. "Naturally occurring oestrogens in plant foodstuffs — a review." *J Food Protect.* 42:577-583, 1979

(39) Letters column, *Science News.* 148:35. July 15, 1995

(40) Svoboda, R.E. *Kundalini Aghora II.* Albuquerque, NM: Brotherhood of Life. 1993

(41) Ibid.

(42) Walker, B. *The Crone: Woman of Age, Wisdom, and Power.* San Francisco, CA: Harper. 1986

(43) Brennan, B.A. *Hands of Light, a Guide to Healing Through the Human Energy Field.* New York, NY: Bantam. 1987

(44) *UC Berkeley Wellness Letter.* March 2001

(45) *American Journal of Psychology.* 157:715, 2000

(46) Fallon, Sally. *Nourishing Traditions.* New Trends, 1999

(47) *Scientific American.* September, 1997.

(48) Cooper, et al. "Lack of dermal absorption of Pro-Gest cream in menopausal women." *The Lancet.* April 25, 1998

(49) Bergner, P. "Botanical Medicine: Fact and fancy about plant estrogens." *J Nutr Dietary Cons.* 8-18, April,1993

(50) Lee, John R. "FAQs About Progesterone Cream."*Medical Letter.* February 21, 2001

(51) Interview with Carolyn De Marco, *Women's Health Alternative Medicine Report.* March, 1999

(52) Nandi, Sattabrata, et al. Proceedings of the National Academy of Sciences. March 2, 1999

(53) Lee, John, MD. *What Your Doctor May Not Tell You About Menopause.* Warner Books. 1996

(54) Schairer, Catherine. *JAMA.* January 26, 2000

(55) Leonetti, H.B., et al. "Transdermal progesterone cream for vasomotor symptoms and postmenopausal bone loss." *Am J Obstet Gynecol.* 94:225-228, 1999

(56) *Health Facts.* November, 1999.

(57) Leonetti, ibid.

(58) Love, Susan, MD. *Dr. Susan Love's Hormone Book.* New York: Random House. 1997

(59) Wolk A., et al. *Archives of Int Med* (January 12,1997) reported in *Science News.* 153:37, 1997

(60) Carper, Jean. *Food Pharmacy Guide to Good Eating.* New York, NY: Bantam. 1991

(61) Trichopoulou, A., et al. "Consumption of Olive Oil and Specific Food Groups in Relation to Breast Cancer Risk in Greece." *J Natl Cancer Inst.* 87:110-116, 1995

(62) Wolk, A., ibid.

(63) Freudenstein, H., et al. "Influence of an isopropanolic aqueous extract of Cimicifugae racemosae rhizoma on the proliferation of MCF-7 cells." Abstract of 23rd Int'l LOF-Symposium on phytoestrogens. January, 1999

(64) Bohnert, K.J. The use of Vitex agnus castus for hyperprolactinemia." *Q Rec Nat Med. Spring,* 1997

(65) *British Medical Journal.* January 20, 2001

(66) Warnecke, G. "Psychosomatic disorders in female climacterium: Clinical efficacy and tolerance of kava extract." *Fortsch Med.* 109:119-122, 1991.

(67) Miksicek, R. "Estrogenic flavonoida: structural requirements for biological activity." *Proc Soc Expert Biol Med.* 208:44-50, 1995

(68) Bergner, Paul. *The Healing Power of Ginseng.* Prima, 1996

(69) Chang, H.M., et al. "Pharmacology and Applications of Chinese Materia Medica." *World Scientific Press,* 1986

(70) Hoffman, David. Proceedings of the Third International Herbal Symposium. Wheaton, MA. 1994

(71) Dolbaum, C.M. "Lab analyses of salivary DHEA and progesterone following ingestion of yam-containing products." *Townsend Letter for Doctors.* 104, 1996

(72) Hasselbring, Bobbie. "Chronic Vaginitis." *Medical Self Care.* February, 1988

(73) "Vaginitis," *Harvard Medical School Health Letter.* February, 1984

(74) Jasionowski, E., MD. "Topical progesterone in treatment of vulvar dystrophy." *American Journal of Obstet. Gynecol.* 127:667, 1977

(75) "Incontinence," *Hot Flash Newsletter.* Vol. #5, No. 2

(76) "Chronic UTIs." *National Women's Health Network News.* May, 1985 & Jan. 1987

(77) Hoffman, S. "UTIs." *American Health.* April, 1989

(78) Ford, Anne Tochon. "Living with Interstitial Cystitis." *A Friend Indeed.* Vol. 16, No. 1, 1999

(79) *American Journal of Clinical Nutrition.* 69:827, 890, 1999

(80) *American Journal of Epidemiology.* January 15, 1999

(81) *New England Journal of Medicine.* 342:836, 2000

(82) *Science News.* 155:278, 1999

(83) Ibid.

(84) *Science News.* 157:236, 2000

(85) *Science News.* 155:181, 1999

(86) *Journal of the American Medical Association.* January 23, 2000

(87) *Science News.* 138:18, November, 1990

(88) "Healthy Bones Year After Year." *National Osteoporosis Foundation Prevention.* November, 1990

(89) Munger, F.G., et al. "Prospective study of dietary protein intake and risk of hip fracture in postmenopausal women." *American Journal of Clinical Nutrition.* 69: 147-52, 1999

(90) *Journal of Bone and Mineral Research.* 15:2504, 2000

(91) Vermeer, C., et al. "Role of vitamin K in bone metabolism." *Annual Review of Nutrition.* 15:1-22, 1995

(92) *American Journal of Clinical Nutrition.* January 2001

(93) Nelson, Miriam, et al. *American Journal of Clinical Nutrition.* May, 1991

(94) Kanis, J.A., et al. "Calcium supplementation of the diet." *British Medical Journal.* January, 1989

(95) *American Journal of Epidemiology.* October, 1990

(96) Lee, J.R., MD. *Hormonal and Nutritional Aspects of Osteoporosis.* 1991

(97) Prior, MD, et al. "Progesterone and the Prevention of Osteoporosis." *Canadian Journal of Ob/Gyn.* Vol. 3, No. 4, 1991

(98) Ehmke, Karen. "Osteoporosis: More Calcium is not the Answer." Ontario's *Common Ground Magazine.* Summer, 1990

(99) *New England Journal of Medicine.* 1990.

(100) *American Journal of Epidemiology.* April, 1991

(101) Whatley, Marianne; DuHamel, Meredith. "Osteoporosis Screening: Pro and Con." *National Women's Health Network News.* February, 1989

(102) Antonopoulos, S.; Demopoulos, C.A.; Andrikopoulos, N.K. "Lipid separation from Urtica dioica." *Journal of Agricultural and Food Chemistry.* 44(10):3052-3056, 1996

Index

Foreign Name Index